Trapped Charged Particles

A Graduate Textbook with Problems and Solutions

Advanced Textbooks in Physics

ISSN: 2059-7711

Published

Trapped Charged Particles: A Graduate Textbook with Problems and Solutions
edited by Richard C Thompson, Niels Madsen & Martina Knoop

Forthcoming

Symmetry, Groups, and Representations in Physics: Solutions Manual
Dimitri D Vvedensky & Timothy S Evans

Studying Distant Galaxies: A Handbook of Methods and Analyses
François Hammer, Mathieu Puech, Hector Flores & Myriam Rodrigues

An Introduction to Particle Dark Matter
Stefano Profumo

An Introducion to String Theory and D-Brane Dynamics: With Problems and Solutions (3rd Edition)
by Richard J Szabo

Advanced Textbooks in Physics

Trapped Charged Particles

A Graduate Textbook with Problems and Solutions

Editors

Martina Knoop
CNRS/Aix-Marseille University, France

Niels Madsen
Swansea University, UK

Richard C Thompson
Imperial College London, UK

World Scientific

NEW JERSEY • LONDON • SINGAPORE • BEIJING • SHANGHAI • HONG KONG • TAIPEI • CHENNAI • TOKYO

Published by

World Scientific Publishing Europe Ltd.
57 Shelton Street, Covent Garden, London WC2H 9HE
Head office: 5 Toh Tuck Link, Singapore 596224
USA office: 27 Warren Street, Suite 401-402, Hackensack, NJ 07601

Library of Congress Cataloging-in-Publication Data
Names: Thompson, Richard (Richard Charles), 1955– editor. | Madsen, Niels, editor. | Knoop, Martina, editor.
Title: Trapped charged particles : a graduate textbook with problems and solutions / editors Richard C. Thompson (Imperial College London, UK), Niels Madsen (Swansea University, UK) & Martina Knoop (Aix Marseille Université, France).
Description: Singapore ; Hackensack, NJ : World Scientific Publishing Co. Pte. Ltd., [2016] | 2016 | Series: Advanced textbooks in physics
Identifiers: LCCN 2015049844| ISBN 9781786340115 (hc ; alk. paper) | ISBN 1786340119 (hc ; alk. paper) | ISBN 9781786340122 (pbk ; alk. paper) | ISBN 1786340127 (pbk ; alk. paper)
Subjects: LCSH: Trapped ions. | Particles (Nuclear physics)
Classification: LCC QC702.7.T73 P49 2016 | DDC 539.7/2--dc23
LC record available at http://lccn.loc.gov/2015049844

British Library Cataloguing-in-Publication Data
A catalogue record for this book is available from the British Library.

Desk Editors: Suraj Kumar/Mary Simpson

Typeset by Stallion Press
Email: enquiries@stallionpress.com

Printed in Singapore by Mainland Press Pte Ltd.

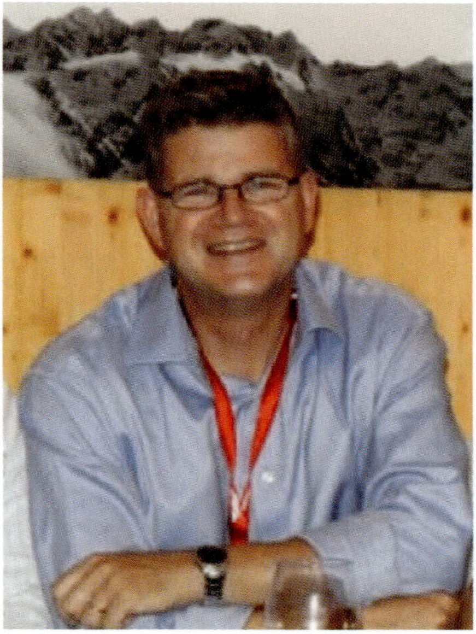

Danny Segal

27/8/1960 to 23/9/2015

This book is dedicated to Professor Danny Segal, who was an active member of the ion trapping community for many years, based at Imperial College London. Danny was one of the organizers of the first European Conference on Trapped Ions (ECTI) in 2010 and lectured at the first Winter School on Physics with Trapped Charged Particles in 2012. He was due to lecture at the second Winter School, which provided the material for this textbook, but his illness prevented him from attending.

Danny was an exceptional scientist, lecturer and colleague and he will be missed greatly.

PREFACE

Trapped charged particles are used in many areas of physics for various purposes ranging from high to low energies, and from fundamental physics through quantum engineering to simulations of space plasmas or solid state systems. Novel applications emerge very rapidly as electromagnetic trapping has turned out to be a versatile precision tool for the manipulation of charged particles. With this book based on lectures given at the 2015 Les Houches Winter School on Physics with Trapped Charged Particles, we hope to contribute a comprehensive text that discusses all the fundamental aspects of both the physics of trapped charged particles and physics with trapped charged particles. The level of comprehension is targeted towards physicists new to the field who wish to deepen their understanding and develop specific applications in the field. All chapters have associated problems for probing the understanding of certain aspects of the subjects discussed and the volume should serve as a good reference for a graduate or advanced undergraduate course.

We would like to thank all the contributing authors and speakers who have helped make this volume as well as the winter school possible. We are aware that besides the lectures, students also benefit from the personal networking aspect, and we therefore look forward to revisit the subjects with a third winter school in 2018.

The Editors

CONTENTS

CHAPTER ONE

PENNING TRAPS

Richard C. Thompson

Blackett Laboratory, Department of Physics,
Imperial College London, London SW7 2AZ, UK
r.thompson@imperial.ac.uk.

Penning traps have been in use for a wide range of experiments in mass spectrometry, plasma physics, atomic spectroscopy, quantum information, and quantum optics for over 40 years. In this chapter, we give an account of the principles of operation of Penning traps, together with a discussion of practical aspects of their use and their advantages for particular types of experiments. A brief survey of recent experiments using Penning traps demonstrates their wide applicability and continuing importance in many fields.

1. Introduction

A Penning trap confines the motion of charged particles by the use of static electric and magnetic fields. In essence, a quadrupole electrostatic field confines particles along a particular direction (the axis of the trap) and the magnetic field, which is parallel to this axis, confines their motion perpendicular to the trap axis. In this way, the particles are trapped in all three dimensions. The Penning trap can be used for electrons, positrons, or atomic and molecular ions, including highly-charged ions. The principles of its operation are straightforward and it has found application in a very wide range of areas of physics.

We start this chapter with a brief historical introduction to Penning traps, then we discuss the operating principles of the trap (Section 2). In Section 3, we introduce a rotating frame in which the behavior of the trapped particles can be visualized in an intuitive manner. We then discuss the particular advantages and disadvantages associated with the Penning trap, and illustrate some of these advantages with brief discussions of some relevant experiments (Section 4). We then look at various practical aspects of the operation of the Penning trap (Section 5) including cooling techniques. In Section 6, we look in more detail at laser cooling in the Penning trap. Finally, we draw some overall conclusions about the Penning trap in Section 7.

The name "Penning Trap" was first introduced by Hans Dehmelt [1,2] in the early 1960s. He later received the Nobel Prize for his work with ion traps [3]. The trap was named after Franz Penning, who performed experiments in the 1930s on electric discharges between coaxial cylinders and noticed that the lifetime of the electrons was increased in the presence of an axial magnetic field [4]. Dehmelt used the Penning trap for radiofrequency (RF) spectroscopy of He^{+} ions and demonstrated that the temperature of trapped ions could be measured by monitoring the induced current in an external circuit connected to the Penning trap electrodes (the so-called "Bolometric technique" [5]).

Other groups were also using Penning traps around the same time, for example, in Edinburgh, a Penning trap was used in the development of a source of polarized electrons [6]. In Mainz, measurements were made of the anomalous magnetic moment (i.e. the g-factor) of electrons in a trap [7,8], and an impressive precision of around three parts in 10^8 was obtained.

One of the most significant steps in the application of Penning traps in atomic physics was made in 1978 when laser cooling of trapped ions was first demonstrated [9]. This work also used the bolometric technique referred to above. Later experiments used fluorescence light for observing this process, as will be discussed later in this chapter.

2. Principles of Operation

2.1. *Motion of a single ion*

Charged particles interact strongly with both electric and magnetic fields and one attractive way to trap such particles would be to put them in a region where there is a three-dimensional (3D) minimum of the electrostatic potential, so that there is a force toward the center of the trap from all directions. However, this is disallowed by Earnshaw's theorem, which follows from the Poisson equation for the electrostatic potential ϕ in the absence of free charges, $\nabla^2\phi(x,y,z) = 0$. As a result, electrostatic fields can be used to trap along at most two axes, and in order to make a 3D trap, some other mechanism must be used to confine the motion in the remaining direction(s). One way of achieving this is to add a uniform magnetic field

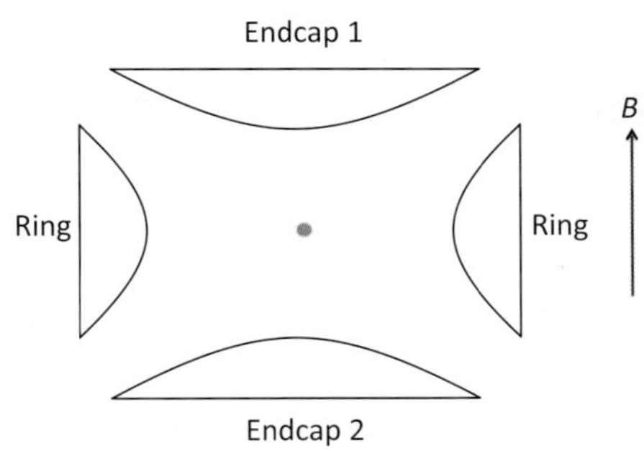

Fig. 1. Cross-section through the electrodes of a Penning trap. The two endcap electrodes are connected together. A DC potential applied between the endcaps and the ring creates a 3D quadrupole potential in the region between the electrodes. This traps particles along the vertical z-direction. The addition of a uniform magnetic field $\mathbf{B} = B\hat{\mathbf{z}}$ along the trap axis ensures 3D trapping. The separation of the endcaps is $2z_0$ and the internal diameter of the ring is $2r_0$, which is typically of the order of 1 cm (see text).

$\mathbf{B} = B\hat{\mathbf{z}}$ which can effectively confine the motion in the radial (x, y) directions by forcing the particle into circular orbits. If this is combined with a quadratic electrostatic potential,

$$\phi(x, y, z) = V_0(2z^2 - x^2 - y^2)/R^2, \tag{1}$$

a stable 3D trap is formed. Here V_0 is the applied trap potential and R^2 is a parameter related to the size of the trap. The potential described by this equation can be generated by a set of three electrodes having the cross-section shown in Figure 1, in which case R^2 is equal to $r_0^2 + 2z_0^2$, where r_0 and z_0 are the distances from the trap center to the ring and endcap electrodes, respectively. This potential has a saddle point at the center of the trap. Axial trapping is provided by the electric field of the saddle potential, which always provides a restoring force in the axial direction. Radial trapping is achieved with the help of the magnetic field, which provides an inward force for an orbiting particle that is stronger than the outward force in the radial plane arising from the saddle potential.

The equation of motion follows from the Lorentz force, $\mathbf{F} = m\ddot{\mathbf{r}} = e(-\nabla\phi + \mathbf{v} \times \mathbf{B})$, for a particle with mass m and charge e. The axial (z) motion then corresponds to simple harmonic motion (SHM) with an angular oscillation frequency $\omega_z = \sqrt{4eV_0/mR^2}$.

The equations of motion for the radial (x, y) motion are more complicated due to the presence of the magnetic field, which couples the two

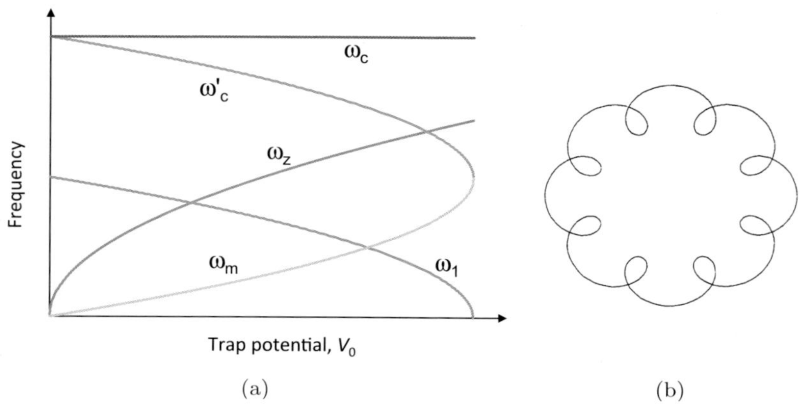

Fig. 2. (a) Plot of the values of the various oscillation frequencies in the Penning trap as a function of the applied trap potential. (b) Typical radial orbit showing a small, fast cyclotron motion superimposed on a larger, slow magnetron orbit.

equations. However, by defining a complex variable $u = x + iy$, they can be combined in a single equation,

$$\ddot{u} - i\omega_c\dot{u} - (\omega_z^2/2)u = 0. \tag{2}$$

Here, $\omega_c = eB/m$ is the cyclotron frequency. The solution to the radial equation of motion is a superposition of two circular motions, one at the *modified cyclotron frequency*, $\omega_c' = \omega_c/2 + \omega_1$, and the other at the *magnetron frequency*, $\omega_m = \omega_c/2 - \omega_1$. The frequency ω_1 is equal to $\sqrt{\omega_c^2/4 - \omega_z^2/2}$ and we will see later that it has a simple physical interpretation.

The dependence of the trap oscillation frequencies on the applied trapping potential is shown in Figure 2(a). Note that all three trap oscillation frequencies (ω_z, ω_m, and ω_c') are always less than the cyclotron frequency ω_c and that the trap becomes unstable when the trapping potential is such that $\omega_z > \omega_c/\sqrt{2}$. At this point, the radial electric field, which pushes the ions away from the trap center, is strong enough to overcome the confining effect due to the magnetic field, so the ions are no longer confined radially. Figure 2(b) shows the path taken by an ion in the radial plane for the particular case that $\omega_c' = 9\omega_m$.

In many experiments (e.g. high precision mass spectrometry), it is necessary to find the value of the cyclotron frequency accurately. It can be seen that this is given by the sum of the magnetron and modified cyclotron frequencies, i.e. $\omega_c = \omega_m + \omega_c'$. However, this relation is exact only when the trap is perfect (that is, the potential is described exactly by Equation (1)).

It can be shown in Ref. [10] that the relation,

$$\omega_c^2 = \omega_c'^2 + \omega_z^2 + \omega_m^2 \tag{3}$$

remains exact even in the presence of misalignments and quadratic imperfections of the field. This equation can therefore be used to obtain accurate values of the cyclotron frequency for real traps that are not perfect.

It is worth noting here that although the axial motion is straightforward SHM, there are anomalies associated with the modified cyclotron and magnetron motions. As a result, the principle of equipartition of energy does not apply to these motions. The anomalies stem from the fact that the radial potential energy, given by $V = -\frac{1}{4}m\omega_z^2 r^2$, is negative, whereas in conventional SHM the potential energy is always positive. For the cyclotron motion, the kinetic energy, $K = \frac{1}{2}m\omega_c'^2 r_c^2$, which of course can only be positive, is always large enough to make the total energy of this motion positive. On the other hand, the kinetic energy associated with the magnetron motion, $K = \frac{1}{2}m\omega_m^2 r_m^2$, is smaller in magnitude than its potential energy, due to the low value of the magnetron frequency. Therefore, the total energy of this motion remains negative, and this has several consequences. One of the important consequences is that removal of energy from this motion results in an *increase* in the magnetron radius. So, if this motion is to be "cooled" (i.e. made smaller in amplitude), energy has to be supplied rather than removed. This means that cooling techniques have to be adapted for this motion.

2.2. *Interaction between ions*

If there are two ions present in the trap, the equations of motion are modified by including the force due to the Coulomb interaction, which introduces a term $e^2/4\pi\epsilon_0 r_{12}^2$, where r_{12} is the distance between the two ions. This couples the motion of both ions and also couples the x, y, and z motions. However, the new equations of motion can be separated into a *center of mass* motion and a *relative* motion. The center of mass motion is identical to that of a single ion, so the solutions are the same motions as we derived above. The relative motion depends on the Coulomb interaction and is no longer simple harmonic because of the nonlinear nature of the interaction. However, if the amplitude of the relative motion is small (i.e. if the temperature is low), a linear expansion of the Coulomb force can be made and the equations then become solvable.

There is a small number of types of motion that are of particular interest [11]. The first is when the two ions are both located on the trap axis at locations $\pm z_1$, where $z_1^3 = e^2/16\pi\epsilon_0 m\omega_z^2$ (found by requiring the ions to be in static equilibrium). Then, the ions are essentially stationary apart from small oscillations due to the thermal motion of the center of mass motion and the relative motion (which for the axial direction can be shown to be at a frequency of $\sqrt{3}\omega_z$). Alternatively, the ions can be in equilibrium in the radial plane with a constant separation, but in this case, they are always moving in an orbit around the center of the trap. The separation can take different values, and this affects the frequency of the orbital motion. When the ions are well separated, they behave as if they are moving independently, so the frequencies of the relative motion approach the single particle values and the rotation around the trap center is generally close to ω_m. However, as the ions get closer together, the orbital frequency ω_R rises from ω_m to a value of $\omega_c/2$. At this point, the separation of the ions has its minimum value, which is $2r_1$, where $r_1^3 = e^2/16\pi\epsilon_0 m\omega_1^2$.

When there is a large number of ions in the trap, it becomes more appropriate to think of the motion in terms of a plasma rather than as individual particles. This type of plasma is referred to as a *single component plasma* or a *non-neutral plasma*. A detailed discussion of such a plasma is given in Chapter 9. Here, it is sufficient to note that at low temperatures, the plasma has an ellipsoidal shape with a constant number density n, a sharp edge and a well-defined aspect ratio. Due to the presence of the magnetic field, the whole plasma rotates at a frequency ω_R, where ω_R is related to n through

$$n = 2\epsilon_0 m\omega_R(\omega_c - \omega_R)/e^2. \tag{4}$$

In a manner similar to the case of two ions, when the ions have large separations (i.e. for low n), the value of ω_R is approximately ω_m, but when the ion density takes its maximum possible value, ω_R becomes equal to $\omega_c/2$. This situation, when the plasma density is maximum, is referred to as *Brillouin flow*.

3. Rotating Frame

We now show that the dynamics discussed above can be understood in a more intuitive manner by moving into a frame of reference that is rotating at $\omega_c/2$ [11]. The equations of motion for a single ion in a rotating frame acquire additional terms due to the centripetal force and the Coriolis force. However, by choosing the rotation frequency to be equal to $\omega_c/2$, the centripetal force exactly balances the Lorentz force due to the magnetic field, and this simplifies the equations of motion considerably. In particular, it removes the coupling between the x and y motions, so each becomes SHM at a new frequency which is dependent on the effective potential resulting from the centripetal force. This oscillation frequency takes the value $\sqrt{\omega_c^2/4 - \omega_z^2/2}$ and it will be seen that this is identical to the value of ω_1 given above. The radial motion of a single ion in a Penning trap can therefore be interpreted as motion in a two-dimensional (2D) simple harmonic potential well (with an oscillation frequency ω_1) in a frame which is rotating at $\omega_c/2$ relative to the laboratory frame. An orbit at a frequency $+\omega_1$ in the rotating frame corresponds to the modified cyclotron motion ($\omega_c' = \omega_c/2 + \omega_1$) in the laboratory frame, while an orbit at $-\omega_1$ corresponds to the magnetron motion ($\omega_m = \omega_c/2 - \omega_1$) in the laboratory frame.

This simple way of interpreting the motion of a single ion also applies in the case of two ions and in the case of a large ion plasma. Consider the motion of two ions in a radial potential characterized by an oscillation frequency ω_1. The ions experience a Coulomb interaction as well as the force from the confining potential. However, when the ions are far apart, the Coulomb interaction is very weak and therefore, they behave essentially independently, so they both move at the single ion frequency in this frame, ω_1. If, on the other hand, the ions are stationary in the rotating frame, they will be in equilibrium close to the minimum of the potential, with a separation $2r_1$ where $r_1^3 = e^2/16\pi\epsilon_0 m\omega_1^2$, so the outward Coulomb force on each ion is exactly balanced by the inward force due to the confining potential. When this arrangement is viewed from the laboratory frame, the ions will be rotating at $\omega_c/2$ as we discussed above.

Similarly, the limits of low and high ion density for a plasma containing many ions can be treated simply in this rotating frame. The general case is when a uniform density plasma is rotating as a solid body at a rate ω_R' in the rotating frame. If the ions were stationary in that frame ($\omega_R' = 0$), they would have a density,

$$n = m(\omega_z^2 + 2\omega_1^2)\epsilon_0/e^2 = m\omega_c^2\epsilon_0/2e^2. \tag{5}$$

If however the plasma is rotating at ω_R', each ion experiences an additional outward centrifugal force due to the rotation, which is equal to $m\omega_R'^2 r$, and reduces the inward force from the trapping potential, $m\omega_1^2 r$. This is equivalent to a reduction of the trap oscillation frequency from ω_1 to $\omega_2 = \sqrt{\omega_1^2 - \omega_R'^2}$. If we substitute this new value into the expression for n, Equation (5), we obtain the new value for the number density,

$$n = m(\omega_z^2 + 2\omega_2^2)\epsilon_0/e^2 = 2m\omega_R(\omega_c - \omega_R)\epsilon_0/e^2. \tag{6}$$

This is identical to the general expression for the number density in the Penning trap, Equation (4), so the variation of number density with plasma rotation frequency can simply be seen as the consequence of the centrifugal force in the rotating frame.

4. Advantages of Penning Traps

In this section, we discuss several features of Penning traps that make them particularly suitable for certain types of experiment. We also show how these advantages are exploited in particular experiments.

4.1. *Isolated and stable environment*

Ions in any type of ion trap are well isolated from their environment: their motion is confined to a particular region by the use of electromagnetic fields, so there are no collisions with the walls of the container. Also, trapping is generally carried out under ultrahigh vacuum (UHV) conditions, so there are no collisions with background gas either. Although ions can collide with each other, their mutual Coulomb repulsion means that they never get close to each other and the internal electronic state is not affected by collisions, and the same is even true for the rotational and vibrational states of trapped molecular ions.

In a Penning trap, the confining fields are static, so there is no micromotion (which can lead to heating) as it occurs in the case of RF traps (see Chapter 2). This means that 3D plasmas containing many thousands of ions can be held under stable conditions in which there are no significant heating effects.

The nature of the confinement in the Penning trap means that ions are isolated from many perturbations and this allows various types of experiment to be performed that are otherwise not possible. For example, a microwave frequency standard based on a cloud of laser-cooled Be^+ ions in a Penning trap was able to achieve very long interaction times, which in turn gives narrow line-width and high frequency stability. In one experiment, Ramsey fringes were observed with an interaction time of 550 s, which gives a central fringe width of only 1 mHz on a transition frequency (between Zeeman states of the hyperfine structure of the ion) of around 300 MHz [12]. Of course, one potential problem with an experiment like this is the unavoidable presence of the magnetic field because any fluctuations of the magnetic field strength will lead to frequency shifts of the transition being studied. However, it is often possible to find a magnetic field at which the RF becomes independent of field to first order, and this allows the effect of magnetic field fluctuations to be strongly suppressed.

An extreme example of the advantage of isolation of trapped particles in a Penning trap is the use of trapped antiprotons and trapped positrons to create antihydrogen. Storage and accumulation of antiparticles would be impossible in other systems because as soon as the particles encounter normal matter, they will annihilate. Therefore, positrons and antiprotons are both routinely stored in Penning traps in the experiments to create and study antihydrogen carried out at the CERN antiproton decelerator. Complex arrangements in these experiments are used to trap both species in the same trap structure, which consists of a long string of cylindrical electrodes with independently-controllable potentials. Regions designed to trap the positively charged positrons have a potential minimum, whereas regions for antiproton storage have a potential maximum. Using careful control of the potentials on each electrode, these regions can be overlapped in order to merge the clouds of positrons and antiprotons for the creation of antihydrogen (see Chapter 14).

4.2. *Tight localization of a single particle*

When a single atomic ion is held in a Penning trap and laser cooled, the typical temperature achieved (the Doppler limit) is around 1 mK. For standard trapping parameters, the residual thermal motion at this temperature is confined to a region having dimensions of the order of 1 μm. This opens up the possibility of very long interaction times between an ion and a laser beam, knowing that the ion will be within the laser beam the whole time and that the Doppler effect due to the residual motion of the ion will be very small. Thus, many delicate experiments have been performed where a single particle is observed continuously — for example in the observation of quantum jumps, where an ion jumps between two electronic levels, one of which interacts resonantly with the Doppler cooling laser, and therefore emits a continuous stream of fluorescence, while the other is 'dark'. When the ion is in this state, it does not interact with the laser and therefore, there is no fluorescence.

4.3. *Strong magnetic field*

Penning traps always involve the application of a strong magnetic field, typically of the order of a few tesla and usually provided by a superconducting magnet. In some cases, this is a disadvantage — for example, the resulting Zeeman splitting of energy levels in laser cooling experiments may lead to the requirement to have more laser frequencies available — but for some experiments, it is a distinct advantage. This is particularly true for measurements of mass and of magnetic moments (see Chapter 17).

For the measurement of mass to high precision, it is convenient to measure the cyclotron frequency in a magnetic field because the cyclotron frequency is directly related to the mass ($\omega_c = eB/m$) and if the field is uniform and stable, it is possible to obtain high precision. There are therefore many examples of experiments that give very precise mass measurements using Penning traps. They are often used at facilities where a wide range of isotopes (including short-lived radioactive isotopes) can be produced, e.g. ISOLTRAP at the CERN ISOLDE facility [13]. In practice, mass measurements are made by a comparison of the cyclotron frequency of the particle of interest to that of a particle whose mass is already well known. If these measurements are made in the same magnetic field, the ratio of the masses is equal to the ratio of the cyclotron frequencies. The pure cyclotron frequency is determined from measurements of the three center of mass modes and combined using Equation (3). Accuracies of better than one part in 10^8 are achievable even for short-lived isotopes. These measurements are important because they allow the determination of nuclear binding energies for a wide range of isotopes, which is necessary for the understanding of nuclear structure physics. For the highest accuracy, a single particle is used and many repeated measurements are made. The proton mass has been determined this way to a precision approaching one part in 10^{10} [14].

Mass spectrometry to lower precision is carried out routinely in a technique known as *Fourier Transform Ion Cyclotron Resonance* (FT-ICR) [15]. This is essentially based around the measurement of the cyclotron frequency of molecular ions in a Penning trap, but it can be used not just for one species but for the analysis of samples containing many different species. The basic design of the 'cell' is similar to a Penning trap, but there is often no attempt made to design the electrodes to match the ideal quadrupolar shape closely. The analysis is performed by radially exciting the sample held in the cell and then taking the Fourier transform of the signal induced in an external circuit resulting from the motion of the ions after excitation. The Fourier transform yields a mass spectrum directly.

In order to measure a magnetic moment, it is necessary to compare the cyclotron frequency of a particle with its spin flip frequency in the same magnetic field. For an electron, these two frequencies are very close because the spin flip frequency ω_s is equal to $g\mu_B B/\hbar = geB/2m$, where the gyromagnetic ratio of the electron $g = 2.00232$. The occurrence of spin flips is detected by introducing a quadratic variation of magnetic field strength with axial position. This changes the axial oscillation frequency slightly for the two different orientations of the spin of the particle, allowing its spin direction to be determined. In this way, the electron's gyromagnetic ratio has been determined to better than one part in 10^{12} [16]. This gives an accurate test of the theory of quantum electrodynamics (QED), which predicts a value of g to high precision given the value of the fine structure constant α.

The magnetic moments of other particles can also be measured in a Penning trap. For instance, the magnetic moment of the proton has recently been measured to very high precision [17]. This experiment, which reaches a precision of around three parts in 10^9, is much more difficult than the electron experiment because the magnetic moment is so small, and this means that a much stronger variation of magnetic field is necessary, which in turn requires that in order to obtain high precision, the excitation of the spin flip and the detection of the spin state of the particle have to be carried out in different locations. There is currently much interest in applying the same technique to measure the magnetic moment of the anti proton. This would allow a comparison of the g-factor of the proton and antiproton to be carried out, which can serve as a test of CPT invariance — one of the most fundamental symmetries in physics. This comparison has already been carried out at the level of 1 ppm (10^{-6}) [18], but the latest measurement techniques should allow a comparison at a level approaching 1 ppb (10^{-9}).

So far, we have only discussed the magnetic moment of free particles. However, the magnetic moment of particles in a bound system is also of interest. In particular, the magnetic moment of an electron in an atomic system is affected by the presence of the nucleus and again, this can be used to perform a test of QED calculations for a bound state (as opposed to the case of a free particle). For these experiments, a similar technique to that described above is used. An example is the measurement of $^{16}O^{7+}$, i.e. a single electron bound to an oxygen nucleus (also known as hydrogen-like oxygen) [19]. In this experiment, the g-factor was measured to a precision of around 3 ppb, consistent with bound state QED calculations. The deviation from the free particle value increases with the nuclear charge (Z) and so measurements in high-Z systems allow the higher-order terms in the QED calculation to be tested.

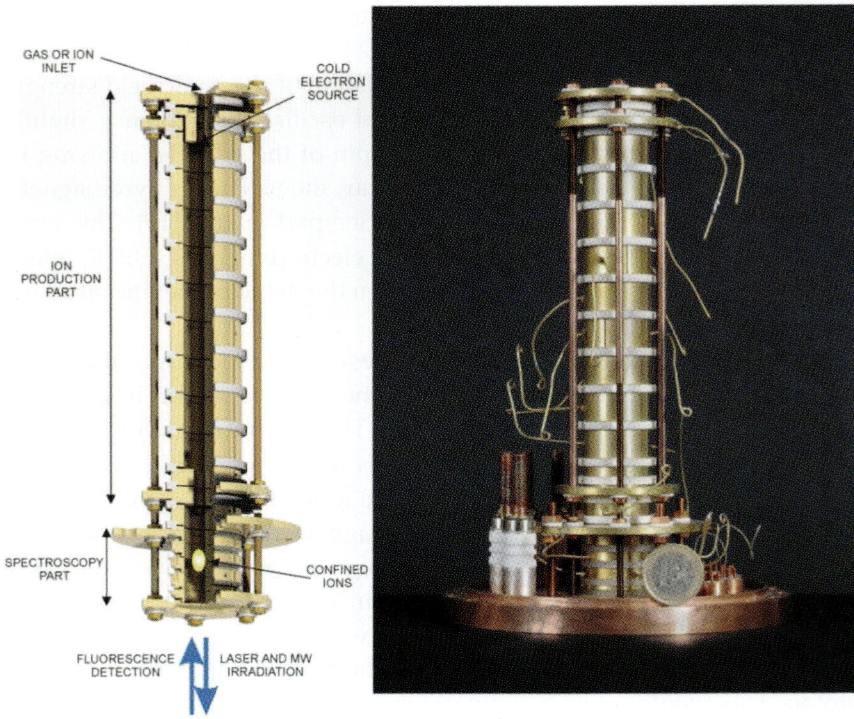

Fig. 3. Cutaway drawing (left) and image (right) of the ion trap for the ARTEMIS experiment at GSI in Darmstadt. The cylindrical electrodes can be configured to give trapping potentials at different locations in the magnetic field. Figure reproduced with permission from GSI.

An example of a trap designed for experiments in this area is shown in Figure 3. The trap is held at cryogenic temperatures when inside the superconducting magnet. The gold-plated hollow cylindrical electrodes can be configured to give trapping potentials at different locations in the axial magnetic field in order to move the ions around. The trap is designed for the measurement of the *g*-factors of medium to heavy hydrogen-like highly charged ions such as $^{28}Si^{13+}$ [20].

4.4. *Cooling of ions*

The ability to cool particles in traps is one of their major advantages over other techniques such as the use of gases, plasmas or atomic beams. Not only is it possible to cool trapped particles, but because they are well isolated from the environment, there is very little unwanted heating, so once they are cooled, the particles will generally remain cold for a long time. There are several different cooling techniques, the most important techniques for Penning traps being laser cooling (discussed in Chapter 6) and resistive cooling (discussed along with other non-laser cooling techniques in Chapter 7). Radiative cooling via synchrotron radiation is also possible but that only applies to the cyclotron motion of electrons or positrons, so it is not discussed any further here.

4.4.1. *Resistive cooling*

In resistive cooling, the motion of ions in the trap gives rise to the induced flow of current in an external electrical circuit and hence to dissipation of energy which comes originally from the motion of the ions (see Chapter 7). An equilibrium is reached where the temperature of the ions is equal to that of the external circuit. If the trap and electronics are at cryogenic temperatures, this means that the temperature of the ion motion can also be in this region. In general, resonant circuits are used, where the trap itself forms part of the circuit and is connected in such a way that it is sensitive to either the axial or the radial motion of the ions. The resonant frequency of the circuit is chosen to coincide with the corresponding oscillation frequency. Although the axial and modified cyclotron motions can be cooled very effectively using this technique, the magnetron motion cannot be cooled this way because the extraction of energy leads to an *increase* of the size of the orbit. The magnetron motion therefore has to be cooled in a different way. Often, this is done by coupling the magnetron motion to the modified cyclotron motion with an applied field oscillating at their sum frequency (ω_c). This can be shown to give rise to a reduction in the size of the orbits of both motions when the modified cyclotron motion is subject to resistive cooling. This technique is called *axialization* [21] or *radial centering*. Resistive cooling is very effective for all species of trapped particles, but it is limited to the temperature of the apparatus, so it is not possible to cool to lower than a few K in general. It is used extensively in precision experiments on trapped ions.

4.4.2. *Laser cooling*

In laser cooling, momentum is exchanged between a laser beam and the ions. Laser cooling of trapped ions is discussed in Chapter 6 (see also, for example, [22]). This technique is only applicable to a small number of species of atomic ion because it needs a suitable atomic energy level structure including a strong optical transition from the ground state of the ion to an excited state which mainly decays back to the ground state. Any other state to which the ion can decay needs to be emptied with a separate laser to return the ion into the laser cooling cycle. In a Penning trap, it is most convenient to work with a system that has no other states into which the ion can decay as otherwise the Zeeman splitting of the states leads to a requirement for many separate laser frequencies. Magnesium and beryllium are the only species where a single laser is required.

The simplest type of laser cooling is *Doppler cooling*, where the Doppler effect is used to make the interaction with the laser stronger when the ion is moving towards the laser and weaker when it is moving away from the laser. This is achieved by tuning the laser slightly to the lower frequency (red) side of the ion's transition frequency. Each time the ion absorbs a photon from the laser, it slows down slightly. The limiting temperature, referred to as the Doppler limit, is determined by a balance between this cooling process and heating that arises from the random nature of the re-emission of photons when the ion decays back to its electronic ground state from the excited state. The Doppler limit is given by $T_D = \hbar\gamma/k_B$ where γ is the decay rate of the excited state. Typically, the Doppler limit for ions of interest is in the range of 1 mK. Laser cooling in the Penning trap, is complicated by the unstable nature of the magnetron motion and we discuss it in more detail in Section 6.

The advent of Doppler laser cooling has had an enormous impact on the range of experiments that is possible in Penning traps (and of course in RF traps too). Doppler cooling effectively eliminates the Doppler effect and reduces the amplitude of the motion of ions so much that they are nearly stationary in the trap (except that in the Penning trap, a cloud of ions will always rotate due to the presence of the magnetic field, even when the ions are cold).

In order to achieve the lowest temperatures, it is necessary to use *optical sideband cooling*. In this cooling technique, the quantum mechanical nature of the motion of an ion in the trap is addressed directly. It is possible to cool the ion to the ground state of its motion. This requires a more complicated energy level structure than simple Doppler cooling, and in particular, it requires a metastable state to be available. Sideband cooling is also discussed in more detail in Section 6.

4.4.3. *Sympathetic cooling*

Sympathetic cooling is a way of extending some of the advantages of Doppler laser cooling to other species that cannot themselves be laser cooled. It works by trapping a mixture of two species at the same time. If one of them is cooled directly using laser cooling, it will also bring down the temperature of the other species through exchange of energy in thermal collisions. Eventually, both species will end up at an equilibrium temperature close to the Doppler limit [23].

4.5. *Disadvantages of the Penning trap*

There are of course disadvantages to the use of Penning traps as well as advantages. The most important one is probably the need to provide a strong magnetic field. This generally involves the use of a superconducting magnet. These are expensive to buy and expensive to run due to the need for a continual supply of liquid helium and liquid nitrogen. Furthermore, since the size of the bore of the magnet is usually a limitation, access to the ions is generally difficult, especially if optical access for lasers and fluorescence is required. Even using optimized designs for the trap electrodes, they will restrict the access to the trapped particles. Once the trap is installed in the magnet, it is generally not possible to make mechanical adjustments, so mirrors and lenses need to be adjusted beforehand such that they cannot go out of adjustment when the trap is installed in the magnet. The need for UHV conditions further complicates access.

Since a vacuum of at least 10^{-9} mbar is required, strong pumping and very careful preparation of the trap components are necessary if the trap is to be held at room temperature (see Chapter 5). If the trap itself is to be held at cryogenic temperatures (as is the case for many experiments, for example, those measuring the magnetic moments of elementary particles and ions), an extremely good vacuum should be attained easily as any cryogenic surface can effectively act as a pump. However, the design of a cryogenic system adds its own complications due to the need for low heat conductance to the outside world.

Finally, the characteristics of the magnetron motion lead to several complications in the use of the Penning trap. Any collisions with residual gas in the vacuum chamber will lead to an increase of the radius of this motion, so the requirement for UHV conditions is particularly strong for the Penning trap. Also, laser cooling needs to be modified for the magnetron motion and even then the cooling rate for this motion is relatively slow. For an ion cloud in a Penning trap, the equivalent of the magnetron motion is a rotation of the whole cloud, so there is always some residual motion even when the temperature is very low. This also causes complications in some experiments.

5. Practical Aspects

5.1. *Design of Penning traps*

The design of a Penning trap is generally determined by the type of experiment it is to be used for. Most Penning traps are designed for use in a superconducting magnet, so the access to the trap is generally along the bore of the magnet and will be constrained by the size of the bore, typically 10 cm in diameter. The electrodes need to be designed to give a pure quadrupole potential near the center of the trap. Although the ideal shape for Penning trap electrodes is therefore a hyperboloid of revolution with a cross-section as shown in Figure 1, this shape is difficult to manufacture accurately and gives very poor access. However, it has been shown in Ref. [24] that a trap consisting of a set of cylindrical electrodes can be designed such that a very good quadrupole field can be generated by careful choice of the length of each electrode. This principle has been used in many traps and it has several advantages including ease of manufacture, good access along the trap axis, and good control of the higher-order terms in the trapping field.

This type of design can also be adapted to the situation where ions need to be moved between different trapping zones (for example, where ions are prepared in one trapping zone but detected or probed in another). In this case, the trap assembly may have tens of electrodes which can be configured in different ways to move ions around (see, for example, Figure 3).

In contrast to experiments that aim to provide a pure quadrupole potential, many studies that focus on the properties of non-neutral plasmas require a large trapping volume and it may not be important for the potential to be accurately quadratic. The electrodes are also usually cylindrical in this case. The central ring electrode may then be relatively long with shorter endcaps providing axial confinement of a plasma that adopts a long, thin shape like a cigar (a prolate ellipsoid). This type of trap is generally referred to as a Penning–Malmberg trap. For more details, see Chapter 9. Similarly, in the case of FT-ICR, the trap or cell may be constructed from electrodes with a simple geometry without causing problems for the use of the technique.

5.2. *Loading of ions into the trap*

If atomic ions are to be trapped, they can be created inside the trap or transported into the trap from outside. Creation of ions in the trap can be performed by forming a low-pressure vapor of the species to be ionized (e.g.

from a small atomic oven that is heated resistively) and ionizing them either by electron impact (using an electron beam that travels along the magnetic field line from a filament or some other source) or by photo-ionization using a pulsed or cw laser. The advantage of using photo-ionization is that the process can be made resonant, so it is then more selective, and unwanted ions will not be created. An alternative in-trap loading technique is direct ablation of ions from a surface using a pulsed laser.

Ions can also be created outside the trap and guided into it along the magnetic field lines. This is more appropriate for ions created in an accelerator (especially rare isotopes or highly-charged ions) and also for other particles such as electrons or protons. One point to note with externally-created ions is that if they have sufficient energy to enter the trap, they will also have sufficient energy to leave the trap again, so something has to be done to ensure that they stay in the trap. One way to do this is to lower the potential on one endcap to let the ions in and then to raise it again immediately so that when they reflect off the potential on the other endcap, they will no longer be able to leave the trap.

5.3. *Detection of ions*

In the Penning trap, the most common techniques are fluorescence detection, electronic detection or direct (destructive) detection of the charged particles. See Ref. [25] for a wider discussion of detection techniques for trapped ions.

Fluorescence detection is used in experiments where laser cooling is employed. It is a very sensitive detection technique and allows a single particle to be detected with ease once it is cold. Fluorescence levels of tens of thousands of counts per second can be obtained under ideal conditions, but the optical access issues mentioned above need to be dealt with carefully.

Electronic detection is strongly related to resistive cooling as both rely on the use of an external circuit that is resonant with the frequency of oscillation of the ions in the trap. Since resistive cooling dissipates energy via an induced current in the external circuit, detection of the ions is possible by monitoring the current in the circuit. This is used extensively in experiments on single electrons, protons and ions where a sensitive detection of the response of the particle to an external drive is required. In general, the electronic detection circuit for single particles needs to be held at cryogenic temperatures so that the required signal can be detected above the thermal noise.

Finally, direct detection of ions is possible on a microchannel plate (MCP) detector. If ions are released from the trap, they will always travel along the magnetic field lines in a cyclotron motion, so this can be used to guide all the ions to the detector. However, this destructive technique is not ideal because it means that the creation and preparation of the ions has to be repeated many times and this may be a lengthy process. In some cases, however, this may be the only possibility. In the same way, electrons in traps can be directly detected on a phosphor screen on release from the trap.

6. Laser Cooling in the Penning Trap

6.1. *Implementation of Doppler cooling*

We discussed the advantages of using laser-cooled ions in Section 4.4.2 above (see also Chapter 6). Here, we discuss some of the practical aspects of laser cooling as applied in Penning traps and recent progress in cooling ions to their quantum mechanical ground state.

The axial motion of ions in the Penning trap is very similar to that in the RF trap (see Chapter 2), so the same considerations apply. An axial laser cooling beam cools the axial motion directly when it is tuned to the red (low frequency) side of a strong resonance transition in the ion.

The main problem for laser cooling of the radial motion in the Penning trap is the magnetron motion, which does not cool when a cooling laser beam in the radial plane is directed through the center of the trap, as would normally be the case in an RF trap. This is related to the negative total energy of the magnetron motion. Since the total energy of the magnetron motion decreases as the radius of its orbit increases, in general, the interaction with the cooling laser leads to an *increase* of the magnetron radius, not a decrease. Conventional laser cooling with a radial cooling beam therefore heats the magnetron motion while cooling the cyclotron motion (where we define 'cooling' to mean a reduction of radius). The alternative geometry of using just an axial laser beam suffers from a related problem in the same way as resistive cooling, discussed above in Section 4.4.1.

There are several ways of overcoming the problem of cooling the magnetron motion. One is to slightly offset the radial laser cooling beam to the side of the trap so that there is a gradient of laser intensity across the center of the trap. This has the effect of preferentially interacting with the ions when the magnetron motion takes them in the same direction as the laser beam. If the photon scattering process takes place then, the magnetron motion will on average be cooled (though only slowly in most circumstances) [26,27].

Another way around this problem for a single particle is to couple the magnetron and cyclotron motions using the axialization technique with laser cooling [28] in a similar manner to how it is used for resistive cooling (discussed in Section 4.4.1).

For the laser cooling of clouds of ions rather than single ions, a similar problem arises and relates to the rotation of the plasma discussed above in Section 2.2. In the absence of additional precautions, the plasma expands, its rotation frequency drops towards the magnetron frequency, and its radial extent becomes large, eventually leading to loss of particles. The plasma adopts a strongly oblate shape. This problem is overcome by applying angular momentum to the cloud in one of several ways. The simplest is again to offset the radial laser cooling beam, and this leads to a torque that tends to increase the speed of rotation of the rotating plasma, which then increases in density and adopts a less oblate configuration. Alternatively, a 'rotating wall' potential can be applied. This is an additional radial dipole or quadrupole potential which is applied using a ring electrode that is split into a number of segments. The potentials applied to each segment of the ring electrode are configured such that the generated field rotates around the trap axis at some frequency above the magnetron frequency. The field then slightly distorts the shape of the plasma and forces it to rotate at the applied frequency, thus controlling the plasma density and shape. This technique is discussed in detail in Chapter 11. It is widely used in non-neutral plasma experiments with ions and electrons and it is also routinely applied in combination with laser cooling [29,30].

There is a strong link between the techniques of axialization and the rotating wall. The oscillating quadrupole field of the axialization technique can be decomposed into two quadrupole fields, counter-rotating at half the applied frequency. Ignoring the field rotating in the opposite sense (which is generally justified since it is not resonant with any motion of the ions), the remaining rotating field is the same as that of a quadrupole rotating wall. However, it is most appropriate to think of the rotating wall as a technique for the manipulation of dense non-neutral plasmas in traps, whereas axialization is often more appropriate for a single particle or a small number of particles.

6.2. *Physical picture of Doppler cooling in the Penning trap*

We now describe a physical picture of Doppler cooling that helps in the interpretation of some experiments with laser cooled plasmas and Coulomb crystals in the Penning trap. Conventional laser cooling of neutral atoms can be shown to be equivalent to a damping force acting on the particle under certain approximations. In other words, the force on a particle is always directed against its motion and is proportional to its speed. This is the reason why a set-up with three perpendicular pairs of laser beams for laser cooling of neutral atoms is sometimes known as *optical molasses* because the lasers give rise to a viscous force on the atoms.

In an ion trap, only one beam is required in principle because the ion motion is bound. However, the same reasoning as above applies if the beam runs through the center of the trap. If, however, the laser beam is offset from the center of the trap, this changes the dynamics of the force on the ion. The force can now be shown to correspond to a *rotating* damping force. The frequency of rotation of this force (Ω_0) is proportional to the gradient of the laser intensity across the center of the trap, and it also depends on the detuning of the laser from resonance. It can therefore be varied by changing the laser cooling parameters. For typical cooling parameters, this frequency turns out to be of the order of 100 kHz, i.e. comparable with the magnetron frequency in many experiments [31]. The damping force behaves a bit like a whirlpool, i.e. a viscous fluid that is rotating about some axis. However, in this case, the angular velocity of the rotation is independent of the distance from the origin.

Analysis of the laser beam offset requirements for effective laser cooling [26,27,31] shows that a necessary condition is that

$$\omega_m < \Omega_0 < \omega_c'. \tag{7}$$

This means that the rate of rotation of the damping force must fall between the magnetron frequency and the modified cyclotron frequency.

In the rotating frame, this is equivalent to saying that the rate of rotation of the damping force (here equal to $\Omega_0 - \omega_c/2$) must fall between $-\omega_1$ and $+\omega_1$. In a simplified picture, it could be said that the rotating damping force 'tries' to make the ion orbit at the same rate as the damping force. If this is faster (in either the negative or positive sense) than the natural frequency of the simple harmonic well in the rotating frame, then the effect of the force will simply be to drive the particle into ever-increasing orbits, i.e. to heat it. On the other hand, if the rate of rotation of the damping force in this frame is less than the natural frequency of the potential well, the damping will take it to smaller orbits, which indicates ion cooling.

For a plasma consisting of many ions, the situation is different because it is possible for a plasma to rotate at any frequency between the magnetron frequency and the modified cyclotron frequency (in the laboratory frame), depending on its density. The effect of the rotating damping force is therefore now to force the plasma to rotate at Ω_0, adjusting its density so that this is the equilibrium state. But, if Ω_0 is less than ω_m or greater than ω_c', this cannot be achieved and the plasma will be heated up out of the trap.

6.3. *Demonstration of Doppler cooling*

As an example, we discuss the demonstration of Doppler cooling at Imperial College London. This experiment is carried out using calcium ions, which have the energy level structure shown in Figure 4. The laser cooling transition is at 397 nm, but calcium suffers from the disadvantage that there is a metastable level into which the ions can fall when they decay from the

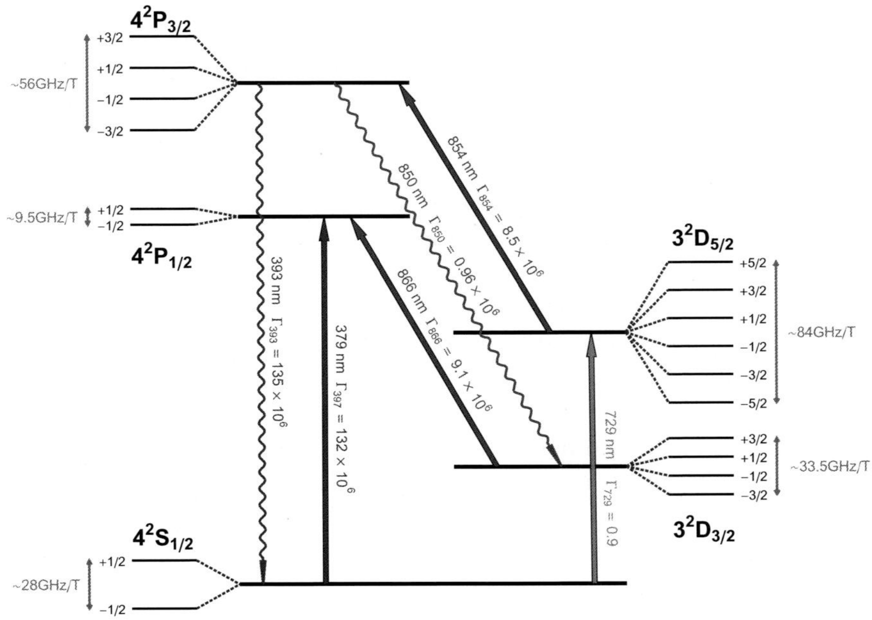

Fig. 4. Energy level diagram for Ca^+. The magnetic field splittings are shown greatly exaggerated. Lasers are required at the wavelengths indicated with solid lines.

$^2P_{1/2}$ excited state. As a result, a separate laser at 866 nm is required, and because of the Zeeman splitting of all levels, laser frequencies addressing all 4 levels of the $^2D_{3/2}$ state as well as both Zeeman levels of the $^2S_{1/2}$ ground state are required.

In this experiment, two sets of Doppler cooling beams are used, one along the trap axis and one in the radial plane so that both axial and radial degrees of freedom (DoF) are strongly cooled. Either the radial beams are offset from the trap axis or an axialization drive is used to ensure that the magnetron motion is cooled.

If the spectrum of a cooled ion is to be recorded by scanning through the resonance transition, there is a problem because as the frequency of the laser cooling beam is changed, the cooling parameters also change, so the temperature of the cooled ion is not constant. In particular, when the laser reaches the line center, it will start laser heating the ion rather than laser cooling it. It can therefore be difficult to interpret the resulting profile as it does not represent a constant temperature. In addition, the natural width of this transition is much larger than the Doppler width at the expected temperature, so it is necessary to deconvolve the Doppler profile from the natural lineshape.

One way around this problem is to record a spectrum of a different transition. In this experiment, the transition from the $^2S_{1/2}$ ground state to the $^2D_{5/2}$ state at 729 nm is recorded. This excited state has a lifetime of around 1 s, so the transition is very narrow and the recorded width represents the Doppler width directly. However, if a narrow laser is used to probe this transition, the lineshape is no longer continuous but consists of a carrier with sidebands (see Figure 5). This is because the ion acts as an oscillator that is frequency modulated at its trap oscillation frequency. For the axial motion, we therefore observe optical sidebands spaced by the axial oscillation frequency (here around 400 kHz). This spectrum demonstrates that the expected Doppler limit temperature of roughly 0.5 mK has been achieved [32]. Although a detailed fit to the quantum dynamics of this spectrum has been used here to determine the temperature, a rough estimate can be obtained simply by measuring the full width at half maximum (FWHM) of the envelope of the observed sideband peaks.

The spectrum of the radial motion is more interesting because it reveals the unusual nature of the motion of an ion in a Penning trap. Such a spectrum is shown in Figure 6. In this spectrum, well-resolved cyclotron sidebands at around 700 kHz can be seen, corresponding to a cyclotron temperature of a few mK. Each cyclotron sideband has structure due to the

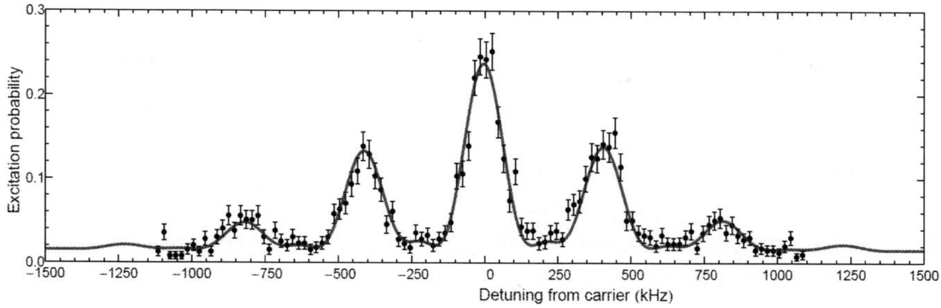

Fig. 5. Optical sideband spectrum of the axial motion of a single ion in a Penning trap after Doppler cooling, recorded at a trap potential of 240 V (giving $\omega_z/2\pi \approx$ 400 kHz). The solid line is a fit to the full quantum dynamics of the system and corresponds to a temperature of $T = 0.47 \pm 0.04$ mK ($\bar{n} = 24 \pm 2$). The error bars reflect the statistical uncertainty in the shelving probability arising from the number of repetitions of the measurement cycle at each frequency step [32].

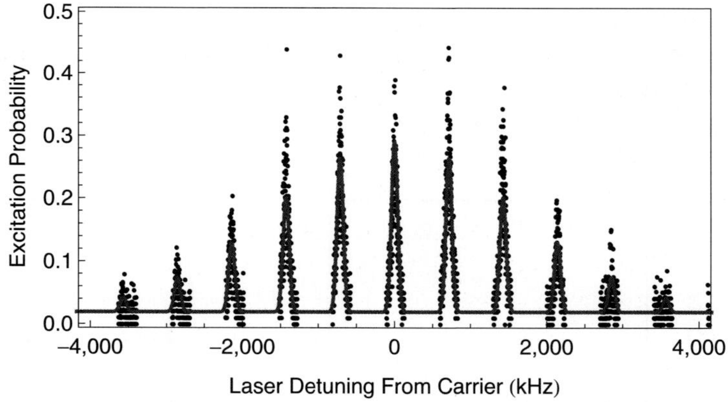

Fig. 6. Radial spectrum showing modified cyclotron sidebands, each of which is broadened due to the magnetron motion. Magnetron sidebands cannot be resolved fully at this trap voltage (5 V) because they are spaced by only 2.5 kHz [32].

magnetron motion, but the sidebands are close together due to the small value of the magnetron frequency, and are therefore unresolved. However, it is clear that the magnetron sidebands have an overall width of only a few tens of kHz, which implies a temperature of only a few tens of μK, much less than the standard Doppler limit. This counter-intuitive result is not unexpected and follows from the fact that the magnetron motion is only cooled very slowly as a result of the laser beam offset discussed above.

Its Doppler limit is therefore much lower than that of the cyclotron motion, which is cooled strongly and has roughly the standard value [32].

6.4. *Optical sideband cooling*

Optical sideband cooling is discussed in Chapter 6. It is best to think of this in terms of the ladder of equally spaced energy levels of the quantum mechanical simple harmonic oscillator represented by the axial motion of the ion in the quadratic trap potential. The steps of the ladder are spectroscopically resolved if they are probed on a narrow optical transition with a highly-stabilized laser. The 729 nm transition, used for the spectroscopic results shown in Figures 5 and 6, is very suitable for this. In sideband cooling, an excitation on the first sideband on the low frequency side of the carrier transition (the 'red sideband') lowers the quantum simple harmonic oscillator state quantum number n by 1 each time the ion is excited. On decay, it is most likely to stay in the same state, so each complete cycle on average lowers the quantum number by 1, and eventually the ion should end up in the ground state ($n = 0$). The sign of this is that the red sideband then disappears because there is no state with a lower value of n that can be excited. This can be seen clearly in Figure 7 which shows the first red and blue sidebands after sideband cooling.

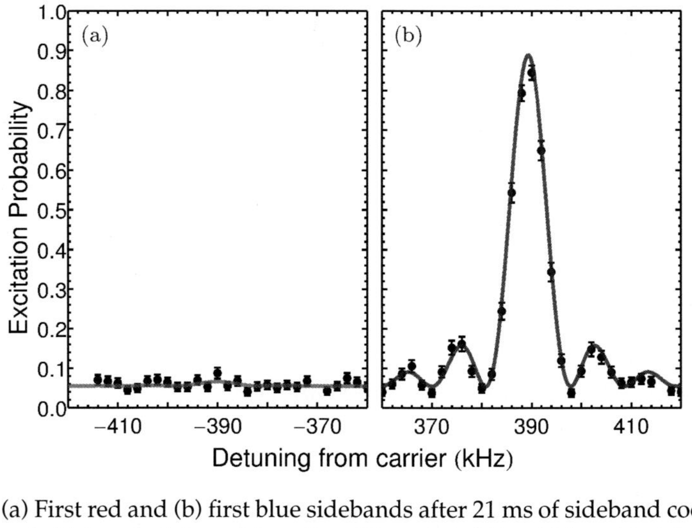

Fig. 7. (a) First red and (b) first blue sidebands after 21 ms of sideband cooling on the first red sideband of the axial motion. The ratio of the sideband heights above the background shows that the average photon number is $\bar{n} = 0.013 \pm 0.009$ [33]. Each plot shows the measured data as points and the fit to the expected coherent dynamics as a solid line.

6.5. *Coulomb crystals*

A striking consequence of the powerful technique of laser cooling is the creation of *ion Coulomb crystals* (ICC) (see Chapter 15). These structures appear when the temperature of a cloud of ions is so low that the Coulomb interaction between particles overcomes thermal effects. The result of this is that the particles form a regular crystal-like structure where the ions have fixed positions relative to each other. The equilibrium distance between particles is determined by a balance between their mutual Coulomb repulsion and the trapping force which pushes them together. Since this distance is typically tens of μm in a Penning trap, the density of such a crystal is many orders of magnitude lower than that of a conventional crystal — in fact, it is usually lower than the density of the residual gas in the vacuum chamber.

Ion Coulomb crystals can be created in both Penning and RF traps [34]. The configuration of an ICC is dependent on the strength of the axial and radial confinement. For very low axial confinement, the equilibrium configuration is a string of ions along the axis of the trap. This type of structure is used for experiments such as quantum information processing in linear RF traps (e.g. [35]). For intermediate ratios of the axial to radial confinement strength, ellipsoidal crystals are formed, and these have been used for a wide range of applications including, for example, cavity QED [36] and the study of ion processes such as ionization and charge exchange [37]. When the radial confinement is weak, crystals can adopt a planar configuration. This is not generally used in linear RF traps because there is a driven *micromotion* for any particles that are not located on the axis of the trap and this becomes much more significant as the radial extent of the crystal increases.

ICC were first observed in Penning traps by the Boulder group [39] and their structure was investigated by direct imaging and also by using Bragg scattering [40]. This group has worked extensively with planar crystals in a Penning trap and has used these for the study of the *drumhead* modes of oscillation of the crystal [41] and for quantum simulation of 2D Ising interactions [38]. An image of such a crystal (as viewed along the axis of the trap) is shown in Figure 8. Since the ion cloud in a Penning trap always rotates around the trap axis, whether it is in the form of a plasma or a crystal, each ion is executing an orbit around this axis. In Figure 8, this is overcome by imaging the crystal with a position-sensitive photomultiplier tube so that the position as well as the time of arrival of each photon is known. Since the rotation frequency of the crystal is also known (because it is driven using the rotating wall technique discussed in Section 6.1), the

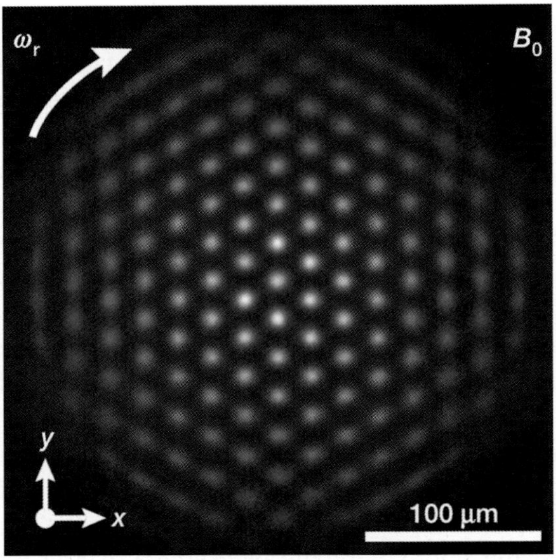

Fig. 8. An image of an ion Coulomb crystal consisting of a single plane of Be^+ ions in a Penning trap [38]. The crystal is rotating, but the image is reconstructed using timing information from a position-sensitive photomultiplier. Reprinted by permission from Macmillan Publishers Ltd: *Nature* **484**, 489, copyright 2012.

rotation of the crystal can effectively be frozen out, so the ions are imaged as points.

The whole range of configurations of a small crystal in a Penning trap, in this case containing 15 ions, can be seen in Figure 9. The ions are imaged here from a direction perpendicular to the trap axis, so the image of each ion is averaged over its radial motion and becomes a horizontal line. The only parameter which is changed between all these images is the trapping potential which ranges in this figure from 10% to 85% of the maximum value it can take for stable trapping.

As explained above, in a Penning trap, the plasma (or in this case, the crystal) is always rotating, and in the presence of laser cooling with a radially offset cooling beam, the speed of rotation is determined by the value of Ω_0, i.e. the rate of rotation of the damping force arising from the laser cooling beam (see Section 6.2). This in turn determines the density of the crystal through Equation (4), and also its aspect ratio (i.e. the ratio of the length to the diameter of the crystal). In the examples shown in Figure 9, each pane shows the experimentally obtained image on the left and a simulated image on the right. This simulated image takes into account the known

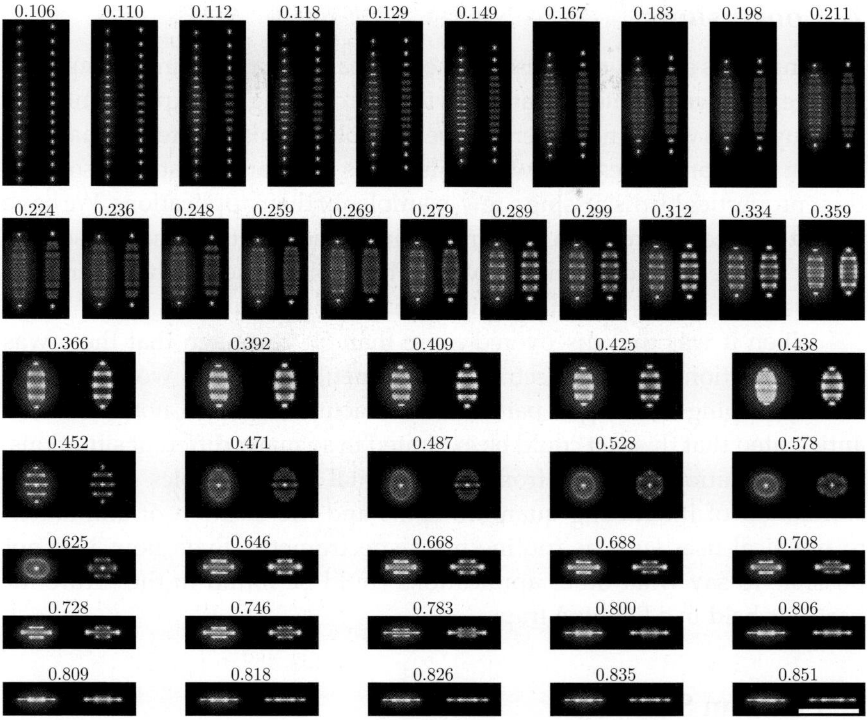

Fig. 9. Conformations of a 15-ion crystal in a Penning trap [42]. Experimentally obtained images (left side of each pane) are compared to computer simulations (right side of each pane). By increasing the axial confinement, a linear string is transformed into a zigzag structure, then a 3-D crystal and finally a planar structure. Each image is labeled with the value of the normalized axial trapping frequency, which increases with the trapping voltage (the trap becomes unstable when this quantity is equal to unity). There is a 100 μm scale bar in the bottom right-hand pane which applies to all the images. Reprinted by permission from Macmillan Publishers Ltd: *Nature Communications* **4**, 2571, copyright 2013.

trapping voltage and is matched by eye to the experimental image only by varying the rate of rotation of the crystal in the simulation. This allows the rate of rotation of the crystal to be determined from the best match of the simulated image to the real image. As expected, this turns out to be consistent with the value of Ω_0 estimated from the parameters of the laser cooling beam, and is found to be roughly constant for all the images in the figure, demonstrating that the crystal rotation always matches the rotation of the damping force created by the laser cooling beam, independent of the crystal configuration [42].

7. Conclusions

Penning traps are now well established in many areas of pure and applied science as powerful and versatile devices for carrying out experiments that in many cases would not otherwise be possible. In this chapter, we have set out the basic principles of how Penning traps work and illustrated some of their properties by discussing a few examples of their applications. We have not attempted to present a comprehensive review of their many uses but rather to give an understanding of their basic properties so that the reader can then investigate specific applications in more detail.

When it was first discovered more than 50 years ago that there was a configuration of static electric and magnetic fields that would lead to stable trapping of charged particles in a vacuum, it could not have been anticipated that this fact could be exploited in so many different situations, with applications ranging from fundamental physics topics such as the simulation of interacting quantum spins and the creation of antimatter, to practical uses such as routine mass spectrometry. Even now, it is not possible to say what other applications could be found in the future for particles held in a Penning trap.

8. Problem Set

Question 1

Starting from the Lorentz force on a charged particle in static electric (**E**) and magnetic (**B**) fields,

$$\mathbf{F} = e(\mathbf{E} + v \times \mathbf{B}) \tag{8}$$

with an electrostatic potential

$$\phi(r) = A(2z^2 - x^2 - y^2), \tag{9}$$

find the three oscillation frequencies (ω_z, ω_c, and ω_m) for a singly charged calcium ion in a magnetic field of 1 T and with $A = 1 \times 10^5$ Vm^{-2}.

Also, find the frequencies for the case of an electron in the same fields.

Question 2

Consider two stationary calcium ions located on the z-axis of the trap in Question 1, at positions $+z_1$ and $-z_1$. By equating the confining force from the trap with the Coulomb repulsion, find the equilibrium value of z_1.

Question 3

Thinking of an ion in the above trap as a quantum mechanical simple harmonic oscillator, calculate the "width" of the ground state wave function for the axial motion. [If you do not remember the formula for this, you can estimate it by calculating the amplitude of the classical motion of an ion having the zero-point energy $\hbar\omega_z/2$.]

Comparing the results of Questions 2 and 3, do you think it is possible to observe effects due to the overlap of ground state ion wavefunctions in a trap?

Question 4

In the book *Angels and Demons*, Dan Brown imagines a device that sounds similar to a Penning trap but stores enough liquid antihydrogen to destroy the Vatican. Imagine instead a real Penning trap (with a 1 T field) containing 1 cm^3 of antiprotons at the maximum possible density (i.e. at the Brillouin limit). What is the number density of antiprotons and how much energy would be released if the antiprotons were allowed to annihilate?

Question 1 solution

The force is

$$\mathbf{F} = e(\mathbf{E} + v \times \mathbf{B}), \tag{10}$$

but $\mathbf{E} = -\nabla\phi$ and $\phi = A(2z^2 - x^2 - y^2)$, so this gives

$$\mathbf{E} = 2Ax\hat{\mathbf{x}} + 2Ay\hat{\mathbf{y}} - 4Az\hat{\mathbf{z}} \tag{11}$$

and $\mathbf{v} \times \mathbf{B} = \dot{y}B\hat{\mathbf{x}} - \dot{x}B\hat{\mathbf{y}}$, so

$$m\ddot{\mathbf{r}} = \mathbf{F} = e[(2Ax + \dot{y}B)\hat{\mathbf{x}} + (2Ay - \dot{x}B)\hat{\mathbf{y}} - 4Az\hat{\mathbf{z}}]. \tag{12}$$

Writing $\omega_c = eB/m$ and $\omega_z^2 = 4eA/m$, we find

$$\ddot{x} - \omega_c\dot{y} - (\omega_z^2/2)x = 0, \tag{13}$$

$$\ddot{y} + \omega_c\dot{x} - (\omega_z^2/2)y = 0, \tag{14}$$

$$\ddot{z} + \omega_z^2 z = 0. \tag{15}$$

The solutions are of the form $C \exp i\omega t$ and Equations (13) and (14) give for the two components of the radial motion,

$$\omega = \omega_c' = \omega_c/2 + \sqrt{\omega_c^2/4 - \omega_z^2/2}, \tag{16}$$

$$\omega = \omega_m = \omega_c/2 - \sqrt{\omega_c^2/4 - \omega_z^2/2}. \tag{17}$$

Equation (15) gives $\omega = \omega_z$ for the axial motion. Putting in the values of $\mathbf{B} = 1$ T and $A = 1 \times 10^5$ Vm^{-2}, we find (for $^{40}Ca^+$) $\omega_c = 2.4 \times 10^6$ s^{-1} [380 kHz], $\omega_z = 9.8 \times 10^5$ s^{-1} [156 kHz], $\omega_c' = 2.2 \times 10^6$ s^{-1} [346 kHz] and $\omega_m = 2.4 \times 10^5$ s^{-1} [35 kHz].

For electrons, we find $\omega_c = 1.76 \times 10^{11}$ s^{-1} [28 GHz], $\omega_z = 2.65 \times 10^8$ s^{-1} [42 MHz], $\omega_c' = 1.76 \times 10^{11}$ s^{-1} [28 GHz] and $\omega_m = 2.0 \times 10^5$ s^{-1} [32 kHz]. Note that ω_m is nearly the same for both species despite the large mass difference.

Question 2 solution

The two particles sit on the z-axis displaced from the origin by equal and opposite amounts. The inwards force on each particle is $mz_1\omega_z^2$ and the outwards force on each particle is $e^2/4\pi\epsilon_0(2z_1)^2$, so in equilibrium, we find

$$mz_1\omega_z^2 = e^2/4\pi\epsilon_0 z_1^2, \tag{18}$$

which gives $z_1^3 = e^2/16\pi\epsilon_0 m\omega_z^2$. For $^{40}Ca^+$, we find $z_1 = 10.1\ \mu$m (for the trap parameters given above). The separation of the particles is therefore just over 20 μm.

Question 3 solution

We can use two different approaches to get a rough estimate. The uncertainty principle says that $\Delta z \Delta p_z \sim (z_0)(m\omega_z z_0) \sim \hbar$, where z_0 represents the approximate size of the ground state wave function. From this, we find $z_0 = \sqrt{\hbar/m\omega_z} = 0.04\ \mu$m. Alternatively, we get the same result by equating the ground state energy $\frac{1}{2}\hbar\omega_z$ to the potential energy $\frac{1}{2}m\omega_z^2 z_0^2$.

Comparing this result with the typical separation of ions derived in Question 2, we can see that under normal circumstances, the wavefunctions are well separated, so we expect no effects due to wavefunction overlap. However, it is possble to engineer situations where there are two different structural configuations of an ion Coulomb crystal that only involve very small displacements of the ions when the configuration changes. Under these circumstances, it is possible in principle to see quantum mechanical effects, though they are technically very challenging to observe. An example is a string of ions having an equilibrium configuration that is very slightly kinked to the left or the right. The wavefunctions of the whole system can have some overlap, so the state with the system in either one or the other configuration is no longer an eigenstate of the system and quantum tunnelling between the two configurations could be observed.

Question 4 solution

With $B = 1$ T, the maximum density of particles is $n = \epsilon_0 B^2/2m = 6.6 \times 10^{13}$ m^{-3}. So 1 cm^3 contains 66 million antiprotons, each of which has a rest mass energy of mc^2, giving a total energy of 0.4 J. It is also interesting to note that the same value can be obtained by calculating the energy density of the magnetic field, $B^2/2\mu_0$, multiplied by the volume of the cloud.

Acknowledgments

This work was supported in part by the European Commission STREP PICC (FP7 2007–2013 Grant number. 249958). We also gratefully acknowledge financial support toward networking activities from COST Action MP 1001 — Ion Traps for Tomorrows Applications.

References

1. H. Dehmelt, Radiofrequency spectroscopy of stored ions I: Storage, *Advances in Atomic and Molecular Physics*, Vol. 3, pp. 53–72. New York, Academic Press (1968).
2. H. Dehmelt, Radiofrequency spectroscopy of stored ions II: Spectroscopy. vol. 5, *Advances in Atomic and Molecular Physics*, pp. 109–154. New York, Academic Press (1969).
3. H. Dehmelt, Experiments with an isolated subatomic particle at rest (Nobel Lecture), *Angew. Chem. Int. Ed. Engl.* **29**(7), 734–738 (1990).
4. F. Penning, Die Glimmentladung bei niedrigem Druck zwischen koaxialen Zylindern in einem axialen Magnetfeld, *Physica* **3**(9), 873–894 (1936).
5. H. G. Dehmelt and F. L. Walls, "Bolometric" technique for the RF spectroscopy of stored ions, *Phys. Rev. Lett.* **21**, 127–131 (1968).
6. J. Byrne and P. S. Farago, On the production of polarized electron beams by spin exchange collisions, *Proc. Phys. Soc.* **86**(4), 801 (1965).
7. G. Gräff *et al.*, Method for measuring the cyclotron and spin resonance of free electrons, *Phys. Rev. Lett.* **21**, 340–342 (1968).
8. G. Gräff *et al.*, Method for measuring the anomalous magnetic moment of free electrons, *Zeitschrift für Physik.* **222**(3), 201–207 (1969).

9. D. J. Wineland *et al.*, Radiation-pressure cooling of bound resonant absorbers, *Phys. Rev. Lett.* **40**, 1639–1642 (1978).
10. L. S. Brown and G. Gabrielse, Geonium theory — physics of a single electron or ion in a Penning trap, *Rev. Modern Phys.* **58**(1), 233–311 (1986).
11. R. C. Thompson and D. C. Wilson, The motion of small numbers of ions in a Penning trap, *Zeitschrift Fur Physik D-Atoms Molecules and Clusters.* **42**(4), 271–277 (1997).
12. J. Bollinger *et al.*, 303-MHz frequency standard based on trapped Be^+ ions, *IEEE Transactions on Instrumentation and Measurement.* **40**(2), 126–128 (1991).
13. M. Mukherjee *et al.*, ISOLTRAP: An on-line Penning trap for mass spectrometry on short-lived nuclides, *Eur. Phys. J. A.* **35**(1), 1–29 (2008).
14. A. Solders *et al.*, Determination of the proton mass from a measurement of the cyclotron frequencies of D^+ and H_2^+ in a Penning trap, *Phys. Rev. A.* **78**, 012514 (2008).
15. A. G. Marshall *et al.*, Fourier transform ion cyclotron resonance mass spectrometry: A primer, *Mass Spectrom. Rev.* **17**(1), 1–35 (1998).
16. D. Hanneke *et al.*, New measurement of the electron magnetic moment and the fine structure constant, *Phys. Rev. Lett.* **100**, 120801 (2008).
17. A. Mooser *et al.*, Direct high-precision measurement of the magnetic moment of the proton, *Nature* **509**(7502), 596–599 (2014).
18. J. DiSciacca *et al.*, One-particle measurement of the antiproton magnetic moment, *Phys. Rev. Lett.* **110**, 130801 (2013).
19. J. Verdú *et al.*, The magnetic moment anomaly of the electron bound in hydrogen-like oxygen $^{16}O^{7+}$, *J. Phys. B: At. Mol. Opt. Phys.* **36**(3), 655 (2003).
20. W. Quint *et al.*, Laser-microwave double-resonance technique for g-factor measurements in highly charged ions, *Phys. Rev. A.* **78**, 032517 (2008).
21. C. Lichtenberg *et al.*, Axialisation, cooling and quenching of ions in a Penning trap, *Eur. Phys. J. D: At. Mol. Opt. Plasma Phys.* **2**(1), 29–32 (1998).
22. D. M. Segal and C. Wunderlich, *Physics with Trapped Charged Particles (Eds M. Knoop, N. Madsen and R. C. Thompson),* Chapter 3 Cooling Techniques for Trapped Ions, pp. 43–81. London, Imperial College Press (2014).
23. M. A. van Eijkelenborg *et al.*, Sympathetic cooling and detection of molecular ions in a Penning trap, *Phys. Rev. A.* **60**, 3903–3910 (1999).
24. G. Gabrielse *et al.*, Open-endcap Penning traps for high precision experiments, *Int. J. Mass Spectrom. Ion Process.* **88**(2–3), 319–332 (1989).
25. M. Knoop, *Physics with Trapped Charged Particles (Eds M. Knoop, N. Madsen, and R. C. Thompson),* Chapter 2 Detection Techniques for Trapped Ions, pp. 25–42. London, Imperial College Press (2014).
26. W. M. Itano and D. J. Wineland, Laser cooling of ions stored in harmonic and Penning traps, *Phys. Rev. A.* **25**, 35–54 (1982).
27. R. C. Thompson and J. Papadimitriou, Simple model for the laser cooling of an ion in a Penning trap, *J. Phys. B: At. Mol. Opt. Phys.* **33**(17), 3393–3405 (2000).
28. H. F. Powell *et al.*, Axialization of laser cooled magnesium ions in a Penning trap, *Phys. Rev. Lett.* **89**, 093003 (2002).
29. X. P. Huang *et al.*, Phase-locked rotation of crystallized non-neutral plasmas by rotating electric fields, *Phys. Rev. Lett.* **80**(1), 73–76 (1998).

30. S. Bharadia *et al.*, Dynamics of laser-cooled Ca^+ ions in a Penning trap with a rotating wall, *Appl. Phys. B: Lasers O.* **107**(4), 1105–1115 (2012).
31. M. Asprusten *et al.*, Theory and simulation of ion Coulomb crystal formation in a Penning trap, *Appl. Phys. B: Lasers O.* **114**(1–2), 157–166 (2014).
32. S. Mavadia *et al.*, Optical sideband spectroscopy of a single ion in a Penning trap, *Phys. Rev. A.* **89**, 032502 (2014).
33. J. G. Goodwin. *Sideband Cooling to the Quantum Ground State in a Penning Trap.* PhD thesis, Imperial College London (2015).
34. R. C. Thompson, Ion Coulomb crystals, *Contemp. Phys.* **56**, 63–79 (2015).
35. T. Monz *et al.*, 14-qubit entanglement: Creation and coherence, *Phys. Rev. Lett.* **106**, 130506 (2011).
36. A. Dantan *et al.*, Large ion Coulomb crystals: A near-ideal medium for coupling optical cavity modes to matter, *Phys. Rev. A.* **80**(4), 4 (2009).
37. M. Drewsen *et al.*, Ion Coulomb crystals: a tool for studying ion processes, *Int. J. Mass Spectrom.* **229**(1–2), 83–91 (2003).
38. J. W. Britton *et al.*, Engineered 2D Ising interactions in a trapped-ion quantum simulator with hundreds of spins, *Nature* **484**(7395), 489–492 (2012).
39. S. L. Gilbert *et al.*, Shell-structure phase of magnetically confined strongly coupled plasmas, *Phys. Rev. Lett.* **60**, 2022–2025 (1988).
40. J. N. Tan *et al.*, Long-range order in laser-cooled, atomic-ion Wigner crystals observed by Bragg scattering, *Phys. Rev. Lett.* **75**(23), 4198–4201 (1995).
41. B. C. Sawyer *et al.*, Spectroscopy and thermometry of drumhead modes in a mesoscopic trapped-ion crystal using entanglement, *Phys. Rev. Lett.* **108**(21), 213003 (2012).
42. S. Mavadia *et al.*, Control of the conformations of ion Coulomb crystals in a Penning trap, *Nat. Commun.* **4**, 2571 (2013).

CHAPTER TWO

RADIOFREQUENCY TRAPS

Martina Knoop

CNRS and Aix-Marseille Université, PIIM, UMR7345,
Centre de Saint Jérôme, Case C21, 13397 Marseille Cedex 20, France
Martina.Knoop@univ-amu.fr

Radiofrequency (RF) traps exist in a large variety of geometries and designs. These devices confine charged species with a vast range of masses from electrons to proteins. Due to their extremely long storage times, RF traps are used today as tools of choice in many high-resolution spectroscopy experiments from quantum information to cold chemistry. This chapter describes their mode of operation and their fundamental characteristics. It will show important parameters of design and describe ways to characterize the properties of a real trap. An overview of geometries exposes existing solutions for various applications.

1. Introduction

Quantum information, frequency metrology, high-precision measurements of fundamental constants, cold chemistry, and single-molecule reactions — when Wolfgang Paul invented the trap that carries his name in 1958 [1], he certainly did not imagine the major impact that this "by-product" of his research would have 50 years later. He was an expert in mass selection questions, and his main research field was nuclear physics. Wolfgang Paul was actively engaged in obtaining the funds and permission to build a 100 MeV electron synchrotron in Bonn, and for this, he concentrated on the question of "strong focussing".[a]

Today, the main interest of the use of ion traps lies in the manipulation and interrogation of ensembles of atomic or molecular ions of various sizes.

[a]See the lecture slides of Jeff Hangst, where you'll discover how this works: the Paul trap is the temporal analogon of the spatial implementation of focussing by quadrupole fields.

The sample can be a single particle or a large cloud, it can be an electron, a charged atom, a charged molecule or even a charged dust particle. Storage times are longer than achieved with any other device in atomic or molecular physics, and this is the main feature which makes the so-called "ion traps" so popular. Radiofrequency (RF) traps and their non-identical twins, Penning traps (see Chapter 1 by Richard Thompson in this volume), are a basic tool for a large variety of applications which you'll find described in detail in other chapters.

2. The Invention of the RF Trap

In 1953, Wolfgang Paul described a precursor of the RF trap: a two-dimensional (2D) mass filter based on quadrupole fields [2]. Very rapidly, the extension to three dimensions followed and was experimentally set-up. The complete theory, set-up and characterization of the "ion cage" is discussed in a fundamental 65-page document [1] which is unfortunately only available in German language. Many developments — in particular in laser manipulation and interrogation — have followed, making RF traps a major tool for precision and high-precision spectroscopy, and you will find various applications in this volume. Paul's work on ion traps has been awarded the Nobel Prize in Physics 1989 (together with Hans G. Dehmelt for Penning traps), the two of them sharing the distinction with Norman F. Ramsey for "the development of atomic precision spectroscopy" [3]. More information on the history of the development and the basic features of the RF trap has been made available during an 2012 exposition on Paul's life and work by the Deutsches Museum Bonn.

3. Operation of RF Traps

The classic "ion cage" is illustrated in Figure 1. It is a structure composed of three metallic electrodes, a ring, and two endcaps, whose geometric shape is hyperbolic, and obeys the relation $r_0^2 = 2z_0^2$. Between these electrodes, a time-varying voltage is applied, resulting in a potential,

$$\Phi(x,y,z,t) = (U_{DC} + V_{AC}\cos\Omega t)\frac{x^2 + y^2 - 2z^2}{2r_0^2}, \tag{1}$$

where U_{DC} and V_{AC} are the static and alternating voltages applied to the electrodes, $\Omega/2\pi$ is the frequency of the applied voltage, and $r = \sqrt{x^2 + y^2}$ and z are the axes of the trap. The variation of the potential is made fast

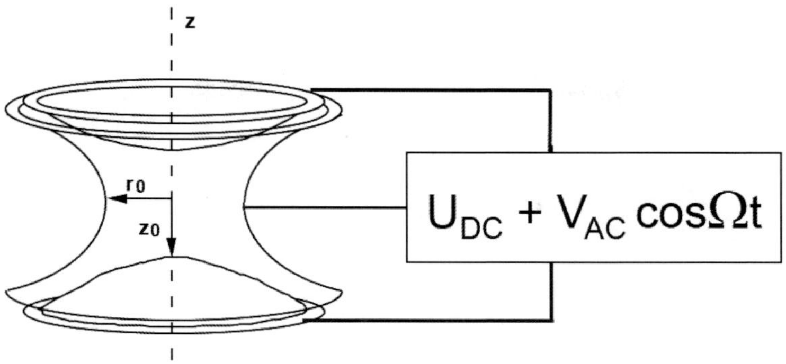

Fig. 1. Set-up of the classic Paul trap, the geometry of the electrodes obeys the relation $r_0^2 = 2z_0^2$.

enough that the charged particle is forced to make an oscillatory movement between the electrodes without being able to ever reach them: the particle is then trapped!

The motion of a particle of charge to mass ratio e/m can be formalized by the following differential equation:

$$\frac{d^2u}{dt^2} + \frac{\Omega^2}{4}(a_u - 2q_u \cos \Omega t)u = 0 \quad \text{with } u = x, y, z, \tag{2}$$

where the parameters a_u and q_u are only defined by the experimental conditions:

$$a_x = -\frac{1}{2} a_z = \frac{1}{2} \frac{8eU_{DC}}{mr_0^2\Omega^2} \quad \text{and} \quad q_x = -\frac{1}{2} q_z = \frac{1}{2} \frac{4eV_{AC}}{mr_0^2\Omega^2}. \tag{3}$$

Fortunately enough, Equation (2) is a well-known differential equation and has been solved by E. Mathieu in the 19th century for the vibration of an elliptic membrane [4].

Stable solutions to Mathieu's equation, corresponding to particle trajectories that are limited to the volume of the trap, are solely determined by the parameters a_u and q_u defined in Equation (3). In order to store a particle in three dimensions, this must be true in x-, y-, and in z-direction simultaneously. Figure 2 shows on the left-hand side the stability diagram for a large interval of a_u and q_u-values. For practical reasons, almost all real-world experimental implementations operate in the first stability zone (depicted on the right-hand side of the same figure).

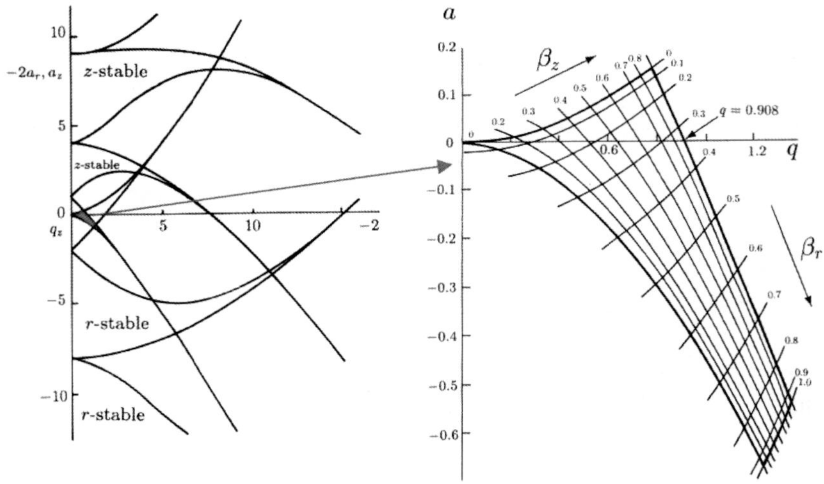

Fig. 2. Stability diagram for the solution of the equation of motion of a single charged particle in a Paul trap. In the vast majority of cases, experimental set-ups operate in the first zone of the stability diagram.

Exact solutions of the Mathieu Equation (2) are given by

$$u(t) = A \sum_{n=-\infty}^{\infty} C_{2n} \cos(\beta + 2n)\frac{\Omega t}{2} + B \sum_{n=-\infty}^{\infty} C_{2n} \sin(\beta + 2n)\frac{\Omega t}{2}, \tag{4}$$

where A and B are constants depending on the initial conditions. The coefficients C_{2n}, which are the amplitudes of the Fourier components of the particle motion, decrease with increasing n. The oscillation of the trapped particle is defined by

$$\omega_u = \beta_u \Omega, \tag{5}$$

where β_u is an iterative fraction of a_u and q_u:

$$\beta_u^2 = a_u + \cfrac{q_u^2}{(\beta_u + 2)^2 - a_u - \cfrac{q_u^2}{(\beta_u + 4)^2 - a_u - \cfrac{q_u^2}{(\beta_u + 6)^2 - a_u - \cdots}}} + \cfrac{q_u^2}{(\beta_u - 2)^2 - a_u - \cfrac{q_u^2}{(\beta_u - 4)^2 - a_u - \cfrac{q_u^2}{(\beta_u - 6)^2 - a_u - \cdots}}} \tag{6}$$

For the determination of experimental parameters, this is not practical, but Dehmelt has shown in the early years of ion trapping [5] that for values of $q_u < 0.4$ and $a_u \ll q_u$, the adiabatic approximation can be used. A simple solution is found in the form,

$$u(t) = R_u \cos \omega_u t \left(1 + \frac{q_u}{2} \cos \Omega t\right) \tag{7}$$

with

$$\beta_u = \sqrt{a_u + \frac{q_u^2}{2}}, \quad \text{and} \quad \omega_u = \beta_u \Omega. \tag{8}$$

The motion of a single particle in an RF trap is a harmonic oscillation, resulting from a superposition of the driven motion at the trapping frequency Ω (*micromotion*) with a slower secular motion ω_u (*macromotion*), quantified by an amplitude of motion R_u. As a matter of fact, R_u increases with increasing distance of the ion from the center of the trap.

It is important to note that β_u-values diverge rapidly from the exact solution outside the indicated interval for the adiabatic approximation. In order to avoid the use of the iterative fraction for the exact value, reasonable values (to within 15% of the exact value) for β_u can also be obtained by the approximative formula given in [6].

3.1. *Strong confinement*

In a potential well of finite size, the energy levels of an oscillating particle are discrete, and this situation is similar to the one of an ion in a trap. The *strong confinement* regime [7] is reached, when the ion's amplitude of oscillation is small compared to the probing wavelength. This condition is easy to fulfil for (*cm*-sized) microwave radiation, but much more difficult to achieve for wavelengths in the optical domain. In this case, the oscillation of the ion has to be damped to a high degree which is in general done by laser-cooling. However, as we have seen in the previous section and in Equation (7), the ion's amplitude of oscillation depends on the distance of the ion from the trap center. Due to Coulomb interaction, only a single particle can reach the strong confinement domain for optical transitions, where the energy spectrum is then decomposed into a central carrier and vibrational sidebands, eliminating the line broadening by the first order Doppler effect. Details about the cooling process and how to reach the ground state of the trap can be found in the chapter by Champenois (Chapter 6).

For high-precision frequency metrology and in particular for quantum information and atomic clock experiments, the strong confinement regime allows extremely high spectral resolution and long decoherence times to be reached. (In cases of particularly low vibrational levels, this mode is known as the Lamb–Dicke regime [8]).

In order to reach this mode of operation experimentally, the trap potential has to be almost "ideal", so that the single ion sits exactly at the potential minimum. Real-world traps need to be compensated to match the trapping site to the potential minimum as asymmetries in the electrical environment (vessel parts, vacuum components, etc.) can induce geometrical shifts in the trapping potential. Different methods for compensation exist, and a very complete review of causes and remedies is given in the article by Berkeland *et al.* [9]. A rough method for compensation is the variation of the amplitude of the trapping RF voltage, and the simultaneous observation of the ion's position in the radial plane. Fine-tuning can then be made by recording the fluorescence signal triggered on the RF-trapping frequency: the observed fluorescence oscillation amplitude is proportional to the micromotion amplitude of the ion and can therefore be used to center the atom in the potential minimum. Details of various techiques can be found in the chapter by Schmidt *et al.* on *Optical Clocks* in this volume (Chapter 18).

3.2. *More than one ion*

We have seen in the previous section that some experiments aiming at long decoherence times require the use of a single ion. A single ion can be detected with very high probability by using Dehmelt's "electron-shelving" technique [5]. For many other applications, more than one ion has to be trapped, cooled or probed, and observed. Several trapped ions of the same sign of charge will feel Coulomb repulsion, and it is this latter which limits the density of a stored ion cloud. Typical inter-ion distances are of the order of a few μm, and as a consequence, the densities reached are about 10^8 particles per cm^3. The space charge of the cloud will modify the potential that the ions experience, and the response of a cloud, in particular its motional frequencies, are therefore slightly shifted to lower values [10].

Günther Werth's group in Mainz, Germany has made many seminal contributions. In 1977, they studied the ion number by looking at the ion's fluorescence and deduced the trapping behavior for different working points throughout the stability diagram [11]. Highest ion numbers are found for Mathieu parameters $q_z \approx 0.55$ and $a_z \approx -0.05$. They could also show experimentally that the spatial distribution of a trapped cloud is Gaussian [12].

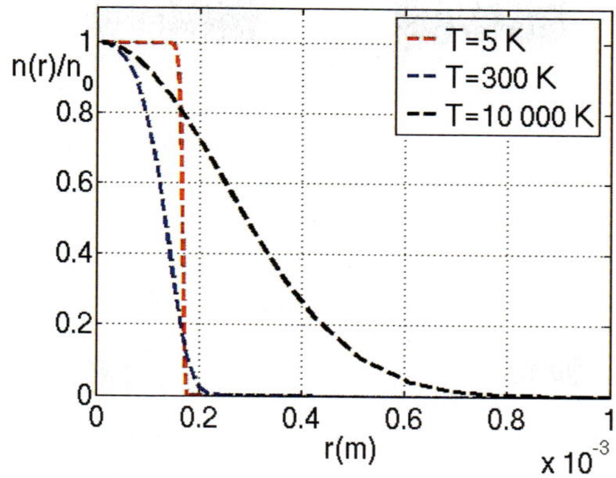

Fig. 3. Particle density in the quadrupole trap as a function of the radial dimensions for different ion temperatures.

For more than roughly 100 ions, the cloud can be considered as a non-neutral plasma, and at low temperatures, it can be modeled as a cold charged fluid [13]. In an RF quadrupole trap, it can be shown (compare Figure 3) that the density profile of the stored ion cloud changes with varying temperatures [14, 15]. Actually, for temperatures below a few kelvin, the profile becomes flat, illustrating a homogeneous density throughout the entire sample. The transition from cloud to residual gas is made on the scale of a Debye length, which is typically smaller than the ion–ion distance.

4. Characterization of RF Traps

Space charge, screening, geometric defects (for example, due to electrodes shorter than infinity!), contact potentials, all these (and other effects) contribute to the fact that a real-world ion trap is non-ideal. Characterization of the dynamics of the stored ion sample with respect to the theoretical prediction is required and reveals the real parameters of the trap. Various techniques can be used which allow the motional frequencies of the trapped ions to be measured. The underlying detection methods are described in a previous volume [16].

Characterizing an RF trap is summarized in a majority of cases by measuring the motional frequencies of the ions. It is straightforward to visualize these frequencies by adding a very small additional oscillating voltage onto one of the trap electrodes. If the frequency of this "tickle" is in resonance with a motional frequency ω_i of the stored ion sample, this can lead to excitation of the sample which potentially changes the sample's response. Using this excitation method, almost every optical or non-optical detection allows the ion's secular frequencies to be observed. In the case of destructive detection on an electron multiplier or MCP by ejection from the trap, the spectra of motional frequencies have to be recorded sequentially. The easiest implementation is the application of the tickle followed by ejection and detection: in the non-resonant case, a signal for a complete ion cloud will be recorded, but in cases where the ions are previously excited by the tickle voltage, a smaller signal will be recorded as ions are already lost during the tickle excitation [17].

For laser-cooled ions, the application of a tickle frequency can excite the ions and consequently change their temperature and thus modify their Doppler broadening. With cooling lasers at fixed frequency, excitation can then be observed by a change in amplitude of the ion's fluorescence.

A very complete study of the ions' response throughout the entire stability diagram has been performed in the mid-90s. In order to scan the trapping behavior of a 3D Paul trap, Alheit *et al.* have created an ion cloud composed of H^+, H_2^+, and H_3^+ ions for many different storage parameters before ejecting it and recording a time-of-flight profile on a multi-channel plate [18]. One of the results regarding the trapping of H_2^+ ions can be seen in Figure 4. Actually, many different lines of very low or vanishing number of trapped ions can be observed. The team has shown that these absences of ion trapping are due to a nonlinear behavior of the trapped ions. In fact, perturbations of order N appear for [19]

$$n_r \frac{\beta_r}{2} + n_z \frac{\beta_z}{2} = \kappa \quad \text{and} \quad |n_r| + |n_z| = N, \tag{9}$$

where n_r, n_z, and κ are integers ≥ 0. These coupling effects have not only been observed between the different components of the macromotion, but also for nonlinearities provoked by the coupling of micro and macromotion.

For many experiments, care has to be taken to avoid these "black canyons" to maintain a reasonable trapping efficiency, but they can also be cleverly exploited. Alheit *et al.* [20] have also proposed to use them for precise isotope separation, as trapping conditions for adjacent masses can differ rapidly for neighboring working points.

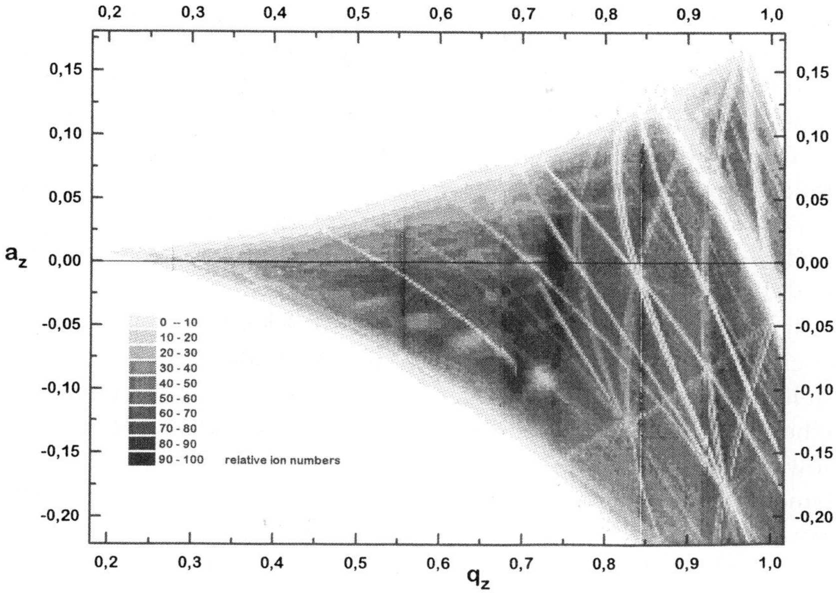

Fig. 4. Scan of the number of trapped hydrogen H_2^+ ions for identical creation conditions (from Ref. [18]). The darker the scale, the more ions are trapped.

5. Various Geometries of RF Traps

Very early in the life of ion traps, the need to introduce charged particles, to create ions in the center of the trap, to interact with electromagnetic radiation, or to optically detect the ion's fluorescence, required modifications of the ideal shape of the trap electrodes. Holes have to be drilled, and electrodes can unfortunately not be infinite and are always truncated.

5.1. *Linear traps*

In order to open the trap to access the trapped particles, it is advantageous to go back to the idea of Paul's original mass filter. The introduction of lasers and other probes is easy in a trap made of four parallel rods [21]. The radial trapping potential is the quadrupole one described above, while the axial confinement (along the z-axis) is made by two additional electrodes at each end of the trapping rods, onto which a DC-voltage is applied. An additional advantage of this geometry is that due to the elongated form, many particles are stored closed to the central zero-line of potential, where they are subject to reduced micromotion. Very few laser-cooled ions will line up as a string of single ions in this trap, allowing more than one ion to be in the strong confinement regime in the radial direction. This major advantage has made the linear trap a candidate of choice in many high-precision experiments from frequency metrology to quantum information.

The stability diagram in a linear trap is the one for directions x and y. Motional frequencies in the z-direction are determined by the potential applied on the endcaps, which is a DC-voltage! Detailed analysis of the stability diagram and effective potentials in a linear trap can be found in Ref. [22].

It has to be added that for reasons of simplicity, the trap electrodes are circular rods in the large majority of experimental realizations. The resulting radial potential will then be no longer perfectly harmonic, and higher-order terms can perturb the operation of the device. It has been shown in Ref. [23] that these additional terms can be minimized if the diameter of the rods d_0 takes a fixed value with respect to the trap radius r_0: $d_0/2 = 1.1468\, r_0$.

Individual addressing of ions is possible and can be made, for example with a clever set-up as developed by the Innsbruck group, using the same high-resolution optics for probing and observation [24]. The distance of single ions along a string in a linear trap is typically of the order of a few micrometer. More specifically, it is determined by the potential along the z-axis, and the number of ions [25].

As the potential varies along the axis, the ion distance varies as well, and the interaction of neighboring ions will not be identical in the center of the chain and at the ends. To overcome this asymmetry, the most elegant solution is to bend the linear trap into a ring, avoiding endcaps or a varying potential. This "race-track" trap has been built in the early 90s by Birkl *et al.* [26], with a radial trap diameter of 5 mm, and a ring diameter of 115 mm. In this storage device, regularly spaced crystals could be observed, and the variation of the radial potential illustrated transitions from a single chain to a multi-shell structure. Other applications of these storage devices have been used for crystalline beams [27] or to resolve isobaric contamination [28].

5.2. *Multipole traps*

Today, quadrupole ion traps can be found in a myriad of high-precision applications due to their extremely long storage times and the existence of the strong confinement regime. Laser-cooled ions can be cooled to the vibrational ground state for more than 99% of the time, and the interaction with the environment is extremely well controlled. However, quadrupole traps do have one main drawback, and that is the micromotion which drives all trapped ions, and whose amplitude increases with the distance of the ion from the center of the trap.

A way around this problem is to modify the geometry of the trapping potential. Gerlich has described the dynamics of higher-order traps and used them for experiments in a cryogenic environment since the beginning of the 90s [29], almost exclusively in the 22-pole version.

Actually, the pseudopotential in the radial plane of an ideal linear multipole trap can be written as

$$V^*_{\text{radial}}(\mathbf{r}) = \frac{qV_0^2}{32\mathcal{E}_k}\left(\frac{r}{r_0}\right)^{2k-2} \tag{10}$$

with q and m, the charge and the mass of the trapped particles, and V_0 and $\Omega/2\pi$, the amplitude and the frequency of the RF trapping field, respectively. $\mathcal{E}_k = m\Omega^2 r_0^2/(2k^2)$ is a characteristic energy. In the following, we consider that there is no static voltage U_s applied to the rods, but we take into account the static potential required for axial confinement, V_{end}, and its effect on the transverse pseudopotential. The total effective potential becomes

$$V^*(\mathbf{r}) = \frac{q^2V_0^2}{32\mathcal{E}_k}\left(\frac{r}{r_0}\right)^{2k-2} + \frac{q\kappa V_{\text{end}}}{2z_0^2}(2z^2 - r^2), \tag{11}$$

where κ is a loss factor depending on the geometry of the end electrodes relative to the rods. It includes all screening effects that can explain the reduction between the potential applied on the end electrodes V_{end} and the one effectively seen by the ions. Figure 5 illustrates the potential in a multipole trap, a detailed description of the dynamics of ions in multipoles can be found in Ref. [15].

The dynamics of ions stored in a multipole trap is nonlinear, and the trajectories of the ions depend on initial conditions. A stability diagram cannot be defined, and the stability parameters are replaced by a local adiabaticity parameter $\eta_{\text{ad}}(r)$ [29], which has been empirically determined to a value of approximately $\eta_{\text{ad}}(r) = 0.36$ [30].

The observed density profiles in a multipole trap are very different from the ones in the quadrupole, in particular for lower temperatures. Ions are "expelled" from the center and the density is increasing towards the walls of the trap. For laser-cooled ions at temperatures well below 10 K, numerical simulations show that the ordered structures formed by crystallized ions in these traps are hollow. A particular application for a reduced

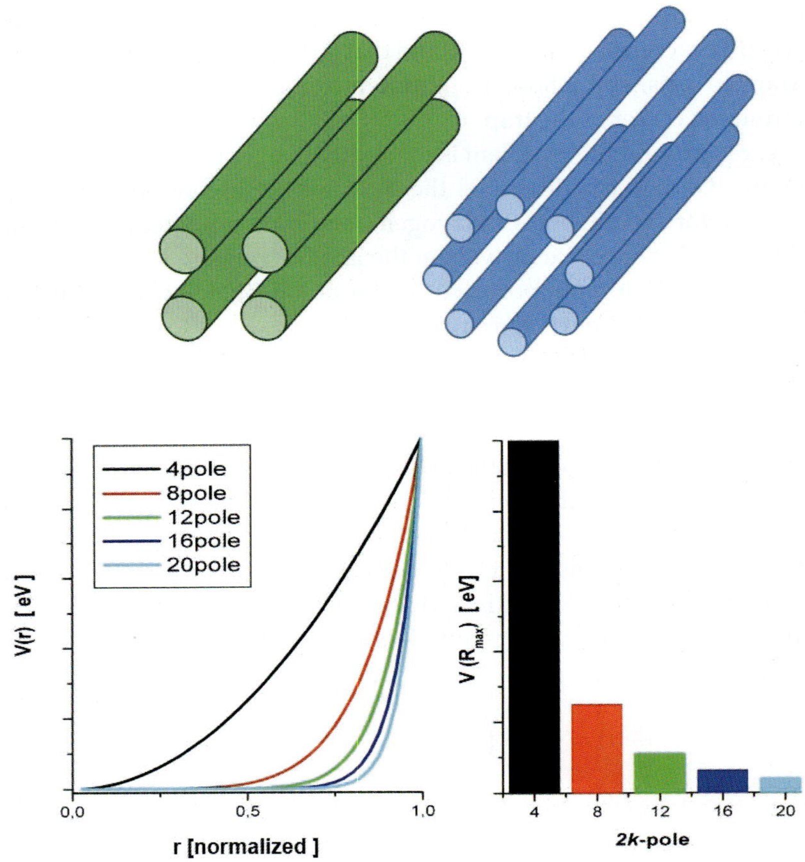

Fig. 5. A linear quadrupole (upper left) and a linear octupole trap (upper right). The lower part of the figure illustrates the geometric variation of the potential for different orders of multipoles (left) and their compared potential well depth for a given RF-voltage (right).

number of ions is to create plane ion rings, which are very well-controlled model systems and could also be used in frequency metrology [31]. We have studied structural transitions of multipole-trapped ion rings [32], and Ref. [33] gives a vast overview about operation and further applications.

Today, two open questions remain for these traps of modified geometry, which have not been yet been definitively answered by the experiments. First, multipole traps require an extraordinary symmetric design, or a large number of compensation electrodes in order to prevent the existence of additional minima of quadrupole geometry [34]. Second, the stability of laser-cooled ion crystals has not been evidenced in a robust way: the modified potential pushes the cooled ions toward the walls of the trap where micromotion issues are important.

5.3. *Miniature traps*

Very practical arguments have led to the reduction of the size of the trap electrodes, in particular, the work on single ions: In a macroscopic trap, with a laser focused to the center of the trap, it can happen that a single ion or single ions are trapped, but they may have a very large oscillation amplitude and not necessarily pass all their time in the laser-beam and scatter photons to be cooled. In a macroscopic trap, not all ions are simultaneously laser-cooled and it can happen that additional ions "pop up" in the fluorescence signal with a time delay.

In the strong confinement regime (see Section 3.1), the excitation spectrum of a single ion shows a central carrier and many sidebands at multiples of the motional frequencies and the trapping frequency [8]. Depending on the experimental set-up and the chosen ion, there might also be hyperfine levels and or Zeeman lines. In order to be able to resolve this forest of lines by laser spectroscopy, it is reasonable to choose high motional frequencies which will be situated far from the carrier. Furthermore, for the harmonic oscillator that is the ion, the kinetic energy is a product of the squares of amplitude and frequency ($E_{\text{kin}} = 1/2m\omega_i^2 r_i^2$). At a given energy (for example, the Doppler cooling limit), the larger the frequency, the smaller will be the oscillating amplitude which is an important criterion for dimensioning a trap experiment.

The larger the trap, the more important will be its electrical capacitance. A typical linear trap of radius $r_0 = 4\,\text{mm}$ has a capacitance of only a few pF. It has to be noted that the electric connection (cables and in particular vacuum feedthroughs) of the trap adds an important capacitance, which will in some cases be even more limiting than the trap itself. Stable confinement at a trapping frequency of several MHz requires large amplitudes (see *Problems*), which can be generated by high-Q resonators [35]. The NIST group has realized a set-up which feeds the trapping frequency signal via an antenna in the UHV vessel, and the amplification is then done in the vessel. Trapping frequencies of around 240 MHz have been reached, leading to motional frequencies above 20 MHz [36].

Reducing the size of the trap will reduce its capacitance, and opens the access to a higher frequency range. For given trapping parameters, a smaller trap radius r_0 will lead to higher q_i values and therefore to larger

ω_i. In miniature traps, a tightly focused laser beam (i.e. a waist of $r_L = 20$ μm) is always larger than the ion trajectory.

Among the very first proposals for a modified miniature trap is the one by Beaty [37]. Schrama *et al.* [38] have simulated and experimentally tested different miniature geometries. They have shown that for the trapping of a single ion, only the very inner part of the trap potential is of critical importance. In many cases, and in order to facilitate access of laser beams and avoid scattered light, miniature traps consist either of endcaps only or of a central ring only. Actually, for these simplified symmetric geometries, the central 10% of the potential are very close to a quadrupole potential. Compared to the oscillation amplitude of a single ion at the center of the structure, the electrodes are already at "infinity" if they are a few hundred micrometers away. Their exact shape is then no longer important and can be largely simplified.

This simplification is paid for by a loss factor $\mathcal{L}$, which is the required multiplication factor for the trapping voltage of a trap with simplified electrodes in order to reach the same potential well depth as an ideal quadrupole trap of identical radius [38]. For a trap made of a cylindrical ring, $\mathcal{L}$ has been measured to be of the order of 6–8 [39].

A very advanced (non-symmetric) version of an endcap trap is the so-called "stylus trap", making use of the extremely open geometry in order to collect fluorescence in a wide solid angle [40].

Due to the fact that these traps are only harmonic in their very center, only single ions or very small clouds can be trapped, and it is in general relatively easy to laser-heat superfluous ions off. It has to be remarked that it can be challenging to detect first fluorescence signals in these simplified traps as the number of experimental parameters including the loss factor $\mathcal{L}$ is relatively high. Moreover, only single or very few ions can be detected, which requires an optimized laser-cooling process as well as an almost perfectly aligned optical detection system. Good luck!

5.4. *Surface traps*

Frequency metrology and other high-precision experiments would maybe have been satisfied with the level of miniaturization achieved by the end of the last millennium. Quantum information processing has been the driving force to go to even smaller structures, and in particular, the proposal to realize a quantum computer with a scalable architecture [41], has made new approaches necessary. In 2005, Chiaverini *et al.* [42] have proposed to simplify the 3D trap to a 2D planar structure which opened the way

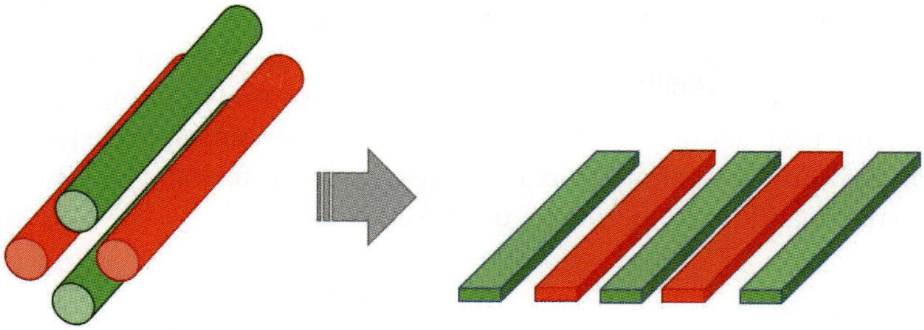

Fig. 6. Projection of a 3D linear trap into a plane (5-wire trap).

to lithographic fabrication (see Figure 6). First planar ion traps have been realized very rapidly [43,44], with all electrodes located in the same plane, and the ions trapped at a distance of a few tens of μm above this plane.

The generated potential well depends on the number and alternation of DC- and RF-electrodes, while the height of the well above the surface of the traps is determined by the width of the electrodes [45]. For $r_0 \ll z_0$, the motional frequencies of the trapped ions will be

$$\omega_r \propto \frac{eV_{AC}}{m\Omega r_0^2}. \tag{12}$$

Many different measurements have shown that these traps are subject to anomalous heating with heating rates much larger than expected from Johnson noise. Patch potentials and other surface contaminations have been found to be a major reason for this behavior [46], and there is a world-wide effort to report best materials, geometries, and dimensions. All data of heating rates in traps have been compiled at a website [47].

Today, two and three layer traps have been fabricated. *In situ* cleaning has shown spectacular advances in reducing the heating rate [48], and many groups have developed original and on-demand geometries which sketch the future of quantum information processing.

6. Outlook

This chapter sketches the operation and implementation of RF-traps. Detailed discussions can be found in the books of March and Hughes [49], or Major *et al.* [50] There is a multitude of realizations today for a wide range of applications. Two very timely examples are the development of RF-traps with integrated optical fibres for detection [51] or as resonant cavity [52], and the large family of hybrid experiments combining traps and cold atoms [53]. Furthermore, many groups have developed macroscopic outreach or training devices, which demonstrate trapping and cooling. Dust particles or glass spheres in a trap under atmospheric pressure form beautiful crystalline structures. These traps are amazing tools to visualize micro and macromotion by the naked eye.

7. Problems

7.1. *Dimensioning a trap drive*

(a) Determine the required V_{AC} for trapping a $^{40}Ca^{+}$-ion in a Paul trap of radius $r_0 = 5\,\mathrm{mm}$, for a miniature Paul trap with $r_0 = 700\,\mu\mathrm{m}$, and for a simplified endcap trap with $r_0 = 700\,\mu\mathrm{m}$ and $\mathcal{L} = 6$ at trapping frequencies of $\Omega_1/2\pi = 1\,\mathrm{MHz}$ and $\Omega_2/2\pi = 20\,\mathrm{MHz}$.

(b) What are the requirements for experimental parameters in order to generate a potential well which is identical in all directions?

Solution (a) See Section 3 for explications and equations. As an example, let $\beta_z = 0.1$, and $U_{DC} = 10\,\mathrm{V}$.

$\Omega/2\pi$	$r_0 = 5\,\mathrm{mm}$	$r_0 = 700\,\mu\mathrm{m}$	$r_0 = 700\,\mu\mathrm{m}$, $\mathcal{L} = 6$
1 MHz	no solution	$V_{AC} = 4.58\,\mathrm{V}$	$V_{AC} = 12.8\,\mathrm{V}$
20 MHz	$V_{AC} = 23,600\,\mathrm{V}$	$V_{AC} = 465\,\mathrm{V}$	$V_{AC} = 2,730\,\mathrm{V}$

(b) Potential well depths, and in consequence, secular frequencies should be identical, $\omega_r = \omega_z$. For the case $r_0 = 700\,\mu\mathrm{m}, \Omega/2\pi = 20\,\mathrm{MHz}$, and $V_{AC} = 465\,\mathrm{V} : U_{DC} = -275\,\mathrm{V}$.

7.2. *Design of an RF trap*

Imagine your favorite spectroscopy experiment: What do you want to measure? To what precision? What is your ion? Its wavelengths? The corresponding line-width? How many ions do you need? What is the expected signal-to- noise ratio? Any special environmental requirements (no B-field no BBR, short-lived nuclides, ...?)

Solution More than a single solution exist.

Depending on the objective of measurement in terms of precision and stability, you should work out the solution along the following points:

(1) Determine the aimed signal-to-noise-ratio,
(2) Estimate the ion number you'll need,
(3) What is your planned detection method (optical, electronical)?
(4) What is your planned excitation method (optical, electronical)?
(5) Determine the trap size including all access possibilities,
(6) Does your ion sample have to attain the strong confinement regime? Is micromotion an issue? Will you need a high ion density? Do your trapping parameters have to be varied over a large interval (β from 0.1 to ?) Do you want to change the shape of your ion cloud?
(7) Determine the trapping parameters of your trap (see Problem 7.1),
(8) Set the external environment (vacuum vessel with antireflection coated windows, pump, residual fields, installation, air condition)
(9) Determine other vacuum parts: ion creation, electronic detection, filtering, ...
(10) Chose your laser for cooling, fluorescence, photo-ionization, repumping, ...
(11) Design your detection: the ion's fluorescence (optical design, instrument, efficiency,. . .).

References

1. W. Paul *et al.*, Ein Ionenkäfig, *Forschungsberichte des Wirtschafts- und Verkehrsministerium Nordrhein-Westfalen, Westdeutscher Verlag Köln-Opladen.* **415**, 1–67 (1958).
2. W. Paul and H. Steinwedel, Ein neues Massenspektrometer ohne Magnetfeld, *Z. Naturforsch. A.* **8**, 448 (1953).
3. W. Paul, Electromagnetic traps for charged and neutral particles, *Rev. Mod. Phys.* **62**, 531 (1990).
4. E. Mathieu, Le mouvement vibratoire d'une membrane de forme elliptique, *J. Math. Pures Appl.* **13**, 137–203 (1868).
5. H. Dehmelt, Radiofrequency spectroscopy of stored ions I: storage, *Adv. At. Mol. Phys.* **3**, 53–72 (1967).
6. J. Carrico, Applications of inhomogeneous oscillatory electric fields in ion physics, *Dyn. Mass Spectrom.* **3**, 1 (1972).
7. R. H. Dicke, The effect of collisions upon the Doppler width of spectral lines, *Phys. Rev.* **89**, 472 (1953).
8. D. J. Wineland and W. M. Itano, Laser cooling of atoms, *Phys. Rev. A.* **20**, 1521 (1979).
9. D. Berkeland *et al.*, Minimization of ion micromotion in a Paul trap, *J. Appl. Phys.* **83**, 5025 (1998).
10. F. Vedel and J. André, Influence of space charge on the computed statistical properties of stored ions cooled by a buffer gas in a quadrupole RF trap, *Phys. Rev. A.* **29**(4), 2098–2101 (1984).

11. R. Ifflaender and G. Werth, Optical detection of ions confined in a RF quadrupole trap, *Metrologia*. **13**, 167–170 (1977).
12. H. Schaaf *et al.*, Trapped ion density distribution in the presence of He-buffer gas, *Appl. Phys.* **25**, 249–251 (1981).
13. S. A. Prasad and T. M. O'Neil, Finite length thermal equilibria of a pure electron plasma column, *Phys. Fluids*, **22**(2), 1958–1988 (1979).
14. L. Cutler *et al.*, Doppler effects due to thermal macromotion of ions in an RF quadrupole trap, *Appl. Phys. B*. **39**(4), 251–259 (1986).
15. C. Champenois, About the dynamics and thermodynamics of trapped ions, *J. Phys. B: At. Mol. Opt. Phy.* **42**(15), 154002 (2009).
16. M. Knoop, *Detection Techniques for Trapped Ions*, In *Physics with Trapped Charged Particles: Lectures from the Les Houches Winter School.* (*Eds R. C. Thompson, M. Knoop, N. Madsen*), pp. 25–42. London, Imperial College Press (2013), ISBN 978-1-78326-404-9.
17. F. Vedel *et al.*, A sensitive method for the detection of stored ions by resonant ejection using a wide-band signal, *Int. J. Mass Spectr. Ion Proc.* **108**, R11–R20 (1991).
18. R. Alheit *et al.*, Observation of instabilities in a Paul trap with higher-order anharmonicities, *Appl. Phys. B*. **61**, 277–283 (1995).
19. Y. Wang *et al.*, The non-linear resonance ion trap. part 2. A general theoretical analysis, *Int. J. of Mass Spectrom. Ion Phys.* **124**, 125–196 (1993).
20. R. Alheit *et al.*, Higher order non-linear resonances in a Paul trap, *Int. J. Mass Spectrom. Ion Processes*. **154**, 155–169 (1996).
21. J. Prestage *et al.*, New ion trap for frequency standard applications, *J. Appl. Phys.* **66**, 1013 (1989).
22. M. Drewsen and A. Brøner, Harmonic linear Paul trap: Stability diagram and effective potentials, *Phys. Rev. A*. **62**, 045401 (2000).
23. A. J. Reuben *et al.*, Ion trajectories in exactly determined quadrupole fields, *Int. J. Mass Spectrom. Ion Process*. **154**(1-2), 43–59 (1996).
24. H. C. Nägerl *et al.*, Laser addressing of individual ions in a linear ion trap, *Phys. Rev. A*. **60**, 145 (1999).
25. D. H. E. Dubin, Theory of structural phase transitions in a trapped Coulomb crystal, *Phys. Rev. Lett.* **71**(17), 2753–2756 (1993).
26. G. Birkl *et al.*, Observation of multi-shell structures in a quadrupole storage ring, *Nature* **357**, 310 (1992).
27. T. Schaetz *et al.*, Crystalline ion beams, *Nature* **412**, 717–720 (2001).
28. E. Minaya Ramirez *et al.*, The ion circus: a novel circular Paul trap to resolve isobaric contamination, *NIM B*. **266**, 4460–4465 (2008).
29. D. Gerlich, Inhomogeneous RF fields: a versatile tool for the study of processes with slow ions, *Adv. Chem. Phys. Ser.* **82**, 1–176 (1992).
30. J. Mikosch *et al.*, Evaporation of trapped anions studied with a 22-pole ion trap in tandem time-of-flight configuration, *Phys. Rev. A*. **78**, 023402 (2008).
31. C. Champenois *et al.*, Ion ring in a linear multipole trap for optical frequency metrology, *Phys. Rev. A*. **81**(4), 043410 (2010).
32. M. Marciante *et al.*, Structural phase transitions in multipole traps, *Appl. Phys. B*. **107**, 1117–1123 (2012).

33. C. Champenois *et al.*, *Ion rings in multipole traps*, In *Ion Traps for Tomorrow's Applications*, In *Proceedings of the Enrico Fermi School (Eds M. Knoop, I. Marzoli, and G. Morigi)*, course 189, pp. 127–138, IOS Press (2015). ISBN 978-1-61499-525-8.
34. R. Otto *et al.*, How can a 22-pole ion trap exhibit ten local minima in the effective potential?, *J. Phys. B: At. Mol. Phys.* **42**(15), 309509 (2009).
35. W. Macalpine and R. Schildknecht, Coaxial Resonators with Helical Inner Conductor, *Proc. IRE.* **47**, 2099–2105 (1959).
36. S. R. Jefferts *et al.*, Coaxial-resonator-driven RF (Paul) trap for strong confinement, *Phys. Rev. A.* **51**, 3112–3116 (1995).
37. E. Beaty, Simple electrodes for quadrupole ion traps, *J. Appl. Phys.* **61**(6), 2118–2122 (1987).
38. C. Schrama *et al.*, Novel miniature ion traps, *Optics Communications.* **101**, 32–36 (1993).
39. C. Champenois *et al.*, Characterization of a miniature Paul-Straubel trap, *Eur. Phys. J. D.* **15**, 105 (2001).
40. R. Maiwald *et al.*, Collecting more than half the fluorescence photons from a single ion, *Phys. Rev. A.* **86**, 043431 (2012).
41. D. Kielpinski *et al.*, Architecture for a large-scale ion-trap quantum computer, *Nature* **417**, 709–711 (2002).
42. J. Chiaverini *et al.*, Surface-electrode architecturefor ion-trap quantum information processing, *Quantum Inf. Comput.* **5**(6), 419–439 (2005).
43. S. Seidelin *et al.*, Microfabricated surface-electrode ion trap for scalable quantum information processing, *Phys. Rev. Lett.* **96**, 253003 (2006).
44. C. E. Pearson *et al.*, Experimental investigation of planar ion traps, *Phys. Rev. A.* **73**, 032307 (2006).
45. M. G. House, Analytic model for electrostatic fields in surface-electrode ion traps, *Phys. Rev. A.* **78**, 033402 (2008).
46. Q. A. Turchette *et al.*, Heating of trapped ions from the quantum ground state, *Phys. Rev. A.* **61**, 063418 (2000).
47. J. Amini. Accumulated heating rates for ion traps (2014). Available on: http://www. quantum.gatech.edu/heating_rate_plot.shtml
48. D. A. Hite *et al.*, 100-fold reduction of electric-field noise in an ion trap cleaned with *In Situ* argon-ion-beam bombardment, *Phys. Rev. Lett.* **109**, 103001 (2012).
49. R. March and R. Hughes, Quadrupole storage mass spectrometry. vol. 102, *Chemical analysis*. New York, John Wiley and Sons (1989).
50. F. G. Major *et al.*, Charged Particle Traps. vol. 37, *Springer Series on Atomic, Optical, and Plasma Physics*. Berlin, Springer Berlin Heidelberg (2005). ISBN 978-3-540-26576-4.
51. A. P. VanDevender *et al.*, Efficient fiber optic detection of trapped ion fluorescence, *Phys. Rev. Lett.* **105**(2), 023001 (2010).
52. M. Steiner *et al.*, Single ion coupled to an optical fiber cavity, *Phys. Rev. Lett.*. **110**(4), 043003 (2013).
53. S. Willitsch, Ion-atom hybrid systems, In *Ion Traps for Tomorrow's Applications*, In Proceedings of the Enrico Fermi School, Course 189, (*Eds. M. Knoop, I. Marzoli, G. Morigi*), IOS Press (2015), pp. 255–268, ISBN 978-1-61499-525-8.

CHAPTER THREE

THE GUIDING CENTER APPROXIMATION

Thomas Sunn Pedersen

Max Planck Institute for Plasma Physics and Greifswald University, Greifswald, Germany
tspe@ipp.mpg.de

The guiding center approximation for charged particles in strong magnetic fields is introduced here. This approximation is very useful in situations where the charged particles are very well magnetized, such that the gyration (Larmor) radius is small compared to relevant length scales of the confinement device, and the gyration is fast relative to relevant timescales in an experiment. The basics of motion in a straight, uniform, static magnetic field are reviewed, and are used as a starting point for analyzing more complicated situations where more forces are present, as well as inhomogeneities in the magnetic field — magnetic curvature as well as gradients in the magnetic field strength. The first and second adiabatic invariant are introduced, and slowly time-varying fields are also covered. As an example of the use of the guiding center approximation, the confinement concept of the cylindrical magnetic mirror is analyzed.

1. Introduction

This chapter covers the following topics:

- motion in a straight uniform *B*-field (basic review),
- the guiding center approximation,
- motion including a static electric field, or gravity,
- motion in inhomogeneous and bent *B*-fields and the first adiabatic invariant,
- time-varying fields,
- the longitudinal invariant.

The chapter begins with a basic review of the well-known case of a charged particle moving in a straight, uniform, static magnetic field. These equations form the basis from which the further derivations proceed. The basic spatial and temporal scales are derived for this simple case, and then, more interesting cases are studied — first, an added electric field, then, a general force, and then the important case of a spatially inhomogeneous magnetic field is analyzed. The use of adiabatic invariants of the particle motion is introduced, and one sees how the identification and use of these invariants enables a relatively simple analysis of important phenomena. Time-varying fields are also heuristically discussed toward the end of the chapter.

2. Charged Particle Motion in a Straight Magnetic Field

We begin by reviewing the well-known text-book situation: a charged particle is in a region with a straight uniform magnetic field and it feels no other forces. This results in screw-like motion, which can be broken into a parallel free-streaming along the magnetic field, and a circular motion in the plane perpendicular to the magnetic field, shown in Figure 1. Although this is truly trivial, it is worth reviewing it here since we will reuse the equations with minor (but important) modifications in the derivations that follow.

We start with Newton's 2nd law and the Lorentz force:

$$\vec{F} = m\vec{a} = q\vec{v} \times \vec{B}. \tag{1}$$

We choose our coordinate system such that the $\hat{z}$-direction lies along $\vec{B}$.

$$\vec{B} = B_0\hat{z}. \tag{2}$$

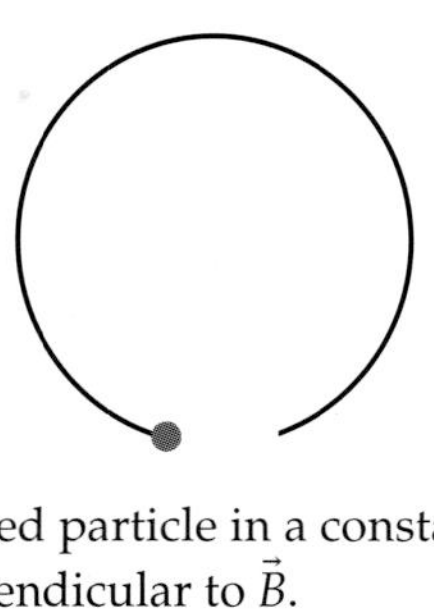

Fig. 1. The motion of a charged particle in a constant uniform magnetic field is a simple circle in the plane perpendicular to $\vec{B}$.

We write Newton's 2nd law coordinate by coordinate:

$$\vec{F} = m\vec{a} = q\vec{v} \times \vec{B} \Rightarrow, \tag{3}$$

$$\frac{dv_x}{dt} = \frac{qB_0}{m} v_y, \tag{4}$$

$$\frac{dv_y}{dt} = -\frac{qB_0}{m} v_x, \tag{5}$$

$$\frac{dv_z}{dt} = 0. \tag{6}$$

It is clear from the equations that qB_0/m is an inverse timescale, so we give it its own symbol, ω_c, the cyclotron frequency allowing us to write Equations (4) and (5):

$$\frac{dv_x}{dt} = \omega_c v_y, \tag{7}$$

$$\frac{dv_y}{dt} = -\omega_c v_x. \tag{8}$$

If we can decouple the v_x and v_y equations, we can solve simple ordinary differential equations (ODEs). This is done by taking the time derivative of Equation (7) and substituting Equation (8) into the resulting equation as follows:

Now, we eliminate v_y from the v_x equation by differentiation and substitution. The v_z equation is trivial to solve.

$$\left.\begin{aligned} \frac{d^2v_x}{dt^2} &= \omega_c \frac{dv_y}{dt} \\ \frac{dv_y}{dt} &= -\omega_c v_x \end{aligned}\right\} \Rightarrow \frac{d^2v_x}{dt^2} = -\omega_c^2 v_x, \tag{9}$$

$$\frac{dv_z}{dt} = 0 \Rightarrow v_z = \text{constant} = v_\parallel. \tag{10}$$

We recognize the simple harmonic oscillator for v_x, and know the solution immediately. We then find v_y by substituting our result for v_x into the previously established relationship:

$$\frac{dv_x}{dt} = \omega_c v_y \Leftrightarrow v_y = \frac{1}{\omega_c}\frac{dv_x}{dt}. \tag{11}$$

This establishes a 90° relationship between v_x and v_y.

$$v_x = v_\perp \cos(\omega_c t + \delta), \tag{12}$$

$$v_y = -v_\perp \sin(\omega_c t + \delta), \tag{13}$$

$$v_z = v_\parallel. \tag{14}$$

We now integrate in time to go from velocity to position:

$$v_x = v_\perp \cos(\omega_c t + \delta) \Rightarrow x = x_{gc} + \frac{v_\perp}{\omega_c} \sin(\omega_c t + \partial), \tag{15}$$

$$v_y = -v_\perp \sin(\omega_c t + \delta) \Rightarrow y = y_{gc} + \frac{v_\perp}{\omega_c} \cos(\omega_c t + \partial), \tag{16}$$

$$v_z = v_\parallel \Rightarrow z = z_0 + v_\parallel t. \tag{17}$$

Here, we have introduced the guiding center (x_{gc}, y_{gc}) around which the particle gyrates, and the Larmor radius:

$$r_L = \left|\frac{v_\perp}{\omega_c}\right| = \left|\frac{mv_\perp}{qB_0}\right|, \tag{18}$$

which is the radius of the circular motion. Note here that since we have (so far) kept the sign of the charge in our definition of ω_c, positive and negative particles will gyrate in opposite directions.

3. The Guiding Center Approximation

If the Larmor radius is on the order of the size of the confining field, then only collisionless orbits are confined, since, after a collision, the particle will have a new velocity vector and therefore a new guiding center. This will lie about one Larmor radius away from the original guiding center. If this new Larmor orbit intersects material walls or extends to regions of much lower B-field, the particle is not confined. Therefore, in order to confine charged particles magnetically for many collision times, the Larmor radius must be very small compared to the confining region.

When the Larmor radius is small compared to other relevant length scales, and the cyclotron frequency is large compared to other relevant frequencies, one can derive analytic formulas for the time evolution of the guiding center (x_{gc}, y_{gc}, z), by averaging over the gyration. Mathematically, what we require is

$$r_L \ll B/\nabla B \tag{19}$$

and

$$\omega_c \gg \frac{\partial B}{\partial t}\frac{1}{B}. \tag{20}$$

The procedure of averaging over the gyration and deriving approximate equations for the the motion of the particle's guiding center is called the *guiding center approximation.*

The guiding center approximation is not just convenient, it is often necessary. We illustrate this with a simple example: for a 100 eV electron in a $B = 1$ T-field, (67 eV perpendicular kinetic energy, 33 eV parallel kinetic energy), the cyclotron frequency is large and the Larmor radius small:

$$\omega_c \approx 1.8 \times 10^{11}\ \mathrm{s}^{-1}, \tag{21}$$

$$r_L \approx 3 \times 10^{-5}\ \mathrm{m}. \tag{22}$$

This could for example be an electron in the edge region of a fusion experiment. In such experiments, the confinement time for the plasma on the closed flux surfaces is in the range 10^{-2} s to several seconds, depending on various parameters. However, just to follow the electron for 1 ms, 10^{-6} s, requires $>10^6$ time-steps if a simple numerical scheme is used. The computational effort is spent almost entirely on calculating the circular motion which was just derived analytically. Averaging over the gyromotion allows fast and accurate calculations of the motion of charged particles in a magnetic field. This is true for both analytic and numerical calculations. One may be surprised that it is more accurate numerically to make an approximation rather than solve the exact equations, but the numbers for our example show us why this could well be the case. Unavoidable numerical errors on the order of the machine accuracy may accumulate and lead to errors on the order of the results themselves, since, for a direct simulation for just a single second of simulation, 10^{12} computational steps are needed. Even an algorithm with each time-step done near machine accuracy of 10^{-12} may not be able to correctly predict the particle orbits for 1 s.

In the guiding center approximation that we will introduce step by step in the following sections, the gyrating particle is effectively replaced by a charged (q), massive (m) ring of current ($I = e\omega_c/2\pi$), with the ring center at the particle's guiding center. Of course, the cases of interest are now ones where one perturbs this idealized situation in order to bring in

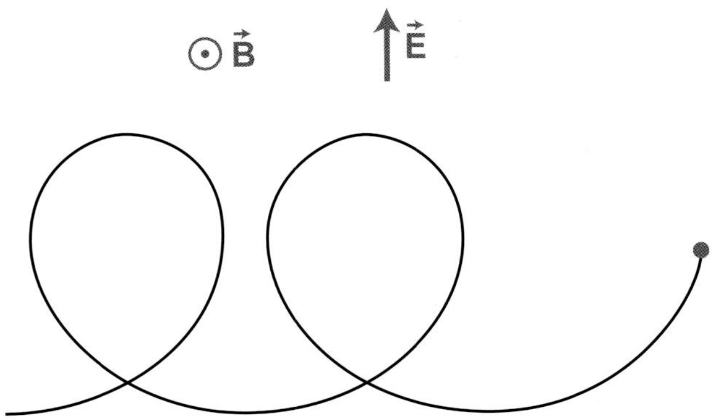

Fig. 2. An electron in crossed $\vec{E}$ and $\vec{B}$ fields will drift in the direction of $\vec{E} \times \vec{B}$.

relevant deviations from the highly idealized situation of a straight uniform magnetic field with no other forces acting on the charged particle. We begin by adding a static, uniform electric field.

4. $\vec{E} \times \vec{B}$ Drift

Since plasma particles are charged, electric fields are present, e.g. through collective phenomena, external confining fields, and single particle Coulomb interactions. The electric field component along B gives simple acceleration or deceleration. The electric field component perpendicular to B is more interesting. In Figure 2, one sees the trajectory of an electron in the plane perpendicular to B when $\vec{E} \perp \vec{B}$.

The net effect is a motion in the $\vec{E} \times \vec{B}$ direction which has a steady state component. We now solve Newton's 2nd law with an added electric field to find the expression for this drift motion. Our equations now read

$$\frac{dv_x}{dt} = \frac{qB_0}{m} v_y, \tag{23}$$

$$\frac{dv_y}{dt} = -\frac{qB_0}{m} v_x + \frac{q}{m} E_y = -\frac{qB_0}{m}\left(v_x - \frac{E_y}{B_0}\right), \tag{24}$$

$$\frac{dv_z}{dt} = 0. \tag{25}$$

E_y/B_0 is a velocity, which we will represent with the symbol v_E; it is constant since we assumed that E and B are constant.

$$\frac{dv_y}{dt} = -\frac{qB_0}{m}(v_x - v_E). \tag{26}$$

Since v_E is constant, we can subtract it inside the d/dt for dv_x/dt

$$\frac{d(v_x - v_E)}{dt} = \frac{qB_0}{m} v_y. \tag{27}$$

Comparing with the original equations we had without an electric field makes us conclude that the new and the original equations have the same form and one only needs to replace v_x by $v_x - v_E$:

$$\frac{d(v_x - v_E)}{dt} = \frac{qB_0}{m} v_y, \qquad \frac{dv_x}{dt} = \frac{qB_0}{m} v_y,$$

$$\frac{dv_y}{dt} = -\frac{qB_0}{m}(v_x - v_E), \qquad \frac{dv_y}{dt} = -\frac{qB_0}{m} v_x,$$

$$\frac{dv_z}{dt} = 0. \qquad \frac{dv_z}{dt} = 0.$$

Now **Earlier**

And we arrive at

$$v_x = \frac{E_y}{B_0} + v_\perp \cos(\omega_c t + \delta), \qquad v_x = v_\perp \cos(\omega_c t + \delta),$$

$$v_y = -v_\perp \sin(\omega_c t + \delta), \qquad v_y = -v_\perp \sin(\omega_c t + \delta),$$

$$v_z = v_\parallel. \qquad v_z = v_\parallel.$$

Now **Earlier**

Here, we re-introduced E/B instead of v_E.

For situations with constant uniform E and B-fields, we can always define a local coordinate system where z is in the B-field direction and y is in the direction of the perpendicular component of E; hence, our derivation is valid in any coordinate system. The coordinate free formula for v_E is

$$\vec{v}_E = \frac{\vec{E} \times \vec{B}}{B^2} = -\frac{\nabla\phi \times \vec{B}}{B^2}. \tag{28}$$

It is clear from the last expression that the drift is along constant electrostatic potential (ϕ) surfaces.

Note that the drift velocity is independent of the particle! There is no reference to q or m in the formula. Thus, electrons and ions drift in the same direction with the same speed.

It seems peculiar that the properties of the particle do not matter. However, this velocity can also be derived entirely without considering particles. If an observer moves at this velocity, the Lorentz transformation shows us that in this inertial frame (moving at the $E \times B$ velocity), there is no electric field. The Lorentz transform is

$$\vec{E}' = \gamma(\vec{E} + \vec{v} \times \vec{B}) + (1 - \gamma)\frac{\vec{v} \cdot \vec{E}}{v^2}\vec{v}, \tag{29}$$

$$\vec{B}' = \gamma\left(\vec{B} - \frac{\vec{v}}{c^2} \times \vec{E}\right) - \frac{\gamma^2}{\gamma + 1}\frac{\vec{v}}{c}\left(\frac{\vec{v}}{c} \cdot \vec{B}\right). \tag{30}$$

In this case, the answer simplifies dramatically — not least because $\vec{v} \perp \vec{E}$ and $\vec{v} \perp \vec{B}$:

$$E' = \gamma(\vec{E} + \vec{v} \times \vec{B}) + (1 - \gamma)\frac{\vec{v} \cdot \vec{E}}{v^2}\vec{v} \tag{31}$$

$$= \gamma\left(\vec{E} + \frac{\vec{E} \times \vec{B}}{B^2} \times \vec{B}\right) = \gamma(\vec{E} - \vec{E}) = 0. \tag{32}$$

A charged particle therefore performs simple cyclotron motion in that frame (as long as $v_E = E/B < c$). The case $E/B > c$ will be treated in an accompanying exercise.

5. $\vec{F}$ x $\vec{B}$ Drift

The derivation we just performed only used Newton's 2nd law and the Lorentz force. There was no reference made to the Lorentz transform or to Maxwell's equations. The Lorentz transform was only introduced after the result was derived — although it clearly could have been used instead, and one can argue that it would have been a more elegant derivation. However, the fact that only Newton's 2nd law was used is an advantage in the following since the derivation can be rather trivially extended to cover other perpendicular forces. Recall the $\vec{E} \times \vec{B}$ drift derivation steps, and compare to a situation where a more general force $\vec{F}$ acts on the particle in a direction perpendicular to the magnetic field vector.

$$\frac{dv_x}{dt} = \frac{qB_0}{m}v_y, \tag{33}$$

$$\frac{dv_y}{dt} = -\frac{qB_0}{m}v_x + \frac{q}{m}E_y \longrightarrow -\frac{qB_0}{m}v_x + \frac{q}{m}\left(\frac{F_y}{q}\right), \tag{34}$$

$$\frac{dv_z}{dt} = 0, \tag{35}$$

$$\vec{v}_E = \frac{\vec{E} \times \vec{B}}{B^2}, \tag{36}$$

$$\vec{v}_F = \frac{\vec{F} \times \vec{B}}{qB^2}. \tag{37}$$

As can be seen, the drift due to a general force generally is sensitive to the particle's charge.

6. Non-uniform *B*-field

Until now, we have assumed $\vec{B}$ to be straight and uniform. But in many types of magnetic traps for charged particles, the magnetic field is non-uniform. First, let us build some intuition on what happens with the particle orbits when the magnetic field strength is no longer spatially uniform. We assume here for simplicity that the B-field remains straight (in the $\hat{z}$-direction) but that the magnetic field strength varies in the $\hat{y}$-direction. It is clear from the expression for the Larmor radius, that the radius is larger in the region with lower B-field strength. Figure 3 shows a numerical simulation of a situation where this is the case. In order to show the effect clearly, the magnetic field changes substantially over a gyration. This breaks the assumptions that we will need in the following, but allows us to show in

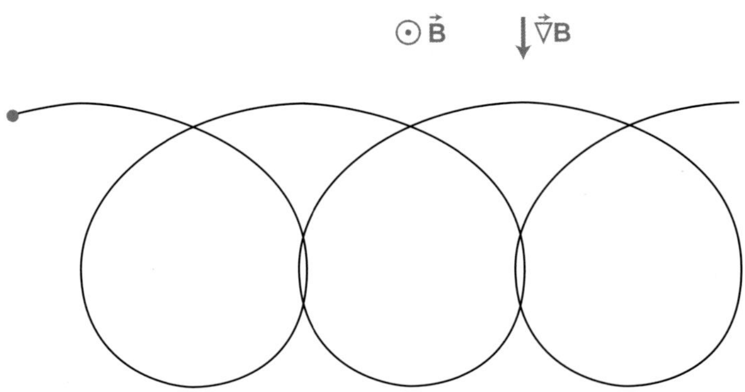

Fig. 3. An electron orbit in a magnetic field whose strength varies significantly in a direction perpendicular to the direction of B itself (gradient pointing downward, i.e. in the negative y-direction). The particle drifts in the negative x-direction.

a couple of gyrations that the particle on average moves in the x-direction — perpendicular to ∇B and perpendicular to $\vec{B}$.

One can derive this drift by Taylor-expanding the B-field, taking advantage of the small value of the Larmor radius (keeping only first order terms):

$$B_z(x, y, z) = B_0 + \frac{\partial B_z}{\partial y}(y - y_{gc}) + O\left(\varepsilon^2\right), \tag{38}$$

$$\varepsilon = \left|\frac{\nabla B}{B}\right| r_L \ll 1. \tag{39}$$

Such a derivation can be found in e.g. *Introduction to Plasma Physics and Controlled Fusion* by Chen. However, it is less algebra-intensive and more useful for the subsequent discussion to derive this drift velocity using the so-called first adiabatic invariant, μ. We therefore introduce the concept of adiabatic invariants now and then return to the derivation of the drift motion for this situation.

7. Adiabatic Invariants

The concept of adiabatic invariants is known from analytic mechanics and has found wide usage in quantum mechanics (Bohr–Sommerfeld–Wilson quantization rule) and also in the context of magnetized particles. We review it briefly here:

Assume that a particle performs periodic motion which can be described by a single coordinate q in a suitably defined spatial coordinate system. For example, a one-dimensional pendulum oscillating in the x-direction would have $q = x$. Then, one can define the action as $\oint p_q dq$. Here, p_q is the generalized momentum associated with q.

If one perturbs the periodic motion by a small amount ε, the action remains conserved to all powers in ε — one says that the action is *exponentially well conserved*.

We have already found one periodic motion for the charged particle in the magnetic field — the gyration. And the conditions for the guiding center approximation guarantee that the perturbation is small — the particle continues in an almost circular path since the magnetic field strength changes only a very small amount over the distance of a Larmor radius since $r_L \ll B/\nabla B$, and the magnetic field barely changes over the timescale of a single gyration, $\omega_c \gg B/(\partial B/\partial t)$. The coordinate for the gyration is Θ, and $p_\Theta = mv_\Theta r$ is the associated generalized momentum (we recognize that this is just the angular momentum in the gyration). Thus, we can define the action for the gyration:

$$\oint p_q dq = \int_0^{2\pi} m v_\Theta r d\Theta = \int_0^{2\pi} m v_\perp r_L d\Theta = 2\pi m v_\perp r_L. \tag{40}$$

Note that one performs the integral over the unperturbed orbit, i.e. for a spatially and temporally constant magnetic field. Thus, the Larmor radius remains constant during the integral. The previously calculated expression for r_L can then be inserted into the formula for the action to yield:

$$\oint p_q dq = 2\pi m v_\perp \frac{m v_\perp}{qB} = \frac{4\pi m}{q} \frac{\frac{1}{2} m v_\perp^2}{B} = \text{constant}. \tag{41}$$

Since π, m, and the charge q are fundamental constants, the following quantity μ is also constant:

$$\mu = \frac{\frac{1}{2} m v_\perp^2}{B} = \text{constant}. \tag{42}$$

One uses this definition since it is more physically meaningful than the raw expression we derived for the action. With this definition, μB is equal to the perpendicular kinetic energy, and we now show that μ itself is the magnetic dipole moment associated with the gyration of the charged particle if we consider the particle as a charged current ring with radius r_L: this ring carries current $I = \frac{q\omega_c}{2\pi}$ since the electron gyrates and therefore carries a circular current. Thus, the magnetic moment $I \times A$ is

$$IA = \frac{q\omega_c}{2\pi} \pi r_L^2 = \frac{q^2 B}{2\pi m} \pi \left(\frac{m v_\perp}{qB} \right)^2 = \frac{m v_\perp^2}{2B} = \mu. \tag{43}$$

This magnetic dipole is antialigned with the magnetic field for both electrons and ions: although electrons gyrate the other way around relative to ions, they have the opposite sign of charge, so the current and the magnetic field generated from it are in the same direction for electrons and ions. This shows that a plasma in a straight magnetic field is diamagnetic, it tends to weaken the magnetic field within which it is embedded.

A magnetic dipole $\vec{\mu}$ embedded in a magnetic field $\vec{B}$ has potential energy $-\vec{\mu} \cdot \vec{B}$. Since the dipole moment of the gyrating particle is antialigned to the magnetic field, it has potential energy μB, so it feels a force equal to $\vec{F} = -\mu \nabla B$. This is called the *mirror force*. As a side remark, this force also works for neutral particles as long as they have a magnetic dipole moment.

This is used to confine antihydrogen away from the material walls, thus avoiding prompt annihilation, see Chapter 14.

If at least some component of the $\mu \nabla B$ force is directed along B, it can provide some confinement along the field lines for charged particles. Particles with sufficient μ and low enough parallel velocity can then be turned around (reflected) away from a region of higher B-field strength. It is as if the particles were reflected off of a mirror — hence the name *mirror force*. The magnetic mirror confinement concept was pursued as a fusion energy confinement concept. However, the mirror confinement concept does not allow one to confine the entire distribution function. In a local thermal equilibrium, and hence, a Maxwellian distribution function, there will always be particles with low enough perpendicular kinetic energy (and therefore low μ) and high enough parallel kinetic energy that they are not reflected. This part of the distribution function then empties out of the trap very rapidly. The losses of plasma will continue even after that as collisions continually repopulate this part of phase space. In Section 9, we will go more into detail.

If the *mirror force* has a component perpendicular to B, it results in a drift. We use now the $F \times B$ formula we derived earlier:

$$\vec{F} = -\mu \nabla B = -\mu \frac{dB_z}{dy} \hat{y}, \tag{44}$$

which we can also write as

$$\vec{v}_{\nabla B} = \frac{\vec{F} \times \vec{B}}{qB^2} = \frac{-\mu \nabla B \times \vec{B}}{qB^2} = \frac{mv_\perp^2}{2B} \frac{\vec{B} \times \nabla B}{qB^2}. \tag{45}$$

8. Non-uniform *B*-field Direction: Curvature Drift

When the magnetic field strength is inhomogeneous, the field is usually curved. Curved fields are also used to confine charged particles: by curving the field, one can make the magnetic field line remain in a finite, closed volume. The curvature of the magnetic field leads to another drift.

In the guiding center approximation, the zeroth order motion of the particle (charged current ring) is the free-streaming along the magnetic field. So, if the magnetic field is curved, the particle moves along this curved path and consequently feels a centrifugal force in the direction of the local radius of curvature of the magnetic field. This force then leads to a drift, which we can calculate using the $F \times B$ drift formula derived earlier. The centrifugal force is

$$\vec{F}_C = \frac{mv_\parallel^2}{R_C}\frac{\vec{R}_C}{R_C} \tag{46}$$

and therefore, the drift velocity is

$$\vec{v}_{R_c} = \frac{\vec{F}_C \times \vec{B}}{qB^2} = \frac{mv_\parallel^2}{R_C^2}\frac{\vec{R}_C \times \vec{B}}{qB^2}. \tag{47}$$

9. Combining the Two Drifts

One can show with a bit of algebra that when there are no volumetric currents, and no strong time-variation of the fields, Maxwell's equations imply that the gradient in the magnetic field strength and the curvature of the magnetic field are related one to one:

$$\left.\begin{array}{r} \nabla \times \vec{B} = \mu_0 \vec{j} = 0 \\ \nabla \cdot \vec{B} = 0 \end{array}\right\} \Rightarrow \frac{\nabla B}{B} = -\frac{\vec{R}_C}{R_C^2}. \tag{48}$$

Therefore, we can combine the two non-uniformity drifts into one formula:

$$\vec{v}_{\nabla B + R_C} = \frac{mv_\parallel^2 + \frac{1}{2}mv_\perp^2}{B}\frac{\vec{B} \times \nabla B}{qB^2}. \tag{49}$$

One sees that the ∇B and curvature drifts cannot cancel or even offset each other. They act in the same direction.

At this point, we should make sure that these drifts are small compared to the gyration velocity $v_\perp$ and the parallel velocity $v_{||}$. Again, we take a 100 eV electron (67 eV perpendicular kinetic energy, 33 eV parallel kinetic energy) in a magnetic field with $B = 1$ T and $R_C = 1$ m:

$v_{Rc+\nabla B} \approx 133$ m/s and the parallel particle velocity is $\approx 3.4 \times 10^6$ m/s. The Larmor radius is also small: $r_L \approx 27 \times \mu$m $\ll 1$ m.

This also serves to illustrate the need to include these drifts. Although these drifts are negligible compared to the particle's thermal velocity, the particle will drift 1 m (the scale length of the magnetic curvature) in 6 ms. Therefore, the deviation from the original field line on which it was gyrating is significant; the drift is important.

10. Mirror Confinement

As mentioned, the *mirror force* $\mu\nabla B$ can also act along the magnetic field direction. This may seem counter-intuitive since the Lorentz force has no component along $\vec{B}$. There is no contradiction — the Lorentz force in a converging magnetic field region does create a force on a gyrating particle pushing it away from the region where the field lines are converging (i.e. where the magnetic field strength is increasing). This is most easily illustrated for a situation where a particle is gyrating around a straight field line pointing in the z-direction, where the field strength is increasing in the z-direction. Applying cylindrical coordinates, with the particle gyration center on the z-axis, an electron is gyrating in the positive θ-direction, with $r = R_L$. A positively charged particle would be gyrating in the negative θ-direction. $\nabla \cdot \vec{B} = 0$ then implies

$$\frac{1}{r}\frac{\partial}{\partial r}(rB_r) + \frac{\partial B_z}{\partial z} = 0 \Leftrightarrow \frac{\partial}{\partial r}(rB_r) = -r\frac{\partial B_z}{\partial z}. \tag{50}$$

Here, we have set $B_\theta = 0$ assuming for simplicity no volumetric currents. Then, integrating the equation from $r' = 0$ to $r' = r$, we get

$$rB_r = -\frac{r^2}{2}\frac{\partial B_z}{\partial z} \Leftrightarrow B_r = -\frac{r}{2}\frac{\partial B_z}{\partial z}, \tag{51}$$

where we have assumed that B_z does not vary significantly over a Larmor radius — since this is the distance over which we need to integrate, given that the particle is gyrating at $r = r_L$. Thus, for increasing B_z, a negative B_r appears. There is a component of the Lorentz force that points in the (negative) z-direction. Note that for both negative and positive particles, the quantity $qv_\perp\hat{\theta}$ is negative since negative particles gyrate in the positive θ-direction and positive particles gyrate in the negative direction.

$$F_z\hat{z} = qv_\perp\hat{\theta} \times B_r\hat{r} = |q|v_\perp\left(-\frac{r_L}{2}\frac{\partial B_z}{\partial z}\right) = -\frac{mv_\perp^2}{2B}\frac{\partial B_z}{\partial z}\hat{z}. \tag{52}$$

Note the vector identity $\hat{\theta} \times \hat{r} = -\hat{z}$ used here. The *mirror force* can be used to confine guiding center particles in the third direction — along $\vec{B}$. Thus, it appears that we have identified a purely magnetic trap that confines particles. In the classical magnetic mirror, a cylindrically symmetric magnetic topology is used, where the magnetic field increases from some low value B_0 in the middle of the trap to a larger value $B_{\max}$ at the two ends of the trap, see Figure 4. Let us investigate this confinement concept. For a static situation, the mechanical energy E of the charged particle is

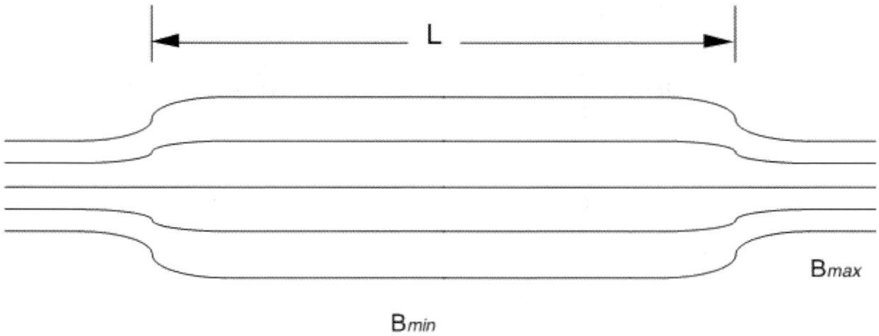

Fig. 4. This figure shows the magnetic field lines in a simple cylindrical magnetic mirror device. Particles with sufficiently high μ and sufficiently low $v_{||}$ are trapped in the low field region and perform, in addition to the tiny gyrations with radius r_L, a periodic bounce motion in the direction parallel to the magnetic field.

conserved. Assuming that the guiding center approximation is valid, μ is also conserved. Thus,

$$E = \frac{1}{2}mv_{\parallel}^2 + \frac{1}{2}mv_{\perp}^2 + q\phi = \frac{1}{2}mv_{\parallel}^2 + \mu B + q\phi \tag{53}$$

is conserved, and μB appears as a potential energy (the potential energy of a magnetic dipole in an external field). Setting $\phi = 0$ at this point (looking at pure magnetic confinement), the particle will be confined in a low-field region if and only if $E < \mu B_{\max}$. A particle located in the low-B-field region ($B = B_0$) with perpendicular velocity $v_{\perp 0}$ and parallel velocity $v_{\parallel 0}$, has

$$\mu = \frac{mv_{\perp 0}^2}{2B_0} \tag{54}$$

and

$$E = \frac{1}{2}mv_{\perp 0}^2 + \frac{1}{2}mv_{\parallel 0}^2 = \frac{1}{2}mv_0^2. \tag{55}$$

So, the particle is confined if and only if

$$E < \mu B_{\max} \Leftrightarrow \frac{1}{2}mv_0^2 < \frac{mv_{\perp 0}^2}{2B_0}B_{\max} \Leftrightarrow \frac{B_0}{B_{\max}} < \frac{v_{\perp 0}^2}{v_0^2} \Leftrightarrow \sqrt{\frac{B_0}{B_{\max}}} < \sin\theta. \tag{56}$$

In the last step, we have introduced the so-called pitch angle θ — the angle between the charged particle's velocity vector and the magnetic field, $v_0 \sin(\theta) = v_{\perp 0}$. Thus, particles with a large pitch angle are confined, and particles with a small pitch angle are not. This means that a full Maxwellian distribution function cannot be confined. A Maxwellian includes all pitch angles, even the very small ones. The criterion in Equation (56) is expressed in the literature in several other forms — these can trivially be derived from Equation (56) using the vector identity $\sin^2\theta + \cos^2\theta = 1$ and the definitions $v_\perp = v\sin\theta$, $v_\parallel = v\cos\theta$, see Refs. [1,2].

11. Other Adiabatic Invariants

If the charged, magnetized particle performs another quasi-periodic motion in addition to the gyration, it will have another adiabatic invariant. The most common case is when the particle performs a periodic motion in its parallel motion. This can happen, for example, when the particle is mirror trapped between two high field regions and bounces between them. The classical case here is the simple cylindrical magnetic mirror, sketched in Figure 4. This invariant is called the longitudinal invariant, usually noted J:

$$J = \oint v_\parallel dl. \tag{57}$$

Another example is that of charged particles in a Penning trap. In this case, particles of one sign of charge are trapped electrostatically in the longitudinal direction by applied repulsive electrostatic potentials. In this case, one can achieve trapping of the entire distribution function at sufficiently large end bias voltages, but only for one sign of charge, see also 1.

12. Time-Varying Fields

12.1. *Conservation of μ for time-varying B-fields*

Due to the aforementioned result from analytic mechanics, μ is conserved also when dB/dt is non-zero, as long as the B-field variation is small in one gyration and has no frequency component near ω_c. This implies that the perpendicular kinetic energy changes. One may wonder if this is really compatible with energy conservation, but the change in energy is due to the induced $\vec{E}$-field:

$$\nabla \times \vec{E} = -\frac{\partial \vec{B}}{\partial t}. \tag{58}$$

This can be proven explicitly with relative ease in situations with simple geometry.

12.2. *Time-varying electric fields — polarization drift*

A time-varying E-field gives rise to a so-called polarization drift (in addition to a time-varying $E \times B$ drift):

$$\vec{v}_D = \frac{m}{qB^2}\frac{\partial \vec{E}}{\partial t} \quad \text{if } \omega \ll \omega_c. \tag{59}$$

The derivation is most easily done using Fourier analysis. That is, assume that the time-variation of the electric field takes a simple sinusoidal form:

$$\vec{E}(t) = \vec{E}_0 \cos(\omega t). \tag{60}$$

We then solve the equations of motion, this time taking into account that the term E/B is time-independent. The assumption $\omega \ll \omega_c$ is not necessary to solve the equations, but when used, it makes the equations collapse into a form that is particularly compact, Equation (59). For $\omega \approx \omega_c$, there is no μ conservation, and the polarization drift formula is no longer valid. The equations show a singularity for $\omega = \omega_c$ — this is the so-called cyclotron resonance, which can be used for plasma heating, or for mass separation experiments (since ω_c depends on the mass of the charged particle).

13. Summary

In order to confine charged particles in a magnetic field for many single particle collisions, the Larmor radius must be small. In this limit, full orbit calculations are very expensive, and generally not necessary. The guiding center approximation is very useful here:

- A charged gyrating particle is approximated as a charged current ring, with constant antialigned magnetic dipole moment, sliding along the magnetic field line in the ring center.
- Such particles have slow drifts away from the magnetic field line they were originally circulating. These drifts can be calculated analytically.
- One can calculate complicated trajectories rather straightforwardly and accurately.

The guiding center approximation can therefore be used to calculate whether orbits are confined or unconfined. This allows a quick identification of configurations that are potentially good traps for charged particles, and in some cases, an assessment of what the confinement time is in the presence of collisions. In the next chapter, we will analyze some toroidal magnetic configurations to determine if and how they confine charged particles.

14. Tutorial Questions and Solutions

14.1. *Problem* 1

In the guiding center approximation, we found that if a charged particle is subject to static, spatially uniform and temporally constant electric and magnetic fields perpendicular to each other, $\vec{E} \perp \vec{B}$, the particle will drift perpendicular to both, at the $\vec{E} \times \vec{B}/B^2$ velocity, and that in that reference frame, the electric field vanishes. This is obviously only valid when the drift velocity is below the speed of light. We will now look at the case $E/B > c$. Note that this occurs even for moderate electric fields as long as the magnetic field strength is low enough.

Consider a charged particle with mass m and charge q, located at $x = 0$ at time $t = 0$ with velocity 0. It is subject to the following constant fields:

$$\vec{E} = E_0\hat{x}, \tag{61}$$

$$\vec{B} = B_0\hat{z}. \tag{62}$$

The particle begins to accelerate for $t > 0$. Answer the following questions, using the relativistic equation of motion,

$$\frac{d}{dt}(\vec{p}) = q(\vec{E} + \vec{v} \times \vec{B}), \tag{63}$$

and the Lorentz transform given earlier, Equation (30):

(a) Will the particle ever return to the $x = 0$ plane? Justify your answer — but you do not need to solve the equation of motion in detail.
(b) Show that there is a reference frame in which the magnetic field disappears and the particle is only subject to an electric field. You may want to consider the previous result for $E/B < c$, and the somewhat symmetric way in which the electric and magnetic fields appear in the Lorentz transform.

14.2. *Solution to problem* 1

Part (a)

The relativistic equation of motion is

$$\frac{d}{dt}(\vec{p}) = q(\vec{E} + \vec{v} \times \vec{B}). \tag{64}$$

The x-component of this equation is

$$\frac{d}{dt}(\gamma m_0 v_x) = q(E + v_y B). \tag{65}$$

If the particle is to come back to $x = 0$, its x-velocity must begin to decrease, then reverse. For this to occur, it must feel a net negative force component in the x-direction, i.e. qv_yB must exceed qE in magnitude:

$$|qv_yB| > |qE| \Leftrightarrow |v_y||B| > |E| \leftrightarrow |v_y| > \left|\frac{E}{B}\right|. \tag{66}$$

But in this case, $\left|\frac{E}{B}\right| > c$, so this cannot happen. The particle will continue to accelerate away from $x = 0$. It never turns around; thus, there is no gyration.

Part (b)

Consistent with our observation, we guess that there is a frame of reference in which $B' = 0$, but $E' \neq 0$. By symmetry with the $\vec{E} \times \vec{B}$ drift, noting that B and E/c appear rather symmetrically (except in some cases for the sign) in the Lorentz transform, we guess

$$\vec{v}_{\text{frame}} = \frac{\vec{E} \times \vec{B}}{E^2} c^2. \tag{67}$$

Note that for this case, $|v_{\text{frame}}| = \frac{B}{E} c^2 < c$, so this frame is subluminous. We now see that this indeed works, noting that $\vec{v} \cdot \vec{B} = 0$:

$$\begin{aligned} \vec{B'} &= \gamma \left(\vec{B} - \frac{\vec{v}}{c^2} \times \vec{E} \right) - \frac{\gamma^2}{\gamma + 1} \frac{\vec{v}}{c} \left(\frac{\vec{v}}{c} \cdot \vec{B} \right) \\ &= \gamma \left(\vec{B} - \frac{\vec{E} \times B}{E^2} \times \vec{E} \right) = \gamma(\vec{B} - \vec{B}) = 0. \end{aligned} \tag{68}$$

The electric field is non-zero but easily calculated since $\vec{v} \cdot \vec{E} = 0$:

$$\vec{E'} = \gamma \left(\vec{E} + \frac{(\vec{E} \times \vec{B}) \times \vec{B}}{E^2} c^2 \right) - \frac{\gamma^2}{\gamma + 1} \frac{\vec{v}}{c} \left(\frac{\vec{v}}{c} \cdot \vec{E} \right) = \gamma^{-1} \vec{E}. \tag{69}$$

14.3. *Problem 2*

This is an initial value problem where one needs to use the drift formulas in a clever way to find out what the particle motion is. One important point is that the $v_\perp$ velocity is the velocity in the circular motion of the guiding center particle. The guiding center drifts are also perpendicular to the magnetic field direction.

Consider a current-carrying infinitely long wire, and a concentric outer conducting cylinder, also infinitely long, surrounding the wire. The wire carries a current of 500 A and for $t < 0$ has zero voltage relative to the grounded external cylinder. The wire radius is 1 mm. An electron is at rest at radius 1 cm.

At $t = 0$, the current carrying wire is charged electrically to 460 V, relative to the grounded outer cylinder. The electron begins to move.

(a) Draw a sketch of the situation (end-on), showing the directions of the electric field, the magnetic field, the ∇B vector, the $\vec{E} \times \vec{B}$ drift, the curvature drift, and the ∇B drift for the electron.
(b) Calculate now also the magnitude (including the sign — although already indicated in part (a)) of the electric field, the magnetic field, at the location of the electron, as well as the $\vec{E} \times \vec{B}$ drift, the curvature drift, and the ∇B drift for the electron. You may use the guiding center approximation but should make sure to verify that this approximation is valid.

14.4. *Solution to problem 2*

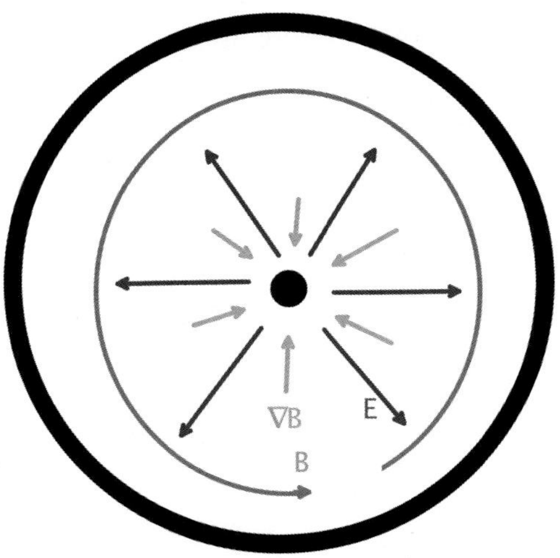

(a) $E = E_r\hat{r}$ positive, as shown in the figure
$I \odot$
The current $I = I\hat{z}$ is directed out of the paper on the figure. The ∇B vector points radially inwards as shown. From that, one finds that the ∇B drifts point into the paper (for an electron or any other negatively charged particle). Since the electron is in a current-free region of space,

the curvature drift points in the same direction, i.e. into the paper. One finds that the $E \times B$ drift points out of the paper — in the same direction as the current, but opposite to the magnetic drifts. We assume in the following that the magnetic drifts are much smaller than the $E \times B$ drift, and verify that subsequently.

(b) We need to determine $\vec{B}, \vec{E}, \nabla B, \frac{1}{2}mv_\perp^2, \frac{1}{2}mv_\parallel^2$
B is easily calculated:

$$2\pi r B = \mu_0 I \Leftrightarrow B = \frac{\mu_0 I}{2\pi r} = \frac{4\pi \cdot 10^{-7} \cdot 5 \cdot 10^2}{2\pi \cdot 10^{-2}} = 10^{-2}\text{Tesla}. \tag{70}$$

The calculation of E follows:

$$\epsilon_0 \nabla \cdot \vec{E} = \rho \Leftrightarrow \epsilon_0 \int E \cdot \mathrm{d}A = Q \Leftrightarrow E \cdot \epsilon_0 \cdot 2\pi r = \frac{Q}{l} \Leftrightarrow E = \frac{Q}{l} \cdot \frac{1}{2\pi\epsilon_0 r}\hat{r}. \tag{71}$$

We now go from $\vec{E} = -\nabla\phi$ to ϕ by integration:

$$\phi(b) - \phi(r) = \frac{Q}{l}\frac{1}{2\pi\varepsilon_0} \cdot \int_r^Q \frac{1}{r}\mathrm{d}r = C \cdot ln\left(\frac{b}{r}\right). \tag{72}$$

Here, C is an integration constant, which we now determine.
$\phi(b) = 0$ and $\phi(a) = -460$ V are given. So,

$$C = \frac{-460V}{\left(\frac{b}{a}\right)},$$

$$\text{so } \phi(r) = \frac{-460V}{ln\left(\frac{b}{a}\right)} \cdot \left(-ln\frac{b}{r}\right) = \frac{-460V}{ln\frac{b}{a}} \cdot ln\frac{r}{b},$$

$$\text{so } E(r) = -\nabla\phi(r) = +100\,V \cdot \frac{1}{r}; \quad E(0.01\,m) = 10^4\frac{V}{m}, \tag{73}$$

$$\text{and then } v_e = \frac{E}{B} = \frac{10^4}{10^{-2}}\frac{m}{s} = 10^6 \cdot \frac{m}{s}$$

Now, for $v_{\nabla B}$ and v_{Rc},
we can calculate $v_\perp$ and $v_\parallel$ approximating B as straight and uniform — this is ok as long as

$$\frac{B}{\nabla B} \gg r_L \quad \text{and} \quad R_c \gg r_L.$$

Let the local coordinates (x, y, z), point in the r-, θ-, z-directions, respectively, at the particle, see Figure 5.

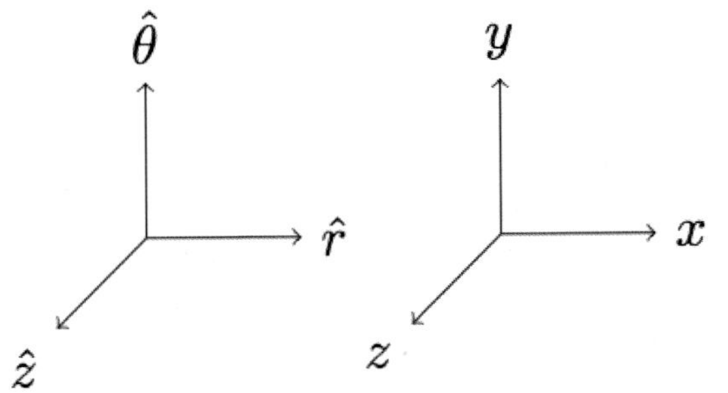

Fig. 5. For the calculation, the cylindrical coordinate system (left) is replaced by a local Cartesian coordinate system (right).

The initial condition is $\vec{v} = 0$. Since there is no force in $\hat{\theta}, v_{\|} = v_\theta = 0$ for all times. In the plane perpendicular to the magnetic field, the particle will perform its gyration plus $E \times B$ drift. In order for the particle to have $\vec{v}(t = 0), v_\perp$ must equal v_E. One can also derive this more rigorously starting from the initial value problem.

$$
\begin{aligned}
\text{So, } v_\perp &= v_E = 10^6 \frac{m}{s}, \\
|v_{\nabla B}| &= \frac{1}{2} m v_\perp^2 \cdot \frac{1}{eBr} = \frac{1}{2} \cdot 9.1 \cdot 10^{-31} \cdot 10^{12} \cdot \frac{1}{1.6 \cdot 10^{-19} \cdot 10^{-2} \cdot 10^{-2}} \\
&= 2.8 \cdot 10^4 \frac{m}{s}, \\
|v_{Rc}| &= 0 \text{ since } v_{\|} = 0.
\end{aligned}
$$

The Larmor radius of the electron is

$$
r_L = \frac{m v_\perp}{eB} = \frac{9.11 \cdot 10^{-31} \cdot 10^6}{1.6 \cdot 10^{-19} \cdot 10^{-2}} \text{meter} \approx 0.6\,\text{mm} \ll 10\,\text{mm}. \tag{74}
$$

Thus, the guiding center approximation is valid.

14.5. *Problem 3*

Consider a charged particle (charge q, mass m), located at $(r, z) = (0, 0)$ in cylindrical coordinates in a magnetic field with $B_z = B_0(1 + z^2/z_0^2)$, $B_\theta = 0$ everywhere. The particle has $v_\perp = v_0$ and $v_{\|} = 0$. You may assume that the magnetic field is strong enough that the guiding center approximation is valid. The particle is also subject to a constant electric field $\vec{E} = E_0\hat{z}$.

Answer the following three questions in any order you see fit:

(a) Show that the particle performs harmonic oscillations in the z-direction, and find the angular frequency of the oscillation, expressed in terms of quantities given in the problem.
(b) What is the oscillation amplitude?
(c) Where would one place a particle which has $v_\perp = v_0$, $v_\parallel = 0$, and its guiding center on the $r = 0$ axis, so that it just stays there gyrating and does not accelerate neither in the positive nor the negative z-direction? (Hint: this is not necessarily the same location as the equilibrium point for the previously calculated oscillation.) Is there always an answer to this question?

14.6. *Solution to problem 3*

The parallel force in the guiding center approximation is

$$F_\parallel = qE_0 - \mu B_0 \frac{2z}{z_0^2}. \tag{75}$$

Here, $\mu = mv_0^2/2B_0$. To show that the particle is performing harmonic oscillations, it pays off to first find the equilibrium point around which the oscillation occurs. This is found as follows:

$$0 = qE_0 - \mu B_0 \frac{2z}{z_0^2} \Leftrightarrow qE_0 = \mu B_0 \frac{2z}{z_0^2} \Leftrightarrow z = \frac{qE_0}{2\mu B_0} z_0^2 = \frac{qE_0}{mv_0^2} z_0^2 \equiv z_{eq}. \tag{76}$$

Now, rewrite the equation of motion using a new azimuthal coordinate $\tilde{z} = z - z_{eq}$ since $\tilde{z} = 0$ is the point around which the oscillation occurs.

$$m\frac{d\tilde{v}_\parallel}{dt} = qE_0 - \mu B_0 \frac{2(\tilde{z} + z_{eq})}{z_0^2} \Leftrightarrow \frac{d^2}{dt^2}\tilde{z} = -\frac{v_0^2}{z_0^2}\tilde{z}. \tag{77}$$

This is the classic harmonic oscillator ODE. Thus,

$$\omega = \frac{v_0}{z_0} = \sqrt{\frac{2\mu B_0}{mz_0^2}}. \tag{78}$$

The particle is at rest at $z = 0$ at $t = 0$, which therefore is an extremum point around the equilibrium point z_{eq}. Thus, the oscillation amplitude is

$$|z_{eq}| = \left| \frac{qE_0 z_0^2}{mv_0^2} \right|. \tag{79}$$

Now to **part (c)**:

As indicated, this equilibrium point is not necessarily the same as what was the case earlier. This is because μ is not the same. In fact, we need to treat μ as an unknown which will be determined self-consistently. Instead, $v_\perp$ is given, at the location of the equilibrium point. We need to set-up the equilibrium condition as follows:

$$qE_0 = \frac{\frac{1}{2}mv_0^2}{B(z)}\nabla_\parallel Bz. \tag{80}$$

Inserting the known expression for the magnetic field strength on axis:

$$qE_0 = \frac{\frac{1}{2}mv_0^2}{B_0(1+z^2/z_0^2)}\frac{2z}{z_0^2}B_0. \tag{81}$$

We can write this as a quadratic equation for the equilibrium point z:

$$qE_0 = \frac{\frac{1}{2}mv_0^2}{B_0(1+z^2/z_0^2)}\frac{2z}{z_0^2}B_0 \Leftrightarrow . \tag{82}$$

$$(z_0^2 + z^2)qE_0 = mv_0^2 z \Leftrightarrow z^2 - \frac{mv_0^2}{qE_0}z + z_0^2 = 0. \tag{83}$$

To make the math look neater, we introduce the symbol z_E:

$$z_E = -\frac{mv_0^2}{qE_0}. \tag{84}$$

Then the equation reads

$$z^2 + z_e z + z_0^2. \tag{85}$$

This is then straightforwardly solved using the standard formula:

$$z = -\frac{1}{2}\left(z_E \pm \sqrt{z_E^2 - 4z_0^2}\right), \tag{86}$$

which is the answer to the problem. As can be seen, there are only solutions to this problem when the term inside the square root is non-negative. That is:

$$z_E^2 \geq 4z_0^2. \tag{87}$$

14.7. *Problem 4*

Consider a charged particle in a cylindrical mirror trap similar to the one depicted in Figure 4. The particle has $v_\perp = 2v_0$ and $v_\parallel = v_0$ in the homogeneous field region where $B = B_{\text{min}}$. The maximum magnetic field strength (in the mirror reflection region) is $B_{\text{max}} = 3B_{\text{min}}$. The mirror reflection region can be considered infinitesimal in length compared to the trap length L (the length over which the magnetic field is $B = B_{\text{min}}$). You may assume that the guiding center approximation is valid.

(a) Confirm that the particle is trapped, and calculate the longitudinal invariant J for this particle.
(b) Now, we slowly increase the magnetic field strength by a factor of two, maintaining the $B_{\text{max}} = 3B_{\text{min}}$ relationship. Does the particle stay trapped?

14.8. *Solution to problem 4*

$\mu = \frac{\frac{1}{2}mv_\perp^2}{B}$ (per definition) so $\mu = \frac{2mv_0^2}{B_{\text{min}}}$ since $v_\perp = 2v_0$ at the location where $B = B_{\text{min}}$

(a) First, we should check that particle is confined at all, before we attempt to define and calculate the second adiabatic invariant:

$$\mu B_{\text{turn}} = \frac{1}{2}mv_\parallel^2 + \frac{1}{2}mv_\perp^2 = \frac{1}{2}mv_0^2 + 2mv_0^2 = \frac{5}{2}mv_0^2,$$

$$\text{so } B_{\text{turn}} = \frac{5}{2}mv_0^2 \cdot \frac{B_{\text{min}}}{2mv_0^2} = \frac{5}{4}B_{\text{min}} < B_{\text{max}} = 3B_{\text{min}}.$$

Thus, the particle is (deeply) trapped.
The velocity $v_\parallel$ is constant along the whole cylinder, except in the infinitesimally short mirror region so

$$J = \oint v_\parallel \, dl = \int_0^L v_0 \, dl + \int_L^0 -v_0 \, dl = 2v_0 L. \tag{88}$$

(b) A slow increase implies that μ and J are conserved; $v_\parallel$ is unchanged, since L is unchanged, and $\mu B = \frac{1}{2}m_\perp^2$ increases. Thus, the particle becomes even more deeply trapped.

14.9. *Problem 5*

μ-conservation implies that the particle gains perpendicular velocity as it enters a region of higher magnetic field. Show that there is a force acting in the θ-direction which changes the perpendicular velocity in such a way as to conserve μ.

14.10. *Solution to problem 5*

In principle there are two terms giving a force in the θ-direction:

$$F_\theta = qv_r B_z(\hat{r} \times \hat{z}) + qv_z B_r(\hat{z} \times \hat{r}) \tag{89}$$

v_r is the rate of change in Larmor radius — since the Larmor radius is very small in the guiding center approximation, its rate of change is also negligible. We therefore focus on the other, much larger term:

$$F_\theta \approx qv_z B_r(\hat{z} \times \hat{r}) = qv_z \left(-\frac{1}{2} r_L \frac{\partial B_z}{\partial z}\right) \Leftrightarrow, \tag{90}$$

$$\frac{\partial v_\perp}{\partial t} = F_\theta/m = \frac{qv_z}{2m} r_L \frac{\partial B_z}{\partial z}. \tag{91}$$

This is consistent with $d\mu/dt = 0$, as shown here:

$$\frac{d}{dt}(\mu B) = \frac{d}{dt}\left(\frac{1}{2}mv_\perp^2\right) \Leftrightarrow \frac{d\mu}{dt}B + \mu\frac{dB}{dt} = mv_\perp \frac{dv_\perp}{dt} \Leftrightarrow, \tag{92}$$

$$\frac{d\mu}{dt}B + \mu\frac{dB}{dz}v_\parallel = mv_\perp \frac{qv_z}{2m} r_L \frac{\partial B_z}{\partial z} \Leftrightarrow, \tag{93}$$

$$\frac{d\mu}{dt}B + \mu\frac{dB}{dz}v_\parallel = \mu\frac{dB}{dz}v_\parallel \Leftrightarrow \frac{d\mu}{dt}B = 0 \Leftrightarrow \frac{d\mu}{dt} = 0. \tag{94}$$

References

1. F. F. Chen, *Introduction to Plasma Physics and Controlled Fusion*. New York, Springer (1984). ISBN 1441932011.
2. R. J. Goldston and P. H. Rutherford, *Introduction to Plasma Physics*. New York, Taylor & Francis (1995). ISBN 075030183X.

CHAPTER FOUR

TOROIDAL SYSTEMS

Thomas Sunn Pedersen*,§, Matthew Stoneking†, and Haruhiko Saitoh‡

*Max Planck Institute for Plasma Physics
and Greifswald University, Germany
†Lawrence University, WI, USA
‡Max Planck Institute for Plasma Physics, Germany
§tspe@ipp.mpg.de

In this chapter, we will derive and discuss the use of toroidal magnetic topologies for the confinement of single charged particles as well as collections of charged particles (plasma). Relative to Penning traps, there are advantages as well as disadvantages to these traps.

1. Introduction

In this chapter, we will look at guiding center drift orbits in toroidal configurations and experimental results from toroidal devices confining non-neutral plasmas. First, we will motivate why these configurations are particularly important to study for confinement of charged particles, and why they are worth studying for confinement of non-neutral plasmas. We will show that the simplest toroidal trap — the pure toroidal field trap — can adequately confine only non-neutral plasmas, and is unable to confine quasi-neutral plasmas. We will then turn to the dipole, and show that for good confinement, the dipolar field must be created from a levitated current-carrying ring. In this case, the configuration can confine non-neutral as well as quasi-neutral plasmas. We will go on to discuss stellarators, where charged particles display more complicated orbits. For all three types of configurations, we will present experimental results from pure electron plasmas, most of which have been obtained in the last 10–15 years.

2. Why Study Non-neutral Plasmas in Toroidal Configurations?

Considering the remarkable confinement results achieved in Penning traps, where plasma has been confined essentially indefinitely, one might ask why one would study non-neutral plasmas in toroidal configurations. The reasons can be summarized as follows:

2.1. *Ability to study partially neutralized plasmas*

Since toroidal configurations provide a fully magnetic confinement, they are capable of confining both signs of charge simultaneously, and for some toroidal topologies, plasmas at an arbitrary degree of neutralization, from single-species to quasi-neutral. Operation at any degree of neutralization has recently been demonstrated in a stellarator [1,2]. The plasma behavior changed appreciably as the degree of neutralization was varied, see Section 10.

2.2. *Elimination of end effects*

The Penning trap works by trapping all particles (of one particular sign of charge). This electrostatic boundary condition turns out to be rather important for the behavior of the plasma. Complete elimination of the ends could potentially simplify the physics and perhaps improve confinement. However, the toroidicity brings in its own complications, as described in the following.

2.3. *Toroidicity introduces new physics and provides connection to fusion energy research*

Toroidicity introduces complicated particle orbits and new physics which is interesting in its own right. Toroidal traps are used for confinement of quasi-neutral plasmas for fusion energy research, and a study of non-neutral plasmas in the same topology addresses the question as to whether the dynamics of these plasmas most resemble toroidal quasi-neutral plasmas (implying that the magnetic topology determines the behavior) or non-neutral plasmas in Penning traps (implying that the non-neutrality determines the behavior). Moreover, radial electric fields, resulting from the slight charge imbalance in a quasi-neutral plasma, can strongly affect confinement in these devices. Studying the effects of the extreme radial electric fields that are generated in non-neutral plasmas could lead to a deeper understanding of the influence of the radial electric field on the confinement of quasi-neutral plasmas in toroidal configurations.

3. A Basic Observation about Non-neutral Plasmas in Toroidal Configurations

Non-neutral plasmas, just as quasi-neutral plasmas, display collective behavior when the Debye length is much smaller than the characteristic scale of the plasma:

$$\lambda_D \ll a \qquad (n\lambda_D^3 \gg 1). \tag{1}$$

For a single component (e.g. pure electron) plasma, this implies that the electric field effects dominate over temperature related effects:

$$\varepsilon_0 \nabla^2 \varphi = en_e \Leftrightarrow \varepsilon_0 \mid \varphi \mid /a^2 \approx en_e \Leftrightarrow \mid \varphi \mid \approx en_e a^2/\varepsilon_0, \tag{2}$$

$$\Leftrightarrow \left|\frac{e\varphi}{T}\right| \approx \frac{e^2 n_e}{\varepsilon_0 T_e} a^2 = \frac{a^2}{\lambda_D^2} \gg 1 \Leftrightarrow \left|\frac{e\varphi}{T}\right| \gg 1. \tag{3}$$

For a quasi-neutral plasma, $\left|\frac{e\varphi}{T}\right| \sim 1$. Thus, in units of the thermal energy, the electrostatic potential is very large, "extreme", in a non-neutral plasma, compared to a quasi-neutral plasma. However, one should be aware that since quasi-neutral plasmas confined for fusion purposes have very large temperatures (keV compared to eV for typical non-neutral plasmas), the electrostatic potential is in fact larger in many fusion plasmas than in many non-neutral plasmas. The comparison to the kinetic energy is, however, relevant. The extreme nature also implies that the $\vec{E} \times \vec{B}$ drift completely dominates over the magnetic drifts. Assume for simplicity that the length scale over which the magnetic field strength changes appreciably is the same as the length scale over which the electrostatic potential changes appreciably. Then,

$$\left|\frac{v_{E\times B}}{v_{\nabla B}}\right| = \frac{|\nabla\varphi|/B}{T \mid \nabla B|/eB^2} \approx \left|\frac{e\varphi}{T}\right| \gg 1. \tag{4}$$

We will show in the next section how this can be very important.

4. The Most Basic Toroidal Trap: Pure Toroidal Field

The most basic toroidal trap is one where a pure toroidal field is used. A pure toroidal field results from either a very large symmetrically arranged set of toroidal field coils, or (as an idealization) from an infinitely long straight current carrying wire.

$$\vec{B} = B_\varphi \widehat{\varphi} = \frac{\mu_0 I}{2\pi R}\widehat{\varphi} \Rightarrow \nabla B = -\frac{\mu_0 I}{2\pi R^2}\widehat{R}.$$

We have an inhomogeneous B-field and therefore magnetic guiding center drifts — in the same direction as the equivalent infinitely long current carrying wire.

$$\vec{v}_{\nabla B + R_C} = \frac{2mv_\parallel^2 + mv_\perp^2}{2B}\frac{\vec{B}\times\nabla B}{qB^2} \rightarrow \frac{T_\parallel + T_\perp}{qRB}\widehat{z}. \quad (5)$$

Thus, a lone electron will drift out of the trap (in the vertical direction in the typical case where the torus is oriented in the horizontal plane). But if one manages to nucleate a pure electron plasma by overwhelming initial losses, the electrons can have very good confinement. This is because the $\vec{E} \times \vec{B}$ drift totally dominates over the magnetic drifts in a pure electron plasma, as was shown in the previous section. This means that the poloidal $E \times B$ drift is much faster than the vertical drift. The charged particle will move poloidally — and then, the vertical drift cancels: on one half of the journey, the particle drifts radially outward, on the other half, it drifts inward — and due to symmetry, the exact same amount, closing the orbit. Once the pure electron plasma has been formed, one must consider if the plasma has an equilibrium. It was shown in 1967 by Daugherty and Levy that an equilibrium exists [3], and in 1994 by O'Neil and Smith [4] that the equilibrium is a maximum energy state and is stable as long as the electrostatic energy cannot be dissipated — similar to the Penning trap. Confinement is predicted to be limited by collisions through magnetic pumping, as described in a paper by Crooks and O'Neil [5].

5. Brief History of Pure Toroidal Field Traps before the Year 2000

The first pure toroidal field non-neutral experiments were performed more than 40 years ago at the Avco Everett company in the United States [6]. The team created pure electron clouds so dense that the electron space charge created a 400 kV electrostatic potential well. The plasmas only had about 60 μs confinement time. Although this means that the electrons circulated toroidally on the order of 1,000 times before being lost, one cannot really speak of good confinement. The authors found that the confinement was limited primarily by ion accumulation. The electron cloud, although very dense, was not cold enough to be considered a plasma. Rather, it was a confined relativistic electron beam with beam energy about equal to the space charge potential, which indirectly implies that the Debye length is not small (Equations (2) and (3)).

In the 1990s, pure electron plasmas were studied in a low aspect ratio experiment at the Institute of Plasma Research in India [7]. They achieved much longer confinement times, of order 3 ms, which verifies single particle confinement, but is orders of magnitudes below the confinement time predicted by Crooks and O'Neil.

The Lawrence non-neutral Torus II (Figure 1) is the latest experiment of this type, and one that has exceeded the confinement results of the previous ones by more than two orders of magnitude. This was done first in a partial torus, and presently in a full torus. The improvements were due to several factors, but first and foremost having a very good vacuum, and therefore avoiding ion contamination. The plasma was also created in such a way so as to ensure a low plasma temperature and therefore a short Debye-length. In 2008, the milestone of above 1 s confinement was reached [8]. The confinement time was measured by detecting an oscillation of the entire plasma, a so-called $m = 1$ diocotron mode, whose frequency is proportional to the total charge content of the plasma. Figure 2 shows the experimental set-up and some representative measurements.

The reported ~3 s confinement time is, however, still not quite as long as that predicted by Crooks and O'Neil. The reason for the discrepancy

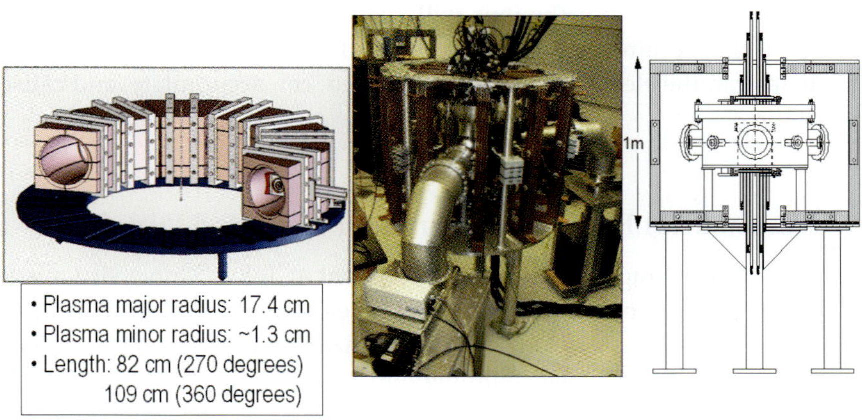

Fig. 1. The Lawrence non-neutral Torus II at Lawrence University in Appleton, WI, USA.

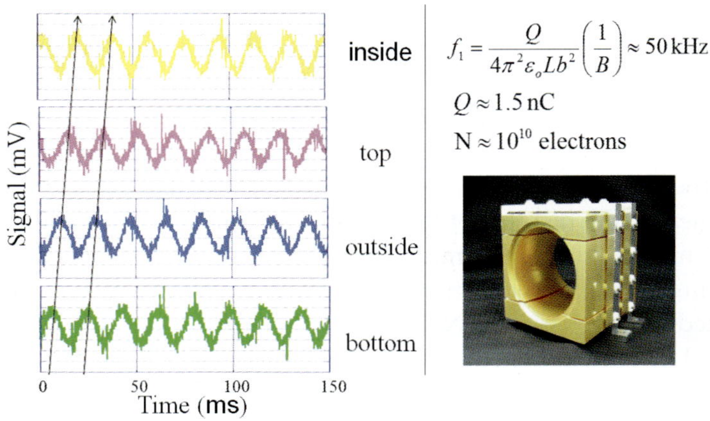

Fig. 2. Measurement of the $m = 1$ diocotron mode allows one to track the charge content of the plasma. The measurements are done by monitoring the image currents on four capacitive probes closely fitting to the plasma (photo on the right). The plasma column is oscillating, inducing periodic image charges in the four segments (left). The frequency of the oscillation is directly proportional to the charge content, as given by the formula at the top right. This confirms a confinement time exceeding 1 s. These data are copyright Prof. M. Stoneking.

is not currently known. Interestingly, the confinement time records were made in a partial torus, and confinement was substantially worse in a full torus. The reason is presumably, that in a partial torus, where the electrons are electrostatically shielded from hitting a material object, ion accumulation is suppressed since the ions will be extracted by the same negative potential that confines the electrons. In a full torus, the ions can circulate freely (as can the electrons), they are confined, can accumulate, and cause instabilities.

6. Non-neutral Plasmas Confined in Levitated Dipoles

In Japan, in the Ring-trap-1 (RT-1) experiment at Tokyo University, a levitated current ring produces an approximately dipolar field in which one can confine plasmas of any degree of neutralization. In recent years, experiments have been performed confining pure electron plasmas in this device. Pure electron plasmas can be confined up to 300 s, i.e. two orders of magnitude higher than in the pure toroidal field trap, and three orders of magnitude higher than in the stellarator (to be discussed in the following) [9].

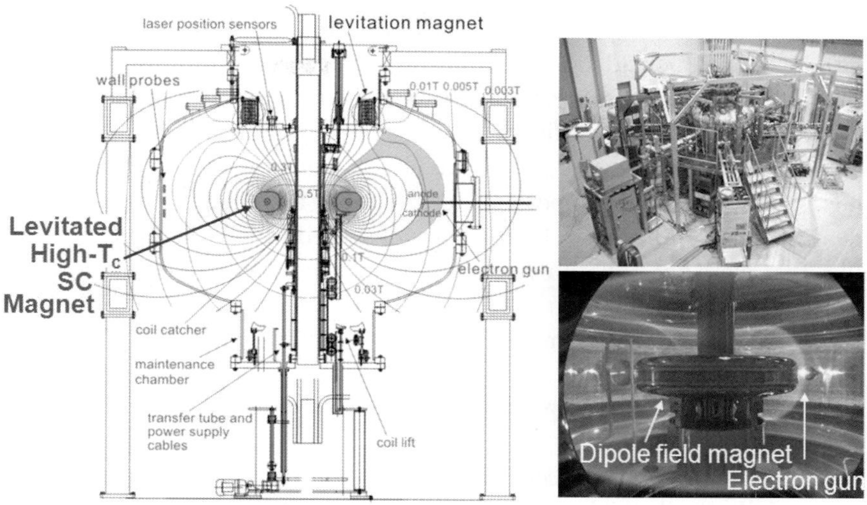

Fig. 3. This figure shows the set-up of the RT-1 experiment. To the left, a CAD drawing shows the engineering details. A high-temperature superconducting circular winding weighing 112 kg is levitated by being attracted to a second, normal-conducting winding located directly above the levitated coil. At the top right, a picture of the facility is shown. At the bottom right, a picture of a neutral plasma being confined is shown. This figure is copyright Dr. H. Saitoh.

As a side note, dipoles also have unique and very attractive confinement properties when it comes to quasi-neutral plasmas. These have been demonstrated both in RT-1 and in the Levitated Dipole Experiment (LDX) operated by Columbia University and MIT [10]. It is, however, outside the scope of this treatment to go into further detail about these properties. We will concentrate our description on confinement of pure electron plasmas, and refer the curious reader to the literature [11,12]. Figure 3 shows the RT-1 set-up used. The levitated coil is a Bi-2223 high-temperature superconductor winding which is inductively charged with current at the bottom of the device, and is then levitated by being attracted to the levitation magnet, placed vertically above it. In this arrangement, the levitation is naturally stable for tilt- and slide motion, but is unstable in the vertical direction. Vertical stability is achieved by feedback stabilization. Laser trackers measure the vertical location of the coil, and a feedback algorithm adjusts the current in the levitation magnet accordingly to control and stabilize the vertical motion. The system can levitate for hours at a time, limited by the slow warm-up of the levitated coil.

6.1. *Injection and formation of pure electron plasmas in RT-1*

The RT-1 group decided to eliminate external objects from their plasmas from the beginning, and only fuel the plasma from the edge of the confinement region. In other confinement devices — Penning traps and stellarators — fueling from the edge leads to hollow density profiles. But a dipole has a natural tendency to peak its density in the high magnetic field region near the coil. And indeed, the plasmas observed in RT-1 had density profiles that were not hollow, even when the plasma was created by injection from the edge.

The discharges were created as follows:

- Electrons are injected with a gun located at edge of the confinement region.
- Soon after the start of beam injection, an electron cloud is created, which partially repels the beam and diminishes the injection current to about 10^{-5}A.
- The injection of electrons is stopped.
- The plasma is observed to become turbulent transiently. Then, it relaxes into a quiescent state.
- In the quiescent phase, the plasma exhibits periodic oscillations.
- The plasma decays.

The confinement time depends strongly on the neutral pressure in RT-1. The confinement time decreases as the neutral pressure is increased as one might expect. However, the relationship is quite complicated — there appear to be two separate scaling regimes. For the longest confinement times (up to 300 s), the plasma remains stable for almost the entire plasma lifetime, then abruptly disappears [13]. A possible explanation could be that ions build up slowly until they reach a critical density, at which time an ion-related instability sets in. This instability then dissipates the electrostatic energy by removing the excess electron charge, either by eliminating the plasma content all-together, or by converting it into a quasi-neutral plasma. Since the diagnostics on RT-1 for these experiments are purely electrostatic, one cannot distinguish easily between the two possibilities.

7. Non-neutral Plasmas in a Stellarator

The idea to use stellarators for confinement of pure electron plasmas was proposed in 2002 [14], and first results on pure electron plasma confinement

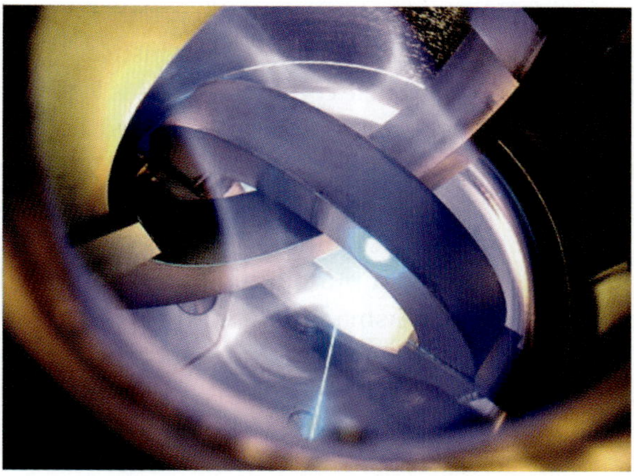

Fig. 4. The magnetic topology of the CNT stellarator is illustrated here by letting an electron beam interact with nitrogen gas.

in the Columbia Non-neutral Torus (CNT) stellarator were published in 2006 [15].

A stellarator is a magnetic surface configuration, also called a flux surface configuration, and reference "flux surface" to this page: Each magnetic field line wraps around a toroidal surface, never leaving the surface. On most surfaces, the field line covers the entire surface, allowing the plasma to flow from any part of the surface to any other part of the surface purely by parallel free streaming. The magnetic topology of the stellarator is illustrated in Figure 4.

The twist of the magnetic field lines also has the effect that when the particles move along the magnetic field, they rotate poloidally as well as toroidally. This cancels out magnetic drifts — even in the absence of $E \times B$ drift. Thus, stellarators, like dipoles, confine single component plasmas as well as quasi-neutral plasmas, as well as anything in between. The stellarator concept was invented already in the early 1950s by Spitzer, who published the concept in 1958 [16]. The stellarator was invented as a confinement device for hot quasi-neutral plasmas for the production of fusion energy. The reader is referred to the vast literature on stellarator confinement of hot quasi-neutral plasmas. In particular, two fairly recent review articles can serve to introduce the concept [17,18].

While the dipole has the engineering disadvantage of having a levitated current ring in the middle of the plasma, a stellarator configuration can be created from external coils that require no levitation. However, stellarators do not have an obvious symmetry that guarantees particle confinement;

dipoles and tokamaks have toroidal symmetry, and Penning traps have cylindrical symmetry. Instead, one must use sophisticated theoretical and numerical tools to optimize particle confinement. This leads to complicated coils. However, a simple-coil stellarator may be used for confinement of pure electron plasmas as we will show in the following.

One idea put forward was that the electric field and the associated $E \times B$ drift would close the orbits that would otherwise be unconfined, similar to how the orbits are closed in a pure toroidal field trap holding a small-Debye-length pure electron plasma. But, before we proceed with this, we should note that although the dedicated studies of pure electron plasmas in stellarators were started in 2004, such plasmas were likely created unintentionally more than 10 years earlier without the experimenters being aware of it.

Experiments in the Auburn Torsatron in the USA [19] and similar experiments in the former USSR [20] were performed in the 1980s with heated filaments emitting electrons in order to measure the magnetic flux surfaces. The experiments were done in a way that closely resembles those done in CNT, but the experimenters did not mention in their papers that the somewhat confusing and disappointing results they achieved with respect to flux surface mapping were likely caused by the space charge and other collective effects of a non-neutral plasma.

The CNT stellarator was taken into operation in 2004. It has a uniquely simple-coil configuration, creating the magnetic surfaces from just four circular coils [21–23]. CNT is a so-called "classical" stellarator; that is, it has not been optimized for good particle confinement. In fact, about half of the particles in a Maxwellian population would be poorly confined if no strong electric field were to be present. The magnetic field strength in CNT varies strongly toroidally and poloidally, and therefore, about half the particles are magnetically trapped and do not circulate over the entire magnetic surface; in particular, they do not circulate poloidally. Instead, they drift out on timescales of 10^{-4} s. However, if the electric field is strong enough, they will circulate poloidally due to the $\vec{E} \times \vec{B}$ drift. Numerical simulations confirm that the confinement should be good although the entire story about particle confinement in CNT turned out to be much more complicated than originally thought as will be described in the following sections. Thus, the CNT stellarator uses the same "trick" to confine these orbits as the pure toroidal field trap does. The difference is that the stellarator confines a large fraction of particles (those that are not magnetically trapped) fully, even in the absence of space charge, whereas the pure toroidal field trap does not have closed orbits until sufficient charge density and associated radial electric field are present.

The theoretical expectation for confinement laid out in Ref. [14] was very optimistic owing to the expectation that a large $\vec{E} \times \vec{B}$ drift would dominate over the ∇B and curvature drifts. Indeed, the plasmas in CNT had $\Delta\phi \sim 200\,\mathrm{V}$ and $T_e \sim 4\,\mathrm{eV}$ so that $\left|\frac{v_{E\times B}}{v_{\nabla B}}\right| \approx \left|\frac{e\varphi}{T_e}\right| \approx 50$. The confinement times were expected to exceed 1 s since all particle orbits would be closed and would only deviate by a very small amount from the magnetic surfaces. However, several other effects degraded confinement as will be summarized in the following.

7.1. *Internal rods degrade confinement*

First results [15] showed that confinement times were up to 20 ms, much below the original theoretical predictions. Radial transport was directly related to the presence of internal rods, on which measurement probes and the electron source were mounted. More rods inserted led to faster transport and lower confinement. The rods were made of insulating materials and were therefore not direct sinks for the electron plasma. They would transiently collect electrons before being charged up negatively enough to repel all other incoming electrons. These negatively biased rods would then act as electrostatic perturbations — effectively creating an $\vec{E} \times \vec{B}$ drift "conveyor belt" from the central region across the magnetic surface to the edge, as schematically illustrated in Figure 5. This process was experimentally and theoretically quite well understood early on in the operation of CNT [24].

7.2. *Neutrals degrade confinement*

It was to be expected that collisions with neutrals would lead to diffusive losses for the electron plasma. For well-confined orbits, this effect would not prevent the long confinement times mentioned earlier as long as the neutral pressure was held reasonably low. CNT was built as an ultrahigh vacuum device, and was able to operate in the $p_n = 10^{-10} - 10^{-8}$ Torr range where confinement times were expected to be well over 1 s. The electron loss rate due to neutral collisions was measured by varying the neutral pressure and measuring the loss rate. The loss rate showed an offset linear relationship with the neutral pressure, where the offset can be attributed to the rod(s) and the slope to the neutral collisions. The result was that the electron confinement time was on the order of one electron-neutral collision

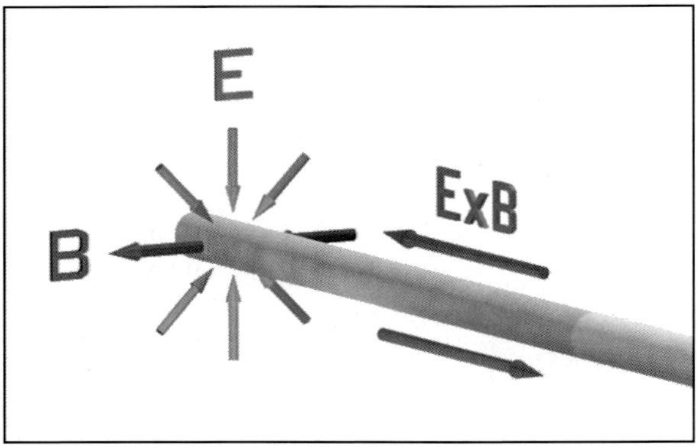

Fig. 5. The insulated rods charge up and produce $\vec{E} \times \vec{B}$ drift patterns that convect the electrons across the magnetic surfaces to the edge.

time. This indicated that the orbit quality was much worse than expected despite the large $\vec{E} \times \vec{B}$ drift [24].

That finding prompted a numerical study of the particle orbits in CNT [25], a study that included the effects of the rather complicated electrostatic boundary condition that was present in CNT at the time, where the electrically grounded structures would be very close to the outer magnetic surface at some locations and far away from them at other locations.

8. The Effects of a Non-conforming Boundary Condition

Until 2008, the internal coils and vacuum chamber in CNT set the electrostatic boundary condition. Since these components do not conform geometrically to the magnetic surfaces, but are all grounded, thus defining equipotential surfaces, they cause large electrostatic potential perturbations, especially in the edge region. One should particularly note that the inner side of the toroidal magnetic surface is very close to a grounded structure (the two interlocking magnets) and the outer side is quite far away from such surfaces. Since, for static or quasi-static situations $\vec{E} = \nabla\phi$, it follows that the $\vec{E} \times \vec{B}$ drift lies on constant-potential surfaces:

$$\vec{v}_E = \frac{\vec{E} \times \vec{B}}{B^2} = \frac{\nabla\phi \times \vec{B}}{B^2} \perp \nabla\phi. \tag{6}$$

Thus, the $\vec{E} \times \vec{B}$ drift takes a charged particle, e.g. our electron, along on an electrostatic potential contour. The parallel free-streaming of the charged

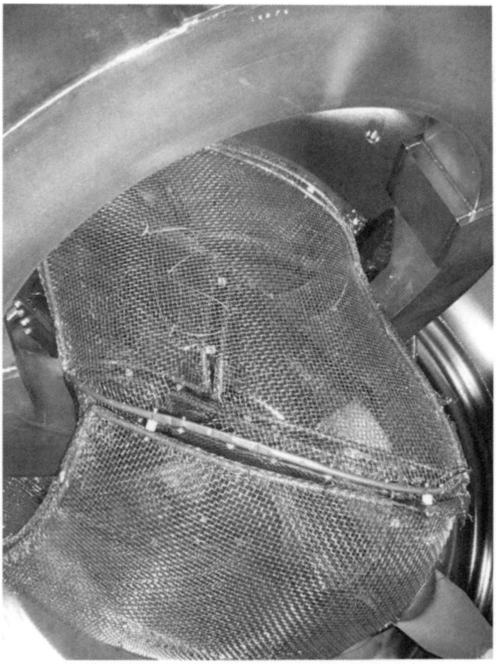

Fig. 6. A flux surface conforming grounded mesh was installed in 2007–2010. The reader can compare to the similar view of a glowing magnetic flux surface in Figure 4.

particle makes it move along on its magnetic surface. Thus, when the electrostatic potential contours and the magnetic surfaces do not coincide, the particle can make enormous radial excursions.

A conceptually simple way to mitigate this problem is to install an electrostatic boundary closely surrounding the plasma, one that has the shape of the outermost flux surface. Such a mesh was installed from 2007 to 2010, Figure 6 shows the mesh installed. The mesh did not, unfortunately, quite conform in shape to the outermost magnetic surface [26], although it provided a much more surface-aligned electrostatic boundary condition than the previous one.

Despite the lack of perfect matching, the mesh led to significant improvement in confinement. In fact, with the mesh installed, confinement times as long as 0.32 s were measured [27]. However, this vastly improved confinement time was mainly due to things other than improved particle orbits. The confinement time improvements were experimentally determined to be due to

- a better vacuum,
- a higher B-field,
- a smaller Debye length,
- an improved orbit quality.

The improved orbit quality only accounted for a small part of the total improvement although code results had indicated that the confinement should be vastly improved. The method with which this analysis was made, and the detailed results can be found in Ref. [27].

8.1. *Experiments with a retractable emitter*

In 2008, an electron emitter capable of retraction in 20 ms was installed [28] (see Figure 7). Since confinement times up to and exceeding 20 ms were achieved already in the first two years of operation, dominated by the presence of internal rods, it was expected that the plasma would remain after retraction of the electron emitter since this would also eliminate the

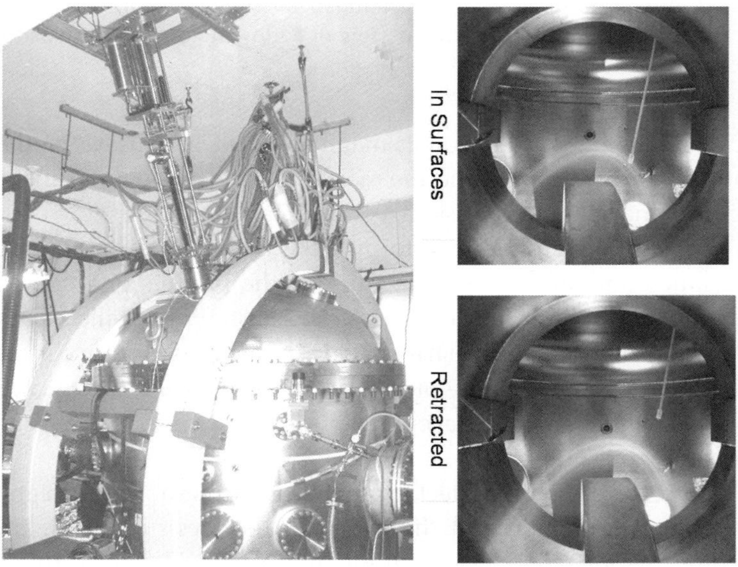

Fig. 7. Photographs of the retractable emitter in CNT, also showing that it can reach the central confinement region as well as be retracted well outside the confinement region.

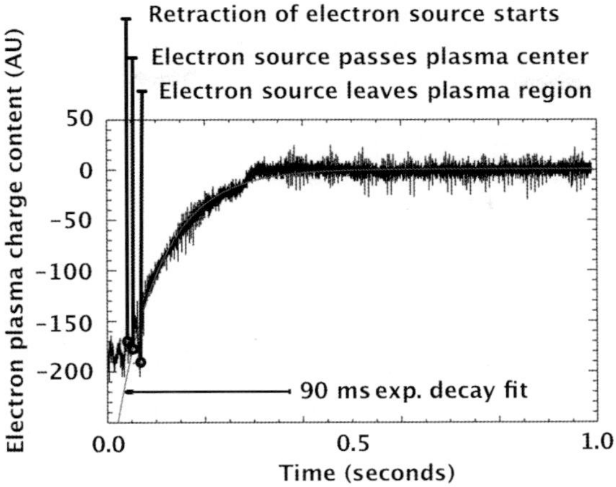

Fig. 8. The charge content of a plasma decays slowly after retraction of the electron emitter for the shot with record confinement of 90 ms. These data and a similar figure appeared first in Ref. [30].

rod-driven transport. Instead, there seemed to be no plasma left after retraction. At that time, external diagnostics had been developed, capable of measuring the presumably slow decay of a pure electron plasma by virtue of measuring the space charge electric field present just outside the plasma. Once these diagnostics had been upgraded and benchmarked to the point where they could measure fast-decaying plasmas down to decay times of about 1 ms [29], a picture emerged as to what was causing the fast decay times: It was determined that ion contamination was the culprit [30].

Once the cause was known, a dedicated campaign was made to improve the neutral pressure in CNT. A $\sim$ 90 ms exponential decay time of the plasma was achieved for a plasma with $B = 0.055$ T, $p_n = 1.8 \times 10^{-9}$ Torr (Figure 8).

9. Pure Electron Plasmas Confined without Internal Objects

It is seen clearly that the plasma remains after retraction. The fact that ion contamination is the limiting factor, rather than neutral collisions, was established in two independent ways: by using gases with different ionization energies, helium (24.6 eV), and nitrogen (14.5 eV). For nitrogen-dominated discharges, the decay is so fast that no confinement can be measured if the neutral pressure is 10 nTorr or higher, i.e. the confinement is well below 5 ms. For conditions where the nitrogen and oxygen partial pressures are below 3 nTorr, and the helium partial pressure dominates, confinement can exceed 20 ms, even if the total neutral pressure is 20 nTorr. This shows that the ionization causes the fast collapse, not the electron-neutral collisions. Further verification of the hypothesis comes from pure electron plasmas at comparably low densities and therefore low space charge electric fields. From previous experiments, these plasmas are known to have lower temperatures than the denser plasmas, and the tail of the electron distribution function therefore does not extend into the energies needed for ionization. Low density plasmas therefore stay below the ionization threshold, do not create ions, and consequently, they decay only slowly, at the rate expected from earlier experiments with internal electron sources. In the end, they last longer than plasmas that start with a much larger electron inventory.

These results, and further details can be found in Ref. [30], including some considerations and arguments regarding why the experiments with internal emitters do not suffer from ion contamination but only show neutral-driven transport.

10. Partially Neutralized Plasmas

Although we described in the previous section that ion contamination is detrimental for confinement of pure electron plasmas, there is much physics to be learned from adding ions. In particular, a purely magnetic confinement concept, such as the stellarator, allows for the creation and study of plasmas at any degree of neutralization, at least in principle. This is in contrast to Penning traps, whose confinement concept only allows for confinement of one sign of charge. Experiments were performed in CNT to determine if it is indeed possible to create and stably confine small Debye-length plasmas at any degree of neutralization. The answer is affirmative: plasmas of arbitrary degree of neutralization (ranging from pure electron to quasi-neutral) can be confined in a stellarator. A recent paper in Plasma Phys. Control. Fusion [2] shows that it is experimentally possible to create, sustain, and study plasmas at any degree of neutralization in a stellarator. This represents a first step in the characterization of plasmas of arbitrary degree of neutrality. As the degree of neutralization was varied from pure electron plasma to quasi-neutral plasma, it was found that the character of instabilities changed from diocotron-like modes (with poloidal mode number $m = 1$, not field-aligned) to drift-wave-like modes that were field-aligned (in this case, poloidal mode number $m = 3$). In between the two extremes, the partially neutralized plasma showed a mixed, multi-mode behavior. The confinement of plasma charge degraded continuously as the degree of neutralization was increased. In addition to the full article just mentioned, we also refer the reader to the shorter summary published in the open-access and non-peer-reviewed journal Stellarator News [31].

11. Concluding Remarks

Toroidal plasma traps have been used successfully to confine pure electron plasmas, partially neutralized plasmas, and quasi-neutral plasmas. Although confinement times and many physics effects are different between the studied configurations, a few common features appear:

- the confinement times of pure electron plasmas exceed those obtained with quasi-neutral plasmas but are generally lower than those in a Penning trap,
- ion accumulation is a serious threat to confinement of otherwise pure electron plasmas in these traps,
- dynamics of these plasmas often resemble dynamics seen in Penning traps,
- these traps have been used to study plasmas of arbitrary neutrality, for the first time,
- as the degree of neutralization is varied, the plasma behavior changes significantly.

Toroidal traps can be used also to confine exotic plasmas such as electron–positron plasmas.

References

1. X. Sarasola, *Plasmas of Arbitrary Neutrality*. PhD thesis, Columbia University (2011).
2. X. Sarasola *et al.*, First observations of partially neutralized and quasineutral plasmas in the Columbia Non-neutral Torus, *Contrib. Plasma Phys.* **50**(6–7), 673–677 (2010).
3. J. D. Daugherty *et al.*, Experiments on the injection and containment of electron clouds in a toroidal apparatus, *Phys. Fluids.* **10**, 155 (1967).
4. T. M. O'Neil and R. A. Smith, Stability theorem for off-axis states of a non-neutral plasma column, *Phys. Fluids B.* **4**, 2720 (1992).
5. S. Crooks and T. O'Neil, Transport in a toroidally confined pure electron plasma, *Phys. Plasmas.* **3**, 2533 (1996).

6. J. D. Daugherty *et al.*, Experiments on the injection and containment of electron clouds in a toroidal apparatus, *Phys. Fluids.* **12**(12), 2677–2693 (1969).
7. P. Zaveri *et al.*, Low-aspect-ratio toroidal equilibria of electron clouds, *Phys. Rev. Lett.* **68**, 3295–3298 (1992).
8. J. P. Marler and M. R. Stoneking, Confinement time exceeding one second for a toroidal electron plasma, *Phys. Rev. Lett.* **100**, 155001 (2008).
9. H. Saitoh *et al.*, High-β plasma formation and observation of peaked density profile in RT-1, *Nucl. Fusion.* **51**, 063034 (2011).
10. D. T. Garnier *et al.*, Design and initial operation of the LDX facility, *Fusion Eng. and Des.* **81**(20–22), 2371–2380 (2006).
11. A. Hasegawa *et al.*, A D-He3 fusion reactor based on a dipole magnetic field, *Nucl. Fusion.* **30**, 2405–2413 (1990).
12. A. C. Boxer *et al.*, Turbulent inward pinch of plasma confined by a levitated dipole magnet, *Nature Phys.* **6**, 207–212 (2010).
13. Z. Yoshida *et al.*, Magnetospheric vortex formation: self-organized confinement of charged particles, *Phys. Rev. Lett.* **104**, 235004 (2010).
14. T. S. Pedersen and A. H. Boozer, Confinement of nonneutral plasmas on magnetic surfaces, *Phys. Rev. Lett.* **88**, 205002 (2002).
15. J. P. Kremer *et al.*, Experimental confirmation of stable, small-Debye-length, pure-electron-plasma equilibria in a stellarator, *Phys. Rev. Lett.* **97**, 095003 (2006).
16. J. Lyman Spitzer, The stellarator concept, *Phys. Fluids.* **1**(4), 253–264 (1958).
17. A. H. Boozer, What is a stellarator?, *Phys. Plasmas.* **5**(5), 1647–1655 (1998).
18. P. Helander *et al.*, Stellarator and tokamak plasmas: a comparison, *Plasma Phys. Control. Fusion.* **54**, 124009 (2012).
19. R. F. Gandy *et al.*, Magnetic surface mapping with an emissive filament technique on the Auburn torsatron, *Rev. Sci. Instrum.* **58**, 509 (1987).
20. A. G. Dikij *et al.*, A new research method of the vacuum magnetic configuration in stellarators, *Sov. J. Plasma Phys.* **14**, 160 (1988).
21. T. S. Pedersen *et al.*, The Columbia Nonneutral Torus: A new experiment to confine nonneutral and positron-electron plasmas in a stellarator, *Fusion Sci. Tech.* **46**, 200 (2004).
22. T. S. Pedersen *et al.*, Construction and initial operation of the Columbia Nonneutral Torus, *Fusion Sci. Technol.* **50**, 372 (2006).
23. T. S. Pedersen *et al.*, Experimental demonstration of a compact stellarator magnetic trap using four circular coils, *Phys. Plasmas.* **13**, 012502 (2006).
24. J. W. Berkery *et al.*, Confinement of pure electron plasmas in the Columbia Non-neutral Torus, *Phys. Plasmas.* **14**, 062503 (2007).
25. B. D. de Gevigney *et al.*, Debye screening and injection of positrons across the magnetic surfaces of a pure electron plasma in a stellarator, *Phys. Plasmas.* **18**, 013508 (2011).
26. P. W. Brenner *et al.*, Magnetic surface visualizations in the CNT stellarator, *IEEE Trans. Plasma Sci.* **36**, 1108 (2008).
27. P. W. Brenner *et al.*, Confinement studies in the Columbia Non-neutral Torus, *Contri. Plasma Phys.* **50**, 678 (2010).
28. J. W. Berkery *et al.*, A retractable electron emitter for the creation of unperturbed pure electron plasmas, *Rev. Sci. Instrum.* **78**(1), 013504 (2007).

29. P. Brenner. *Confinement of Non-Neutral Plasmas in Stellarator Magnetic Surfaces*. PhD thesis, Columbia University (2011).
30. P. W. Brenner and T. Sunn Pedersen, Pure electron plasmas confined for 90 ms in a stellarator without electron sources or internal objects, *Phys. Plasmas*. **19**, 050701 (2012).
31. X. Sarasola and T. S. Pedersen, Plasmas of an arbitrary degree of neutrality confined in a stellarator, *Stellarator News*. **140**, 1–2 (2013).

CHAPTER FIVE

ULTRAHIGH VACUUM FOR TRAPPED IONS

Jeroen C. J. Koelemeij*,‡ and Martina Knoop†,§

*LaserLaB and Department of Physics & Astronomy, VU Amsterdam, de Boelelaan 1081, 1081 HV Amsterdam, The Netherlands

†CNRS and Aix-Marseille Université, PIIM, UMR7345, Centre de Saint Jérôme, Case C21, 13397 Marseille Cedex 20, France
‡j.c.j.koelemeij@vu.nl
§Martina.Knoop@univ-amu.fr

Trapped-ion experiments aim to realize quantum systems under well-controlled conditions, which require minimizing interactions with the environment. Ultrahigh vacuum (UHV) therefore is a critical experimental requirement. In this chapter, we review the most essential features of UHV, and we provide practical guidelines for its production and characterization.

1. Introduction

Trapping single ions is a beautiful technique for realizing high-resolution spectroscopy experiments, and probing the fundamentals of (quantum) physics. In such experiments, performed on samples which can range from single ions to clouds of thousands of ions, atomic transitions are probed with lasers at the highest resolution in order to reach the smallest linewidths, and to produce quantum states with the longest coherence times. To avoid line broadening and decoherence, the influence of interactions with the environment, in particular collisions, should be minimized. Ultrahigh vacuum (UHV) is the experimental solution to avoiding interactions with residual gas, which otherwise severely limit the lifetime of internal and motional quantum states of trapped ions by non-radiative transfer, as well as the storage time itself. In this chapter, we present the most important features of UHV in the context of trapped-ion experiments, and provide guidelines for its production and characterization. First, we explain what UHV is, and what its main features are. We subsequently describe general aspects of producing and characterizing UHV conditions. Finally, we give practical guidelines to designing, building, commissioning and maintaining UHV apparatus. In the literature, several standard works exist [1–4]; additional specific articles are cited in the text. Detailed technical information about vacuum equipment, its properties and applications can also be found on the websites and application notes of the larger vacuum equipment manufacturers.

2. UHV Vacuum: What and Why

The SI unit for pressure measurement is the pascal (Pa), 1 Pa being defined as 1 Pa $\equiv$ 1 N/m^2. This is the unit figuring in the ideal gas law $p = nk_BT$. Despite the SI convention, in laboratory measurement equipment, the units of mbar or Torr are commonly encountered. Normal pressure is 1013 mbar or 760 Torr, which corresponds to atmospheric pressure at sea level. 1 mbar is the equivalent of 100 Pa, while 1 Torr equals approximately 133.3 Pa.

2.1. *Vacuum regimes*

Pumping down a vacuum vessel from atmospheric pressure will first take us through the so-called low vacuum range, which is located between 1,000 and 30 mbar. Pumping down further takes us to the medium vacuum, ranging from 30 mbar down to 10^{-3} mbar. Pressures at even lower values (10^{-3}–10^{-9} mbar) are called high or secondary vacuum. Only below 10^{-9} mbar, the UHV range is attained, which gives place to extremely high vacuum at values below 10^{-12} mbar.

Within these different vacuum ranges, we distinguish two main regimes, depending on the ratio of the mean free path of residual gas particles to the apparatus dimensions. If this ratio, also known as the Knudsen number, is smaller than unity, we speak of laminar flow. Conversely, if the mean free path is larger than the apparatus dimensions, the so-called molecular flow regime applies. This regime is reached for all vessels of diameter inferior to 1 m at a pressure below 10^{-4} mbar (assuming a residual gas composed primarily of nitrogen).

2.2. *Ion-neutral collisions*

Collisions with background-gas constituents form the main reason to minimize the residual gas pressure in the ion trap chamber. Let us remark that in a vacuum at a pressure of 10^{-9} mbar, the particle density is still about 3×10^7 particles per cm^3, which is comparable to the ion-cloud density and leads us to suspect that the probability of collisions may be non-negligible. In the following, only collisions between a trapped ion and a neutral atom (or molecule) from the residual gas background are considered. Ion–ion collisions do not play a role in vacuum considerations as their frequency is orders of magnitude below that of ion-neutral collisions.

If collisions with residual gas atoms only transfer kinetic energy between the collisional partners, they are called elastic collisions. If energy is transferred between the motional and internal degrees of freedom, then collisions are called inelastic. While collisions are generally considered as sources of motional heating, elastic collisions can also be used to deliberately transfer energy so as to cool ions (cf. Chapter 7 by L Hilico). Consider a cloud of ions stored in a Paul trap with a trap depth 10 eV, for which it was empirically shown that the steady-state ion kinetic energy roughly equals one tenth of the trap depth, or 1 eV ($\approx$ 12,000 K) under UHV conditions, while collisions with a room-temperature helium 'buffer gas cooling' were observed to substantially reduce the ion temperature [5]. Such thermalization can also be carried out with a cold buffer gas, as performed for example in physico-chemical reactions at cryogenic temperatures [6]. Elastic collisions are mainly produced by simple atoms, with high-lying energy levels such as the noble gases. In particular, helium, but also neon and argon, exchange energy with trapped ions almost exclusively through elastic collisions.

By contrast, molecules can readily match the energy amount of any atomic transition by virtue of their many rovibrational levels, so that in ion-molecule collisions internal energy may be transferred non-radiatively with high probability. This reduces the lifetime of both the internal and motional (quantum) states of the trapped ions and results in phase changes, and therefore has an adverse effect on the achievable quantum coherence times, atomic line-widths, and frequency shifts. These collisions can also mix close-lying energy levels (j-mixing). Measurements and details on the influence of elastic and inelastic collisions can be found for example in Refs. [7–12].

The described collisions can be formalized in the Langevin picture, characterized by a long-range potential $V(r) \propto -1/r^4$ (corresponding to the interaction between a Coulomb charge and the dipole moment induced in the neutral collisional partner by the Coulomb charge), and an impact parameter b corresponding to the lateral distance between both partners. See also Chapter 7 by Laurent Hilico on non-laser cooling techniques, and Ref. [13] for more details on Langevin collisional cross-sections.

Inelastic collisions can have an even more destructive impact on trapped ions if they involve chemical reactions or charge exchange, such as reactions of the type $X^+ + H_2 \rightarrow XH^+ + H$. Reactions can be exothermic or endothermic depending on whether they release or require energy, which can often be deduced from a comparison of the total (binding) energies before and after the reaction. In case the experiment uses laser-cooling or laser-induced excitation, one should be aware that an ion which just absorbed a photon may contain sufficient energy to turn an endothermic reaction pathway into an exothermic one. Such extra internal energy can also serve to trigger other (unwanted) reactions. References [14–16] provide concrete examples.

3. Producing UHV

The final pressure in a vacuum chamber corresponds to an equilibrium reached between the pumping speed (or throughput) of the vacuum pump(s), the backflow which comes from the finite compression ratio of the pumps and possible leaks, and the outgassing from the walls of the chamber and any part or component present inside the vessel. In the following, we review the different types of vacuum pumps commonly encountered in trapped ion UHV set-ups.

3.1. *Pumps*

For a room-temperature vacuum apparatus, no single pump allows UHV conditions to be reached from atmospheric pressure. Different stages of pumping and different types of pumps are necessary to reach pressure values well below 10^{-9} mbar. The pumps discussed in the following section are typically used starting from a secondary vacuum around 10^{-4}–10^{-6} mbar produced by a forepump. Such pressure levels can be obtained with various types of pumps, and in some cases, such pumps can be shared between multiple set-ups as they will only serve during the first few days of the initial pump-down procedure. No matter what vacuum equipment you use for pre-pumping (often, the choice is limited to the 'historical' inventory of the laboratory), always keep in mind that a pump has a compression ratio which is never infinite, and that even tiny traces of oil (such as those from rotary vane pumps or oil-diffusion pumps) can make your ion trap set-up non-ideal, or in the worst case render it useless. A cryogenic baffle should be used with any pump containing oil or grease to avoid spurious contamination. Regardless of the type of secondary pump that is used, the UHV chamber must also contain a valve to allow replacement of the secondary pump while preserving UHV.

Four types of pumps are able to reach and/or maintain UHV conditions:

Turbomolecular pumps (TMPs) use fast-spinning blades to channel atoms away from the main vacuum volume. These blades have a geometric asymmetry to assure a unidirectional gas flow. They can be supported by magnetic bearings, which provide an almost frictionless mode of operation. This results in longer lifetimes of the equipment but can generate some unwanted interactions with your spectroscopy experiment. For example, magnetic bearings may cause magnetic field (gradients) inside the trap apparatus.

Apart from their pump speed, TMPs are essentially defined by their compression ratio, which lies in the range of $10^7 - 10^{11}$. The finite compression ratio is due to a small backflow through the pump with lower ratios corresponding to gas constituents with smaller masses. TMPs with a so-called drag or Holweck section, which reduces backflow, offer the highest compression ratios, and are well suited to deal with high loads of noble gases (e.g. helium). In order to spin up to its ultimate rotation speed, a TMP requires an initial pressure well below 10 mbar (achieved by a fore-pump connected to its exhaust), after which pressure values below 10^{-9} mbar can be obtained. Although TMPs exist which operate at a backing pressure of several mbar (achievable with simple diaphragm pumps), it has been observed that the compression ratio in this case may limit the ultimate pressure to several 10^{-11} mbar. Therefore, to achieve pressures in the low 10^{-11} mbar range, it is advisable to provide a backing pressure below 1 mbar.

TMPs should be equipped with a mesh to protect the blades which rotate at high speed (60,000 revolutions per minute). The concomitant reduction in pump speed, given by the mesh open area ratio, is a small price to pay to prevent shattered TMP blades due to some component falling unexpectedly into the TMP! Alternatively, if maximum pump speed is crucial, most TMPs may be mounted sideways.

Due to their 'mechanical' mode of operation, TMPs produce vibrations, which is a point of consideration when designing vibration-sensitive experiments. TMPs also have to be permanently plugged in and should not be moved while spinning, which limits their use in mobile set-ups. Notwithstanding the mechanical vibrations and possible magnetic field gradients, TMPs have been used to successfully create UHV conditions for, e.g. high-precision spectroscopy of trapped ions. The risk of inadvertent venting of the apparatus due to power outages is readily mitigated using 'smart' valves at the backing side of the TMP, which shut automatically at power down, and which will re-open after power up only after a certain time delay.

Titanium Sublimation Pumps (TSPs) consist of titanium-covered filaments which can be resistively heated such that the titanium sublimates and covers the surrounding surfaces, where it acts as a getter material. In order to avoid rapid oxidation of the filament as well as rapid depletion of the deposited titanium layer, the TSP should be operated under high vacuum conditions ($< 10^{-8}$ mbar to avoid rapid depletion). For water (H_2O), a TSP offers a pumping speed of 3 $ls^{-1}cm^{-2}$, while the pumping speed for CO is 9 $ls^{-1}cm^{-2}$. Depending on the molecular species, these values increase typically by a factor of 2–4 when cooling from room temperature to liquid-nitrogen temperature. When mounting a TSP, direct lines of sight from the filaments to the trap structure and other electrical components (e.g. vacuum feedthroughs) should be avoided, yet without severely constraining the surface area exposed to the TSP filaments.

Ion Pumps employ a discharge, which ionizes residual gas atoms and accelerates them towards the electrodes where they get stuck. This operation is enhanced by adding a magnetic field of a few tenths of a tesla, which forces ions and electrons into a spiralling trajectory, thus improving the interaction path length and the ionization efficiency. For a typical ion pump, it takes a few thousand volts applied to the electrodes to ignite the discharge. The subsequent discharge current is proportional to the density of ionized atoms, and can therefore be used to estimate the value of the pressure reached. A typical value for the ratio of discharge current to pressure is about 1,000 A/Torr. In the most common type of ion pump, the above principle of operation is combined with walls permanently coated by a getter material (ion getter pump). For the best performance, ion pumps should be part of the UHV chamber (see also the discussion on conductance in Section 4.1).

Getter pumps are available in various forms and can provide additional pump speed. For example, Akerman *et al.* reported the use of non-evaporable getter strips which are thermally activated at 300°C, and which helped in achieving a pressure in the low 10^{-12} mbar range [17].

A typical ion trap vacuum chamber is equipped with a combination of a (removable) TMP pumped by a primary pump at its exhaust (e.g. a drum or diaphragm pump, or dry scroll pump), connected through a bakeable all-metal valve to the chamber, which itself is directly connected to an ion getter pump and in some cases equipped with an additional TSP and/or a non-evaporable getter pump.

It is possible to reach very low vacuum values (below 10^{-13} mbar) by use of a cryogenic vacuum environment. At temperatures below 77 K, most residual-gas molecules condense onto the cold chamber walls. As commercial pressure, gauges do not operate at such low pressure levels, the pressure is most conveniently estimated from the trapped particles themselves (e.g. by monitoring quantum jumps). For example, trapping antiprotons for sufficiently long durations required cryogenic cooling, as first described by Gabrielse *et al.* [18]. Although a detailed overview of cryogenic pumping methods is beyond the scope of this chapter, we point out that cryopumps may lead to additional (and sometimes unexpected) issues such as superconductivity (in particular when cooling to a few kelvin), strain or differential motion of trap components due to different coefficients of thermal expansion of the materials used, and temperature gradients due to ohmic Radiofreqeuncy (RF) heating of trap electrodes in combination with low thermal conductivity to the cryogenic heat sink.

3.2. *Pressure monitoring and leak detection*

Depending on the pressure range, different methods and equipments are available to measure pressure, and we will here review the most common ones used in ion-trap set-ups. It should be kept in mind that in almost all cases, the measured pressure value depends on the composition of the residual gas. Pressure gauges are typically calibrated for 'standard' air or for N_2, so if your chamber has been flooded with helium, the pressure reading might be far off. Your device might have a precise (relative) calibration, but the measurement of absolute pressure values is difficult, as the residual gas composition is different for every vacuum chamber. Moreover, the pressure measurement depends on the geometry of the set-up and the associated pressure gradients. The inaccuracy of the measurement can therefore be of the order of 30%. Better values can be reached by combining two devices, and by individual *in situ* calibration of pressure gauges in the vacuum vessel. Often, pressure gauge manuals provide detailed information on the calibration of these devices.

A first and very coarse indication of the quality of a primary or secondary vacuum can be obtained by ear and by eye from the noise the pump produces (with the noise level indicating the gas load) and from the rotation speed of the (backing) pumps. For pressures above 10^{-4} mbar, accurate pressure readings can be obtained from a Pirani gauge. Pressures down to 10^{-9} mbar can also be measured by a Penning gauge, a cold-cathode gauge whose principle of operation shares elements of ion pumps as well as the Bayard–Alpert gauges explained below.

The workhorse for pressure measurement in UHV set-ups is the Bayard–Alpert or ionization gauge, which spans a pressure range from 10^{-4} to 10^{-12} mbar. A resistively heated filament emits electrons which ionize the background gas, and the current so produced is collected. An ionization gauge often has an extra heating filament which will degas the gauge, but there is also a long-term self-degassing effect if the gauge is operated continuously. Bayard–Alpert gauges are normally calibrated for nitrogen. They should be installed as close as possible to the experiment to enable pressure measurement at the region of interest (normally the trap structure). At the same time, the gauge should be mounted as far away as possible from the experiment as it produces electrons, visible radiation, and heat. A good compromise is to mount the ionization gauge close to the trap, and to operate it only during phases of pressure variation.

For experiments which require knowledge of individual gases or the composition of the background gas, a residual gas analyzer (RGA) is an important device. An RGA typically is a mass filter as proposed by Paul [19], for a given mass range. A 'simple' RGA monitors gases with atomic masses up to 64 amu, allows for individual calibration of different components with 1 amu resolution, and — like the ionization gauge — produces electrons and ions. In situations where a detachable TMP station is used for initial pumping (to be taken over by an ion getter pump at a later stage), it is useful to extend the station with an RGA, which may also be used for helium leak testing (see below).

Spectroscopic measurements are a way to measure pressure and pressure variations in the heart of your ion trap. It is possible to measure lifetimes with different gases with quenching experiments [8–11] or to evaluate them by monitoring quantum jump statistics [20, 21].

If the chamber does not reach UHV conditions even though it was properly designed, mounted, cleaned, and baked (see Section 4), the chamber possibly contains one or several leaks. Leaks can stem from incorrect mounting of vacuum flanges, or from imperfectly soldered, brazed or welded joints. A close visual inspection upon delivery and installation of all UHV components is therefore mandatory. Glass-to-metal soldering is a very delicate process, and defects can lead to leaks located preferentially at glass-to-metal transitions. All other welding seams, in particular at feedthroughs, also require inspection.

A coarse leak test consists of spraying acetone on a suspicious site of a pumped chamber, and to look for changes in the pressure reading (be advised that acetone dissolves plastics and may damage the LCD screens of devices which are typically found nearby a vacuum set-up, such as pressure meters and multimeters). The pressure changes may be positive if acetone is sucked into the chamber and evaporates there, or negative if the leak is small enough for the acetone molecules to temporarily seal the leak. Note that the sprayed acetone evaporates rapidly, leading to thermal shock and a subsequent mechanical effect on the leak. Examples are known of significant leaks at glass-to-metal transitions which were permanently 'cured' by spraying acetone onto them.

A pressurized vessel can be tested with soap water (on the outside!) in which case bubbles indicate possible leaks.

The most sophisticated way to search for leaks is to use a (helium) leak detector. In this case, the chamber (or rather the exhaust of the TMP) is connected to the leak detector which comprises a helium detector or an RGA, and a primary pump. Searching for leaks is done by spraying small amounts of helium gas through a fine nozzle near suspicious parts of the chamber. In the case a leak is present, the helium will make its way into the vacuum apparatus and eventually to the helium detector. As helium floats upwards, the chamber should be tested from top to bottom for unambiguous detection, taking into account the delay required for the helium to travel from the chamber to the detector. Spraying small amounts of helium also enhances the spatial resolution. As such small flows of helium from the nozzle are often not audible in typical noisy laboratory environments, there is a risk of the helium flow ceasing without the operator noticing it (with the ultimate consequence being that a leak goes overlooked). The helium flow should therefore be regularly checked by spraying helium into a beaker filled with a small amount of water, and looking for helium bubbles. The sensitivity of a leak detector is of the order of 10^{-11} mbar l/s, and most leak detectors provide acoustic and/or visual signals proportional to the throughput of the leak detected. To discover even the tiniest leaks, the chamber may be covered with a plastic bag, which is then filled with helium.

4. Designing UHV Apparatus

Conceiving and setting up a new UHV chamber requires a certain amount of preparation and design work. As will be explained below, a good design of the vessel is the starting point to rapidly achieve very good pressure conditions. Typical design choices involve the geometry of the vacuum vessel, the materials used, as well as the preparation, handling and installation of vacuum components, and materials. Proper vacuum design and vacuum processing ultimately make the difference between achieving high vacuum and UHV.

4.1. *Pumping and conductance*

Optimum UHV chamber design entails optimizing the throughput to the primary pump(s) in order to reach the lowest possible pressures. The guiding principle is to maximize conductances towards the pumps and to minimize the exposure to outgassing surfaces and conductances to eventual higher-pressure parts of the vessel.

In the molecular flow regime, the mass flow (throughput) and pressure are essentially governed by Kirchhoff's law for electrical circuits, with pressure differences replacing voltage differences, and with the flow resistance given by the inverse of the vacuum conductance, C. Generally, C is independent of the pressure, and its value is determined by its geometry in a rather intuitive way (i.e. a larger aperture provides a higher conductance). For example, the conductance, C_a, of an aperture with area A is expressed as (see e.g. Ref. [22])

$$C_a = A\,v_{\mathrm{av}}/4, \tag{1}$$

where $v_{\mathrm{av}} = \sqrt{8k_B T/\pi m}$, with T the temperature of the gas, k_B Boltzmann's constant, and m the mass of the gas constituent. To find the conductance C_t of a tube (or nipple), specified by its diameter d and length L, we write $A = \pi(d/2)^2$ and subsequently multiply Equation (1) with $4d/3l$ (valid for long tubes with L substantially longer than d) to find [22]

$$C_t = \frac{\pi d^3}{12L} v_{\mathrm{av}}. \tag{2}$$

Note that the above equations give C in units of m^3/s, whereas conductance is commonly specified in liters per second (l/s). For example, for air ($m \approx$ 28.8 amu) at 293 K, and inserting d and L in units of cm, we find $C_t \approx 12.15\, d^3/L$ [l/s].

The mass flow Q between two chambers with pressures p_1 and p_2, connected by a vacuum component with conductance C, is given by $Q = (p_2 - p_1) \times C$, which resembles Ohm's law. Note that Q is often given in units of mbar l/s. Similar to electrical resistances, the equivalent conductance of two conductances C_1 and C_2 placed in series is found by adding the inverse values (resistances), i.e. $C_{\text{eff}} = (1/C_1 + 1/C_2)^{-1}$. The same procedure applies if one of the conductances is actually a pump speed. As an example, the effective pump speed of a 300 l/s-pump connected to a chamber by a 10 cm-diameter tube of 15 cm length (conductance approximately 810 l/s) is reduced to 219 l/s. It is therefore preferable to mount the input flange of pumps directly onto the chamber without additional reducing elements. Of course, this depends on the pump speed that is ultimately required, and in chambers with low outgassing rates, this requirement may be relaxed.

In some situations, it is desirable to have a high flow resistance between different chambers. Experiments which combine ion traps with molecular beams, for example, typically consist of a source chamber in which the beam is formed (which often limits the pressure to the high vacuum range), and a UHV chamber where the beam is overlapped with the ion trap. Connecting the chambers with a long, skinny tube with a low conductance allows for the desired large pressure drop between the chambers, a method generally referred to as differential pumping. In Figure 1, an example of an apparatus consisting of three differentially pumped stages is shown.

5. Commissioning, Operating, and Maintaining UHV Apparatus

5.1. *Choice of UHV-compatible materials*

The above-mentioned mass flow to the primary pump of a vacuum chamber may originate from adjacent higher pressure segments of the vessel, but a major contribution in every vacuum vessel stems from the release of adsorbed molecules from all surfaces, a process referred to as outgassing. As the outgassing rate depends on the type of material and on how it was treated, the choice of materials and subsequent handling is crucial. In addition, all parts and components should have a low to very low vapor pressure. Standard chambers are either made of glass or fused quartz, or of

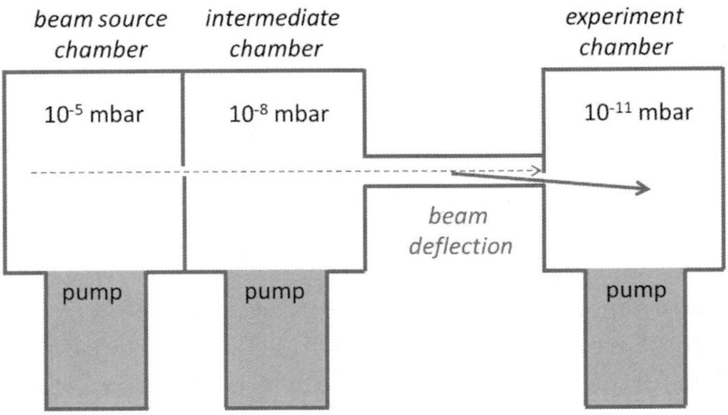

Fig. 1. Schematic drawing of a differentially pumped vacuum system for producing a molecular beam (dashed arrow) to be used in a UHV experiment. Typical pressure values are indicated for each section. In cases where only a small fraction of the beam will be used, such as state-prepared molecules or ions of a certain mass, a lower UHV pressure may be achieved by deflecting the species of interest while blocking the main beam's access to the UHV chamber.

regular stainless steel (304 type). For more demanding conditions, in particular regarding the magnetic field, they can be made of 'non-magnetic' stainless steel (316 L), aluminium, or titanium. Polishing all inner surfaces helps in reducing the effective surface area from which outgassing may occur.

Outgassing data of materials and components are readily found on the websites of Space agencies (ESA, NASA). In recent years, many UHV compatible materials have been discovered by the ion trapping community, and today, UHV-compatible solders, epoxies, and dielectrics are available.

5.2. *Vacuum apparatus bakeout*

After exposure to air, the walls of a vacuum chamber contain a large amount of adsorbed water molecules. The desorption rate of adsorbed molecules Γ behaves according to an Arrhenius-type Equation ([23]):

$$\Gamma \propto A \nu e^{-\frac{E_a}{k_B T}}, \tag{3}$$

where A is the wall surface area, ν the vibrational frequency of the bond between the H_2O molecule and the wall, and E_a the activation energy needed for desorption. At 300 K and a pressure of 10^{-7} mbar, virtually no change in the abundance of H_2O happens. This changes drastically at elevated temperatures, for which the desorption rate increases exponentially. Therefore, in order to effectively remove H_2O, vacuum vessels need to be baked out, typically at temperatures of 200–400°C. After cooling down, only adsorbed molecules with a higher activation energy E_a remain, which desorb at a much lower rate and therefore have a much smaller impact on the background pressure. Most often, the residual gas consists primarily of H_2, and CO.

In practice, the chamber is heated up slowly (below 15 K/h), after which it is baked for one to several days. Initially, the pressure will rise due to the increased desorption rate as well as the temperature increases itself (as dictated by the ideal gas law). Once a larger fraction of the adsorbed molecules have desorbed and been pumped out of the apparatus, the pressure starts to drop. Once the decrease in pressure is leveling off, typically at pressures of order 10^{-9} mbar, the apparatus is ready to be cooled down, and UHV conditions should be reached. Figure 2 qualitatively shows how the pressure responds to temperature changes during bakeout, and how it develops over time.

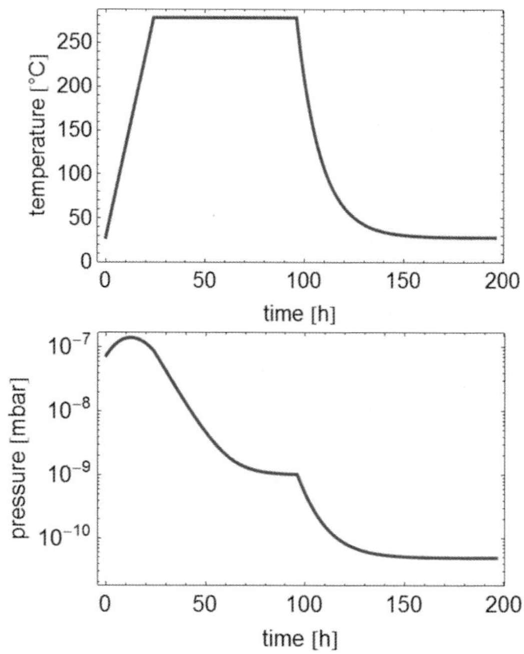

Fig. 2. Qualitative pressure behavior over time (bottom) during bakeout. The top graph shows the temperature of the apparatus during bakeout.

Care must be taken to avoid any hot or cold spots or steep temperature gradients (it is wise to keep gradients in particular across glass-to-metal transitions below 15 K). All materials, components and vacuum seals should be selected for the planned bakeout temperature (for example, one should be aware that bent copper wire will lose its stiffness at elevated temperatures and may deform under the influence of gravity). It can furthermore be advantageous to bake the chamber in air before first use. Under these conditions, an oxide layer is formed (giving stainless steel a characteristic champagne-like color) which reduces H_2 outgassing from the bulk of the chamber walls [24].

5.3. *Preparation of UHV apparatus and components*

Careful preparation of the vacuum chamber and its contents is just as important as the bakeout procedure described above. All in-vacuum parts must be cleaned thoroughly, going through several stages of ultrasonic cleaning in water with dishwashing detergent, ethanol, acetone, and isopropanol, in order to eliminate possible traces of contamination, grease and finger prints. The use of HPLC-grade acetone and isopropanol is highly recommended. All parts should be handled with powder-free gloves and lint-free paper or towels, and protected using clean-room grade aluminium foil. Tools should be equally well cleaned and protected.

Virtual leaks or trapped air pockets should be avoided. A good solution is to use vented screws (having a central bore, or a cut in the screw's outer thread). As such, screws may have become magnetized during machining, it is wise to demagnetize the screws (and other steel components near the trap) by degaussing them before cleaning, or heating them in vacuum to above the Curie temperature.

UHV chambers are normally sealed with copper gaskets which are clamped between the knife edges of the flanges using bolts and nuts. In order to achieve a continuous, leak-free 'cut' of the knife into the copper at a uniform pressure, the bolts should be tightened following a crisscross, starlike pattern. Often, flanges have a small notch giving access to the knife-copper seal for leak testing. When mating two such flanges, and contrary to the drawings in the manuals of some manufacturers, it is best not to align the notches, so that each side of the copper casket can be leak-tested separately.

Copper gaskets are single-use components. If the chamber is not to be baked above 150°C, re-usable Viton O-rings may be used. For specific applications under secondary vacuum conditions, vacuum grease might improve the tightness of O-ring seals. Although vacuum grease has a very low vapor pressure it cannot be baked, and it should be avoided for UHV applications with the exception of cryogenic vessels. Furthermore, it has been found to present a high positron annihilation cross-section.

5.4. *Venting and restoring UHV*

In case the UHV chamber has to be opened for maintenance or repairs, it should be slowly purged with dry nitrogen before being exposed to air. Nitrogen desorbs at a higher rate than water and is readily pumped out, while it helps preventing water molecules of condensing onto the wall. If properly vented ant purged with dry nitrogen, a short and mild bake-out to 80–100°C may restore UHV within one or two days. Note that if venting using a pressurized gas bottle, the pressure inside the vessel must be monitored to avoid over-pressurizing the chamber. To be safe, the chamber could be vented from a gas-filled balloon, or an empty balloon could be used as a pressure monitor at the gas inlet.

6. Conclusion

The vacuum environment of an ion trap has a strong influence on the ultimate performance of the experimental set-up. Design, choice of material, and operation of the vessel is therefore an important issue contributing to the long-term success of the experiment.

Acknowledgment

J.C.J.K. wishes to thank J. Bouma for his inspiring introduction to and expert advice on the subject of UHV.

References

1. J. F. O'Hanlon, *A User's Guide to Vacuum Technology*. John Wiley & Sons, Inc. (2004). ISBN 978-0-471-46716-8.
2. W. Umrath, *Fundamentals of vacuum technology*. Leybold Oerlikon, Cologne (2007). Available at: https://archive.org/details/FundamentalsOfVacuum Technology.
3. K. Jousten, ed., *Handbook of Vacuum Technology*. Wiley-VCH (2008). ISBN 978-3-527-40723-1.
4. J. Moore *et al.*, *Building Scientific Apparatus*. Cambridge University Press (2009). ISBN 978-0-521-87858-6.

5. H. Schaaf *et al.*, Trapped ion density distribution in the presence of He-buffer gas, *Appl. Phys.* **25**, 249 (1981).
6. D. Gerlich, Inhomogeneous RF fields: a versatile tool for the study of processes with slow ions, *Adv. Chem. Phys. Ser.* **82** (1992).
7. R. Bonner and R. March, The effects of charge exchange collisions on the motion of ions in three-dimensional quadrupole electric fields Part II. Program improvements and fundamental results, *Int. J. Mass Spectrom.* **25**(4), 411–431 (1977).
8. A. Madej and J. Sankey, Quantum jumps and the single trapped barium ion: Determination of collisional quenching rates for the $5d^2D_{5/2}$ level, *Phys. Rev. A.* **41**, 2621 (1990).
9. D. Seidel and L. Maleki, YbII lifetime, *Phys. Rev. A.* **51**, R2699–2702 (1995).
10. M. Knoop *et al.*, Lifetime, collisional-quenching, and *j*-mixing measurements of the metastable 3*D* levels of Ca^+, *Phys. Rev. A.* **52**, 3763 (1995).
11. M. Knoop *et al.*, Collisional quenching and *j*-mixing rate constants for the 3*D* levels of Ca^+, *Phys. Rev. A.* **58**, 264 (1998).
12. R. A. Hart *et al.*, A quantum scattering interferometer, *Nature.* **446**, 892–895 (2007).
13. D. J. Wineland *et al.*, Experimental Issues in Coherent Quantum-State Manipulation of Trapped Atomic Ions, *J. Res. Natl. Inst. Stand. Technol.* **103**, 259 (1998).
14. F. Vedel and M. Vedel, Investigations on the kinetic energy of trapped ions by consideration of ion/molecule collisions, *J. Mod. Opt.* **39**(2), 431–443 (1992).
15. A. Bertelsen *et al.*, Photo-dissociation of cold MgH^+ ions: Towards rotational temperature measurements and controlled dissociation, *EPJ D.* **31**, 403 (2004).
16. F. H. J. Hall *et al.*, Light-assisted ion-neutral reactive processes in the cold regime: Radiative molecule formation versus charge exchange, *Phys. Rev. Lett.* **107**, 243202 (2011).
17. N. Akerman *et al.*, Quantum control of $^{88}Sr^+$ in a miniature linear Paul trap, *Appl. Phys. B.* **107**, 1167–1174 (2011).
18. G. Gabrielse *et al.*, Thousandfold improvement in the measured antiproton mass, *Phys. Rev. Lett.* **65**, 1317–1320 (1990).
19. W. Paul and H. Steinwedel, Ein neues Massenspektrometer ohne Magnetfeld, *Z. Naturforsch. A.* **8**, 448 (1953).
20. P. Staanum *et al.*, Lifetime measurement of the metastable $3d^2d_{5/2}$ state in the $40Ca^+$ ion using the shelving technique on a few-ion string, *Phys. Rev. A* **69**, 032503 (2004).
21. M. Knoop *et al.*, Metastable level lifetimes from electron-shelving measurements with ion clouds and single ions, *Eur. Phys. J. D.* **29**, 163–171 (2004).
22. Introduction to Vacuum Technology, Pfeiffer Vacuum, http://www.pfeiffer-vacuum.com/en/know-how/introduction-to-vacuum-technology/.
23. G. A. Somorjai and Y. Li, *Introduction to Surface Chemistry and Catalysis*. John Wiley & Sons, Inc. (2010). ISBN 978-0-470-50823-7.
24. G. Moraw and R. Dobrozemsky, Attainment of outgassing rates below 10^{-13} Torr liters/sec cm^2 for aluminium and stainless steel after bakeout at moderate temperatures, *Jpn. J. Appl. Phys.* **13**, 261–264 (1974).

CHAPTER SIX

LASER COOLING TECHNIQUES APPLICABLE TO TRAPPED IONS

C. Champenois

CNRS and Aix-Marseille Université, PIIM, UMR 7345,
Centre de Saint Jérôme, 13397 Marseille Cedex 20, France
caroline.champenois@univ-amu.fr

This chapter gathers two lectures which were dedicated to processes involved in general laser cooling and to laser cooling technics specific to trapped particles. In this last lecture, assumptions about the atomic motion were made, which were directly inspired by the situation of ions trapped in an Radiofrequency (RF) quadrupole trap. Nevertheless, the motion of ions in Penning traps has a lot to share with the motion in RF quadrupole traps, mostly its harmonic nature. As a consequence, methods explained in this last context can be adapted to ions in Penning traps. The spirit of this chapter is to start from the fundamental basic equations to allow the reader to derive the formulae in his own specific context. One of the goals is to identify the parameters that control the relevant orders of magnitude that need to be estimated before building a laser cooling set-up.

1. The Radiation Pressure Force

To understand the mechanical effects of light on atoms, one must consider the internal structure of atoms and their quantized internal energy. The radiation pressure induced by light relies on the photon momentum transferred to an atom when it absorbs a photon. In such a process, energy and momentum must be conserved and atoms absorb photons if their energy $\hbar\omega_L$ is very close to an energy gap ΔE between two energy levels. The photon momentum $\hbar k_L$ is large enough to induce mechanical effect when the associated wavelength $\lambda_L = 2\pi/k_L$ is in the optical domain. For most atoms, the corresponding energy gap separates different electronic states.[a] In the following, we consider lasers as the source of photons to cool atoms. It implies that these photons carry the same energy and momentum. As a consequence, they hit only one transition ΔE. Therefore, we now consider the atom as a two-level system, provided that these two-levels are determined by the wavelength of the laser. The excited electronic states appropriate for efficient laser–atom coupling have a finite lifetime τ_e of the order of 10 ns. So, once in the excited state, the atom soon relaxes to its ground state and emits a photon to conserve energy.

In 1917, Einstein identifies two different emission processes: spontaneous emission and stimulated emission. Those two ways imply a different coupling with light. Spontaneous emission results from the coupling with the vacuum electromagnetic field and, in free space, the emitted photon wave-vector has a random direction which averages to zero on many absorption/spontaneous emission cycles. The net recoil for the atom on one absorption/spontaneous emission cycle is then *on average* $\Delta \mathbf{p} = \hbar \mathbf{k}_L$. Depending on the atom mass m, the recoil velocity $v_{\mathrm{rec}} = \hbar k_L/m$ ranges from few mm/s to 3 m/s for hydrogen atoms. The stimulated emission (which is at the core of laser) results from the coupling with the excitation laser itself and gives back a photon identical to the absorbed one. The net recoil for the atom on one absorption/stimulated emission cycle is null and does not contribute to the average force experienced by an atom. In the optical domain, one can show, by comparing Einstein coefficient, that spontaneous emission is a lot more probable than stimulated emission, which starts to play a role when the atom is strongly driven by the laser.

The recoil experienced by one atom reduces its velocity if the atom and the photon are counter-propagating. To make this configuration favorable, the momentum and energy conservation laws must be obeyed for this specific geometry. If $\mathbf{p}$ and $\mathbf{p}'$ are the atomic momentum before and after a photon absorption, and $\hbar\omega_0 = \Delta E = E_e - E_g$ is the atomic energy gap, the conservation laws,

$$\mathbf{p}' = \mathbf{p} + \hbar \mathbf{k}_L, \tag{1}$$

$$E_g + \hbar\omega_L + \mathbf{p}^2/2m = E_e + \mathbf{p}'^2/2m, \tag{2}$$

[a]Photons inducing transitions between sub-levels of the same electronic state have a too small wave-vector to have a relevant mechanical effect on atoms.

induce that the Doppler shifted laser frequency $\omega_L^{at} = \omega_L - \mathbf{k}_L.\mathbf{v}$ must obey $\omega_L^{at} = \omega_0 + \hbar\mathbf{k}_L^2/2m$. If $\omega_L < \omega_0$, the laser frequency reaches the atomic resonance for atoms moving against the laser beam ($-\mathbf{k}_L.\mathbf{v} > 0$) and then $||\mathbf{p}'|| < ||\mathbf{p}||$. The frequency difference $\omega_{\text{rec}} = \hbar\mathbf{k}_L^2/2m$ we are forgetting is the recoil kinetic energy (divided by $\hbar$), of the order of a few tens of kHz. This frequency shift is small compared to the spontaneous scattering rate $\gamma = 1/\tau_e$, which, as will be seen later, defines the smallest reachable frequency scale. In the first part of this chapter, we then neglect the role of the recoil energy in the energy budget.

To analyze the atomic velocity evolution when choosing a negative detuning $\delta = \omega_L - \omega_0$, the averaged force on an atom must be estimated. This force $\mathbf{F}$ is the net recoil on one absorption/spontaneous emission cycle ($\hbar\mathbf{k}_L$) $\times$ the number of spontaneously emitted photons per unit time. This number depends on the probability P_e for an atom to be in the excited state and on the probability γ for an atom in the excited state to emit spontaneously a photon. Then, the averaged force is simply $\gamma \times P_e \times \hbar\mathbf{k}$. Once the atom and its cooling transition is chosen, the only parameter that still needs to be controlled is P_e. To that purpose, we need to turn to the precise evolution of the probability P_e with the atom–laser interaction, in the next section.

2. A Two-level Atom Interacting with a Laser Beam

The strongest term in the coupling between an atom and an electromagnetic field in the optical domain is due to the laser electric field, which couples to the transition dipole d_{eg} by

$$\hat{V}_{AL}(\mathbf{r}, t) = -\hat{\mathbf{d}}_{eg}.\mathbf{E}_L(\mathbf{r}, t), \tag{3}$$

where $\mathbf{r}$ is the averaged position of the atom center of mass and the spreading of the atomic wave-function is assumed to be negligible compared to the light wavelength. These assumptions form the core of the dipolar approximation [1,2]. The transition operator can be written like

$$\hat{\mathbf{d}}_{eg} = d_{eg}\mathbf{u}_L(|e\rangle\langle g| - |g\rangle\langle e|), \tag{4}$$

where $\mathbf{u}_L$ is the local electric field polarization and the transition dipole amplitude depends on the electronic orbitals of the two coupled states $|g\rangle, |e\rangle$ through the electron position operator $d_{eg} = q_e\langle e|\hat{\mathbf{r}}_e.\mathbf{u}_L|g\rangle$. Here, selection rules apply and a dipolar transition can only occur between states defined by a kinetic angular momentum L and a total angular momentum

J such that $L_e = L_g \pm 1$ and $J_e = J_g, J_g \pm 1$. The light polarization also induces a selection rule on the implied Zeeman sub-states. For a complete demonstration of these rules, see an Atomic Physics textbook [3,4]. Considering two specific atomic levels, if the transition dipole is null, then the atom-laser coupling must be developed further. Then appear terms leading to magnetic dipole transitions, which belong to a different energy domain, or quadrupole electric transitions, which are used for example in optical atomic clock based on single ion (see Ref. [4]).

Considering the laser wave as a plane wave $\mathbf{E}_L(\mathbf{r}, t) = E_L \mathbf{u}_L \cos(\omega t - \Phi(\mathbf{r}))$, the Rabi frequency scales the interaction strength like

$$\hbar\Omega_1(\mathbf{r}) = -d_{eg} E_L(\mathbf{r}). \tag{5}$$

This interaction and the spontaneous emission drive the evolution of the internal degrees of freedom (DoF), which can be accounted for in the time evolution of the density matrix of the internal state $\hat{\rho}$. It obeys the master equation,

$$\frac{\partial}{\partial t}\hat{\rho} = -\frac{\mathrm{i}}{\hbar}\left[\hat{H}, \hat{\rho}\right] + \hat{\mathcal{L}}\hat{\rho}, \tag{6}$$

where the Hamiltonian $\hat{H}$ is the sum of the free atom Hamiltonian $\hat{H}_0$ and of the atom–laser coupling operator,

$$\hat{V}_{AL}(\mathbf{r}, t) = \hbar\Omega_1(\mathbf{r}(t))(|e\rangle\langle g| - |g\rangle\langle e|)\cos(\omega t - \Phi(\mathbf{r}(t))). \tag{7}$$

$\mathcal{L}\hat{\rho}$ rules the non-Hamiltonian evolution induced by relaxation (spontaneous emission, collisions, etc.). Lindblad operators $\hat{\mathcal{L}}$ have a different form if the relaxation process implies only decoherence (elastic collisions, laser spectral line-width) or also decay from the excited state (spontaneous emission, inelastic collision, etc.). Once projected on the basis $(|g\rangle, |e\rangle)$, the master equation gives a set of first order differential equation called the optical Bloch equations (OBE), where the relative motion of the atom in the wave $\mathbf{r}(t)$ induces a modulation of the laser–atom interaction through the amplitude $\Omega_1(\mathbf{r}(t))$ and the phase $\Phi(\mathbf{r}(t))$. In a first step, we neglect these modulation effects and consider an atom at rest, experiencing a position independent coupling.

2.1. *The radiation pressure force for an atom at rest*

For a fixed position of the atom inside the wave, $\Phi(\mathbf{r}) = \Phi_0$ and $\Omega_1(\mathbf{r}) = \Omega_1$ and the self-Hamiltonian $\hat{H}_0$ reduces to the internal energy $\hbar\omega_0|e\rangle\langle e|$.

Considering that $\rho_{gg} + \rho_{ee} = 1$ and that $\rho_{ge} = \rho_{eg}^*$, the OBE are defined by

$$\begin{aligned}\frac{\mathrm{d}\rho_{ee}}{\mathrm{d}t} &= i(\rho_{eg} - \rho_{ge})\Omega_1 \cos(\omega_L t - \Phi_0) - \gamma_p \rho_{ee},\\ \frac{\mathrm{d}\rho_{eg}}{\mathrm{d}t} &= -i\omega_0 \rho_{eg} - i(\rho_{ee} - \rho_{gg})\Omega_1 \cos(\omega_L t - \Phi_0) - \gamma_d \rho_{eg}.\end{aligned} \tag{8}$$

When setting the relaxation terms γ_p and γ_d to zero, one can see that the coherences ρ_{ge}, ρ_{eg} evolve on the short timescale imposed by the laser frequency. We are interested in the envelope evolution induced by the competition between excitation and decay and can eliminate the rapid evolution by using modified coherence function like

$$\rho_{eg} = \tilde{\rho}_{eg} e^{-i(\omega_L t - \Phi_0)}. \tag{9}$$

Furthermore, the decomposition of $\cos(\omega_L t - \Phi_0)$ into $(\exp(i(\omega_L t - \Phi_0) + \exp(-i(\omega_L t - \Phi_0))/2$ gives two kinds of terms for the mean population time evolution:

$$\frac{\mathrm{d}\rho_{ee}}{\mathrm{d}t} = i\Omega_1 \left(\tilde{\rho}_{eg} e^{-i\omega_L t} - \tilde{\rho}_{ge} e^{i\omega_L t}\right) \frac{e^{(i(\omega_L t - \Phi_0)} + e^{(-i(\omega_L t - \Phi_0)}}{2} - \gamma_p \rho_{ee}. \tag{10}$$

We neglect the fast oscillating terms $\exp(\pm i2\omega_L t)$ and only keep the slow envelope effect. This secular approximation is also named the rotating wave approximation (RWA) and is relevant for excitation by a continuous wave with the typical laser intensities used for atom manipulation by lasers. In the frame of this approximation, the OBE reduce to

$$\begin{aligned}\frac{\mathrm{d}\rho_{ee}}{\mathrm{d}t} &= i(\tilde{\rho}_{eg} - \tilde{\rho}_{ge})\Omega_1/2 - \gamma_p \rho_{ee},\\ \frac{\mathrm{d}\tilde{\rho}_{eg}}{\mathrm{d}t} &= -i(\omega_0 - \omega_L)\tilde{\rho}_{eg} - i(\rho_{ee} - \rho_{gg})\Omega_1/2 - \gamma_d \tilde{\rho}_{eg},\end{aligned} \tag{11}$$

where the time evolution of the three components of the Bloch vector: $u(t) = \Re(\tilde{\rho}_{eg})$, $v(t) = \Im(\tilde{\rho}_{eg})$ and $w(t) = (\rho_{ee} - \rho_{gg})/2 = \rho_{ee} - 1/2$ can be extracted.

$$\begin{aligned}\dot{u}(t) &= \delta_L v(t) - \gamma_d u(t),\\ \dot{v}(t) &= -\delta_L u(t) - \Omega_1 w(t) - \gamma_d v(t),\\ \dot{w}(t) &= \Omega_1 v(t) - \gamma_p (w(t) + 1/2).\end{aligned} \tag{12}$$

If the only source of decoherence and decay is spontaneous emission, $\gamma_p = 2\gamma_d = \gamma$ (the case where the laser spectral line-width cannot be neglected is worked out in Exercices 8.3), the stationary solutions of the OBE write like

$$u_{\rm st} = \frac{\delta_L}{\Omega_1}\frac{s}{1+s}, \quad v_{\rm st} = \frac{\gamma}{2\Omega_1}\frac{s}{1+s}, \quad \rho_{ee} = w_{\rm st} + 1/2 = \frac{1}{2}\frac{s}{1+s}. \tag{13}$$

They depend on a parameter s called the *saturation parameter* which gathers all the relevant parameters of the atom–laser excitation,

$$s = \frac{\Omega_1^2/2}{\delta_L^2 + \gamma^2/4}. \tag{14}$$

For a small saturation parameter ($s \ll 1$), the atom responds linearly with s, which is proportional to the laser local intensity ($\Omega_1^2 \propto E_L^2 \propto I_L$). On resonance ($\delta_L = 0$), s simplifies to $s_0 = 2\Omega_1^2/\gamma^2$. The saturation intensity I_s, defined by $s_0(I_s) = 1$, is a characteristic parameter of the transition strength and a very relevant parameter to scale the requirement in laser intensity for an experiment. It is of the order of few mW/cm^2 for alkalis (sodium, rubidium, cesium, etc.) and alkali-earth ions (Be^+, Ca^+, Sr^+, ...).

Going back to the force on atom, it behaves like

$$P_e = \rho_{ee} = \frac{\Omega_1^2}{4(\Omega_1^2/2 + \delta_L^2 + \gamma^2/4)}, \tag{15}$$

and is maximum (and equal to 1/2) when $\delta_L = 0$. It has a Lorentzian profile when the laser detuning is scanned with a line shape characterized by the spectral width (FWHM) $\Delta\omega = \gamma\sqrt{1+s_0}$. γ is then the smallest observable line-width for a transition and is called its natural line-width. It is broadened if the saturation parameter on resonance is non-negligible compared to 1, which is often called power broadening.

2.2. *Force on a moving atom, in the broadband limit*

The resolution of Equation (8) with a position dependent coupling through $\Phi(\mathbf{r}(t))$ and $\Omega_1(\mathbf{r}(t))$ implies a combined resolution of the time evolution of the internal and external DoF, which requires a numerical resolution for general cases. This can be avoided if the dynamics of the internal state is a lot more rapid than the external dynamics. Then, we can consider that the ρ_{ij} terms adapt instantaneously to $\mathbf{r}$ and $\mathbf{v}$, which can be considered as constant in the OBE. To check this assumption, one has to identify the two involved timescales. It takes $\tau_e = 1/\gamma$ for the internal dynamics to reach its stationary state. The external evolution (motion induced changes) plays a role when the Doppler shift accumulated over a time $T_{\rm ext}$ drives the atom out of the resonance line, such that $k_L \Delta v(T_{\rm ext}) = \gamma/2$. At most, the atom scatters photons with an averaged rate equal to $\gamma/2$, then $\Delta v(T_{\rm ext}) \simeq v_{\rm rec} T_{\rm ext} \gamma/2$ so $T_{\rm ext} \simeq (2\omega_{\rm rec})^{-1}$. Reaching $T_{\rm ext} \gg T_{\rm int}$ requires $\gamma \gg 2\omega_{\rm rec} = \hbar k_L^2/m$. This broadband condition is obeyed for all the strong dipole transitions used for Doppler laser cooling in alkaline atoms or alkaline-earth ions as $\gamma/2\pi$ is of the order of 10 MHz whereas $\omega_{\rm rec}/2\pi$ ranges from 10 to 100 kHz.

In the rest of this first part chapter concerning unbounded atoms, we assume the broadband condition is obeyed and, at time t, the probability for the atom to be in the excited state is simply given by Equation (15), where Ω_1 is replaced by $\Omega_1(\mathbf{r}(t))$ and δ_L is replaced by $\delta_L - \mathbf{k}_L.\mathbf{v}(t)$. The most simple case to imagine is to slow an atomic beam, where it is obvious to chose a counter-propagating laser beam to reduce the atom velocity. Still, to make the force efficient, the detuning needs to be adapted to the atomic beam velocity. This issue is more specifically addressed in an Exercise 8.1.

For an atomic gas in thermal equilibrium, to make sure that the photon recoil results in a reduction of the atom velocity, one has to make sure that absorption of counter-propagating photons is more favorable than absorption of co-propagating ones. This is done by choosing a negative detuning δ_L. Then, the absorption probability is a lot more favorable for a velocity class such that $\delta_L - \mathbf{k}_L.\mathbf{v} \simeq 0$ which implies $\mathbf{k}_L.\mathbf{v} < 0$. To bring the atomic velocity close to zero, it takes two counter-propagating laser beams, with same intensity and detuning, in a configuration called an optical molasses. In the low saturation limit, where the atom response is linear with the intensity, the total force is the sum of the force induced by each laser beam $\mathbf{F} = \mathbf{F}_+ + \mathbf{F}_-$ with

$$\mathbf{F}_\pm = \pm \hbar \mathbf{k}_L \gamma \rho_{ee}^\pm(\mathbf{v}) \tag{16}$$

and $\rho_{ee}^\pm(\mathbf{v}) = s_\pm(\mathbf{v})/2$.

If $k_L v \ll \gamma$, the linear development of F for small $v = ||\mathbf{v}||$ gives a force proportional to the velocity $\mathbf{F} = -m\alpha\mathbf{v}$ with

$$\alpha = \omega_{\rm rec} s \frac{-4\gamma\delta_L}{\delta_L^2 + \gamma^2/4}, \tag{17}$$

where s is the saturation parameter induced by the coupling with each laser beam. This force is an actual damping force if $\delta_L < 0$ like intuitively deduced. Figure 1 shows the contribution by each laser beam and the resulting damping force for different detunings. It illustrates the concept of capture range for such a force. In the low saturation limit, the force keeps a good sign for any velocity value, but its efficiency depends on the

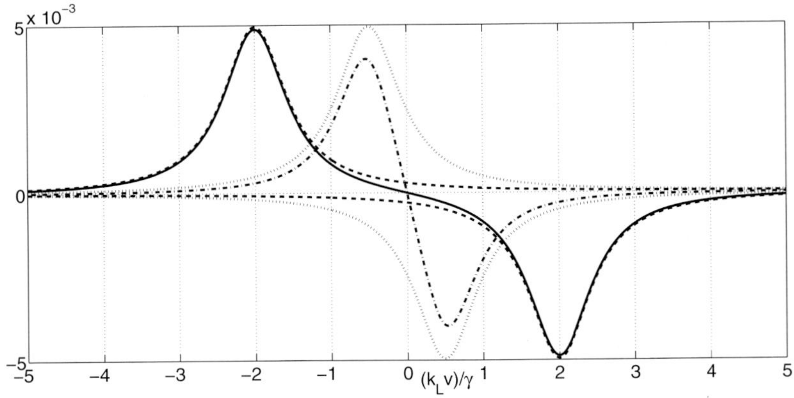

Fig. 1. Force induced by a 1D optical molasse in units of $(\hbar k_L \gamma)$ versus the atomic velocity in units of $k_L.v/\gamma$ in the linear approximation ($s_0 = 0.01$) for two different detunings: $\delta_L = -2\gamma$ (dashed line for the two beam contributions and solid line for the resulting force) and $\delta_L = -\gamma/2$ (dotted line for the two beam contributions and dash-dotted line for the resulting force).

atom velocity relative to the detuning. The two contributions are maximum for $\pm v_{\max} = \pm|\delta_L|/k_L$ and have a FWHM around this maximum equal to $v_c = \gamma/k_L$ in velocity range. One can consider that for $|v - v_{\max}| > 2v_c$, the force is negligible. The choice of the detuning determines the velocity profile of the resulting damping force, as illustrated by the two examples of Figure 1. It results from a compromise between the velocity range that needs to be captured, the time required for cooling and the aimed temperature are as discussed in the following.

The velocity evolution timescale ruled by Doppler cooling is

$$\tau_{\rm DC} = \frac{1}{8\omega_{\rm rec}s}\left(\frac{2|\delta_L|}{\gamma} + \frac{\gamma}{2|\delta_L|}\right). \tag{18}$$

The first point to note is that if δ_L is too close to the resonance, this timescale τ_{DC} tends to infinity. To understand this feature, one must remember that the velocity reduction requires to make unbalanced the absorption by co- and counter-propagating beams. Setting the laser too close to resonance brings these two contributions close to a balance which leads to a high number of scattered photons but no net reduction of the mean velocity. A typically well-unbalanced situation is reached for $\delta_L = -\gamma/2$, for which $\tau_{DC} = 1/(4\omega_{\rm rec}s_0)$. For a typical low saturation parameter $s_0 = 1/10$, $\tau_{DC} = 2.5/\omega_{\rm rec}$ which, for heavy alkalies, is smaller than 1 ms and can be lower than 100 μs. The extrapolation of the 1D scheme to 2D serves, for example, to reduce the divergence of an atomic beam and increase its brightness (see Exercise 8.2). In 3D, you can cool an atomic gas in optical molasses.

2.3. *How cold can the atoms get?*

The development of the radiation pressure as a damping force could let us think that atoms can be cooled down to zero velocity. This is not the case because of the time fluctuations of the force due to the random direction of each individual kick, and which is responsible for a spreading in the momentum distribution, synonymous for a heating process. This spreading due to random kicks is analogous to Brownian motion and is characterized by a diffusion law for the momentum variance $\Delta\mathbf{p}^2$ which is N times the square of the momentum step $\hbar k_L$. During time t, an atom scatters $P_e\gamma t$ photons giving a diffusion induced by spontaneous emission $\Delta\mathbf{p}^2/\Delta t = (\hbar k_L)^2 P_e\gamma$. The absorption process is also responsible for an increase of the momentum variance because of the fluctuations of the differential number of absorbed photons from each laser beam. In the low saturation limit, these numbers are uncorrelated and follow a Poisson statistic: $\Delta^2(N_+ - N_-) = (N_+ + N_-) = N = P_e\gamma t$, each absorption contributing also with a kick length of $\hbar k_L$. The total momentum diffusion in 1D is then $\Delta\mathbf{p}^2 = \hbar^2 k_L^2 2P_e\gamma t$. In the linear (or low saturation) regime, and if s remains the saturation parameter associated with one laser beam, $P_e = s$ in 1D and $P_e = 3s$ in 3D because we assume the Doppler effect is now negligible on P_e. For a more detailed description of the different contribution to the momentum diffusion, see Refs. [3, 5]. In 3D, the global time evolution of the momentum variance, involving laser cooling and heating is ruled by

$$\Delta\mathbf{p}^2/\Delta t = 6(\hbar k_L)^2 s\gamma - 2\alpha\mathbf{p}^2. \tag{19}$$

The equilibrium value defines the reached temperature through

$$\left(\frac{\mathbf{p}^2}{2m}\right)_{\text{eq}} = \frac{3}{2}k_B T_{\text{eq}} = \frac{3(\hbar k_L)^2 s\gamma}{m\alpha}, \tag{20}$$

which simplifies to

$$k_B T_{\text{eq}} = \frac{\hbar\gamma}{4}\left(\frac{2|\delta_L|}{\gamma} + \frac{\gamma}{2|\delta_L|}\right). \tag{21}$$

This temperature depends only on the detuning because we set ourselves in the low saturation regime. It reaches a minimum value which depends only on the lifetime of the excited state by $k_B T_D = \hbar\gamma/2$ for $\delta = -\gamma/2$. For strong dipole transition in alkalies, this minimum temperature, called the Doppler temperature, is in the range of 100 μK. For example, it is 140 μK in Rb ($\tau_e = 27$ ns) and 0.5 mK for Ca^+ ($\tau_e = 7$ ns).

The reached mean squared velocity v_D depends on the atomic mass:

$$v_D = \sqrt{\frac{\hbar\gamma}{2m}} = \sqrt{v_{\rm rec} v_c} \tag{22}$$

and is the geometric mean of the capture velocity $v_c = \hbar\gamma/2k_L$ and the recoil velocity. For Ca^+ ($m = 40$ amu), $v_{rec} = 2.3$ cm/s, $v_c = 4.6$ m/s and $v_D \simeq 0.3$ m/s. This connection between the three relevant velocity scales is very useful to keep in mind and remember that all this demonstration makes sense if $v_D \ll v_c$, which implies $v_{\rm rec} \ll v_c$ which is equivalent to $2\omega_{\rm rec} \ll \gamma$, where we find again the broad line condition!

A quick comparison of Equations (18) and (21) shows that the cooling timescale $\tau_{\rm DC}$ can be re-expressed as

$$\tau_{\rm DC} = \frac{k_B T_{\rm eq}}{\hbar\gamma} \frac{1}{2s\omega_{\rm rec}}. \tag{23}$$

This last expression illustrates the strategy to choose: the laser detuning controls the final temperature and for a given aimed temperature, the timescale is controlled by the saturation parameter, namely the laser intensity. To reach the Doppler limit, $\tau_{\rm DC}$ reduces to $(2s_0\omega_{\rm rec})^{-1}$.

2.4. *Are all atoms a two-level system?*

Actually, an atom is rarely a two-level system and selection rules of dipole transitions must be taken into consideration to build an effective two-level system. These rules connect the light polarization and the Zeeman sublevels concerned with the transition. A genuine two-level system is formed by a $J = 0$ and $J = 1$ state like in Ca if the transition is driven by a polarized light. For more details about selection rules, which should be looked upon closely before designing an experiment, see Ref. [2].

Some commonly trapped ions cannot be reduced to two-level systems. They are the heavy alkaline-earth ions (Ca^+, Sr^+, Ba^+) and share the property to have a D state lying lower in energy than the P excited state coupled to the S ground state by a strong dipole allowed transition, the resonance line (see Figure 2(a)). In neutral alkalies (Rb, Cs), this D state is above the P state and it makes a big difference: $S \to P$ and $D \to P$ are dipole allowed, $S \to D$ is dipole forbidden, but allowed by coupling

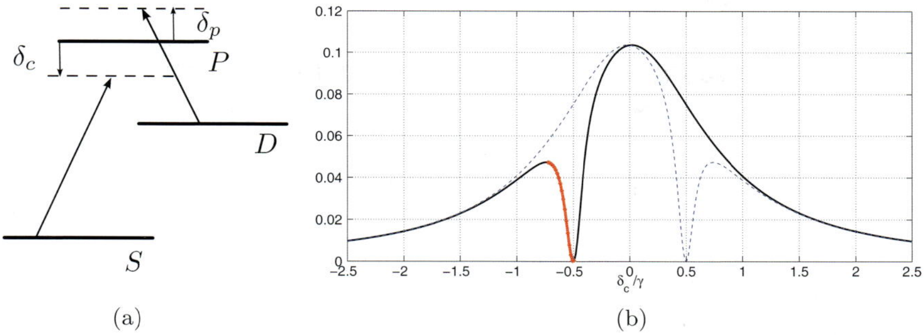

Fig. 2. (a) Laser coupling scheme involved for Doppler laser cooling in heavy alkali-earth ions like Ca^+, Sr^+, Ba^+. (b) Probability of occupation of the P excited state in a Λ-scheme level system versus the detuning δ_c of the main cooling transition $S \to P$. The P level lifetime $1/\gamma$ is 7 ns and the branching ratio to the long-lived state D is 1/15 (Ca^+ typical parameter). The Rabi frequency on the main cooling transition is $\gamma/2$ and is $\gamma/5$ on the repumping one. Blue curve: the pump detuning is positive, $\delta_p = +\gamma/2$. Black curve: the pump detuning is negative, $\delta_p = -\gamma/2$.

with the electric quadrupole. When excited by the main cooling laser on the $S \to P$ transition, the Ca^+-like ions decay to the long-lived state D with a probability ranging from $\simeq 1/15$ for Ca^+ and Sr^+ to $\simeq 1/3$ for Ba^+. A second laser (p) is then required to pump the atom out of the metastable state, building a Λ-shape level scheme (see Figure 2(a)), well known to produce Coherent Population Trapping (CPT) when the two lasers share the same detuning ($\delta_c = \delta_p$). The CPT gives rise to a dark line in the cooling transition spectra, visible in Figure 2(b). There are two main consequences of the effective Λ-scheme involved in Doppler cooling. The first one is that the maximum stationary occupation probability of the excited state is lower than 1/2 (for Ca^+, it is typically 0.27). As efficient Doppler cooling requires low saturation regime, this feature is not a severe drawback. The second feature, related to the modified line shape, is a more severe issue. Indeed, depending on the value of the repumping laser detuning δ_p, choosing $\delta_c < 0$ may not guarantee cooling. This is illustrated in Figure 2(b) where the red brushed part of the curve highlights negative detuning for which $P_e(\delta_b - kv) < P_e(\delta_b + kv)$ for a class of small velocities. Then, absorption of co-propagating photons is more probable than counter-propagating photons, leading to heating. Depending on the relative Rabi frequencies and detuning, the heating detuning range can be narrowed or even shifted to the positive detuning range where it does not interfere with cooling.

3. There is Another Force

The *ad hoc* demonstration we have run, focusing on absorption and emission of photons, left aside a large part of the light–atom interaction which does not reduce to radiation pressure. To take into account the full aspect of the mechanical effect of atom-light interactions, we have to go back to the Heisenberg picture where position and momentum are operators with a time evolution, and $\mathbf{r}(t)$ and $\mathbf{p}(t)$ are the average over the atomic state of these operators. The averaged Heisenberg equations rule the time evolution by

$$\frac{\mathrm{d}\mathbf{r}}{\mathrm{d}t} = \frac{\mathbf{p}}{m}, \tag{24}$$

$$\frac{\mathrm{d}\mathbf{p}}{\mathrm{d}t} = \mathbf{F} = -\langle \nabla V_{AL}(t) \rangle - \langle \nabla V_{AV} \rangle. \tag{25}$$

The averaged force induced by coupling with the electromagnetic field of the vacuum V_{AR}, and responsible for spontaneous emission, is null. The atom–laser coupling is a development over the atomic wave-packet and the first-order term, assessing the atomic wave-packet is small compared to λ_L, is the electric-dipole interaction,

$$\mathbf{F} = \langle \mathbf{d}_{eg} \cdot \mathbf{u}_L \rangle \nabla E_L(\mathbf{r}(t), t). \tag{26}$$

The time evolution of the dipole is known thanks to our study of the internal DoF:

$$\langle \mathbf{d}_{eg}.\mathbf{u}_L \rangle = d_{eg}(\rho_{eg} + \rho_{ge}) \tag{27}$$

$$= 2d_{eg}(u_{\mathrm{st}} \cos{(\omega_L t + \Phi(\mathbf{r}))} - v_{\mathrm{st}} \sin{(\omega_L t - \Phi(\mathbf{r}))}. \tag{28}$$

The real and imaginary parts of the coherence u and v give the dipole contribution in phase and in quadrature with the electric field. Once again, we made the broad line approximation by assuming that the coherence has reached its stationary value $(u_{\mathrm{st}}, v_{\mathrm{st}})$ for each new position. The force on an atom is then explicitly

$$\mathbf{F} = -2\hbar(u_{\mathrm{st}} \cos{(\omega_L t - \Phi(\mathbf{r}))} - v_{\mathrm{st}} \sin{(\omega_L t - \Phi(\mathbf{r}))} \nabla(\Omega_1(\mathbf{r}) \cos{(\omega_L t - \Phi(\mathbf{r}))} \tag{29}$$

and is made of two kinds of oscillating terms. Two terms are products of $\sin{(\omega_L t - \Phi(\mathbf{r}))}$ and $\cos{(\omega_L t - \Phi(\mathbf{r}))}$ and the time average of these products is null. The two remaining terms come from the $\sin^2(\omega_L t - \Phi(\mathbf{r}))$ and the $\cos^2(\omega_L t - \Phi(\mathbf{r}))$ terms and they result in two contributions to the force:

$$\mathbf{F} = -2\hbar\Omega_1(\mathbf{r})\left(u_{\mathrm{st}}\frac{\nabla\Omega_1(\mathbf{r})}{\Omega_1(\mathbf{r})} - v_{\mathrm{st}}\nabla\Phi(\mathbf{r})\right). \tag{30}$$

Let's now take a closer look at these general expressions. For a travelling wave with a uniform intensity (on the atom motion scale), $\Phi(\mathbf{r}) = \mathbf{k}_L.\mathbf{r}$ and $\nabla\Omega_1(\mathbf{r}) = 0$. The force has one contribution we already met as the radiation pressure force:

$$\mathbf{F}_P = \hbar\mathbf{k}_L\Omega_1 v_{\mathrm{st}} = \hbar\mathbf{k}_L\gamma\rho_{ee}. \tag{31}$$

What's new here is the other contribution that could not be extracted from our previous analysis:

$$\mathbf{F}_{\mathrm{dip}} = -\frac{\hbar\delta_L}{2}\frac{\nabla s(\mathbf{r})}{1+s(\mathbf{r})}. \tag{32}$$

This force, called the dipolar force, is conservative and does not imply absorption and emission of photons. It can be derived from a potential energy $U_{\mathrm{dip}}(\mathbf{r})$ of the form,

$$U_{\mathrm{dip}}(\mathbf{r}) = \frac{\hbar\delta_L}{2}\log\left(1+s(\mathbf{r})\right), \tag{33}$$

with a sign depending on the sign of δ_L: By choosing a red or blue detuning, one can control if atoms are attracted or repelled by higher laser intensity. This dipolar potential can reach few mK and is used to trap (nearly exclusively neutral) cold atoms in optical tweezer (for single atoms) or in optical lattices (for an ensemble of ordered atoms) and in practice, it is used with large detuning ($\delta_L \gg \Omega_1$) to cancel radiation pressure from the same laser. The potential then takes a simple form $U_{\mathrm{dip}}(\mathbf{r}) = \hbar\Omega_1^2(\mathbf{r})/(4\delta_L)$ that may ring a bell to those of you who are familiar to the dressed atom picture introduced by Cohen-Tannoudji [6] to formalize the energy shift introduced by photons and atom coupling.

4. What's New with a Bounded Motion?

We would like to insist that in the first sections of this chapter, we have seen that the atom motion modifies the atom–laser interaction through the induced modulation of the strength and phase of the atom–laser interaction,

$$V_{AL}(\mathbf{r}, t) = -d_{eg} \cdot E_L(\mathbf{r}) \cos(\omega t - \Phi(\mathbf{r})). \tag{34}$$

We also showed that in some cases, this motion effect can be taken into account by a Doppler shift in the effective laser detuning. The primordial role of position modulation over velocity Doppler effect was first demonstrated in 1952 by Dicke [7] in *"The Effect of Collisions upon the Doppler Width of Spectral Lines"*. By reducing the mean free path of the atoms in a gas cell by increased pressure, Dicke observed a narrowing of the Doppler broadened spectra without any cooling involved. He further demonstrated that if the mean free path is negligible compared to the wavelength radiation, there is no Doppler broadening, an effect now called Lamb–Dicke effect.

The fact that a large velocity distribution may have no broadening effect does not contradict our previous analysis about motion induced effect if the broadband condition is not fulfilled anymore: if the motion relevant timescale T_{ext} is shortened by any confining effect, it may become of the order of τ_e and our previous timescale separation technique fails to model the atomic system. We then have to keep the original form of the atom–laser interaction and can make assumption about this motion to deduce the form of the line spectrum.

Let's assume the laser propagates along one of the trap axis (Ox for example), and that the motion is well described by $x(t) \simeq X \cos(\omega_x t)$. This can be the case for uncorrelated ions in an Radiofrequency (RF) trap where the contribution of the micromotion is neglected and it is certainly a good approximation for single ions sitting at the node of the RF electric field of a 3D or linear RF trap (see Chapters 1 and 2). Let's treat the motion classically and observe its effect on the line spectrum.

4.1. *Oscillation motion in the classical limit*

We focus on the motion induced phase modulation in the atom–laser interaction and forget about the intensity modulation. A periodic phase modulation gives rise to extra frequencies which can be obtained by the Fourier transform,

$$e^{ik_L x(t)} = e^{ik_L X \cos \omega_x t} = \mathcal{J}_0(k_L X) + i\mathcal{J}_1(k_L X)e^{\pm i\omega_x t} - \mathcal{J}_2(k_L X)e^{\pm i2\omega_x t} \ldots, \tag{35}$$

where the $\mathcal{J}_n$ are Bessel functions and $k_L X$ is the modulation index. From the atom point of view, it is like the laser emits several (coherent) lines with angular frequencies ω_L, $\omega_L \pm \omega_x$, $\omega_L \pm 2\omega_x, \ldots$. The coupling strength on

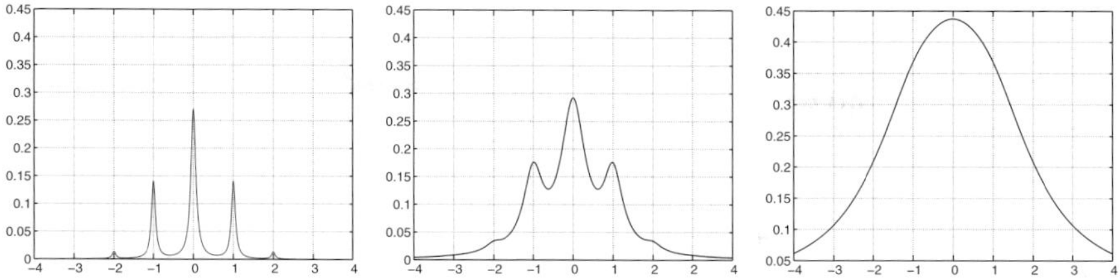

(a) $\gamma = \omega_x/10$ (b) $\gamma = \omega_x/2$ (c) $\gamma = 2\omega_x$

Fig. 3. Line spectra for an oscillating motion with a modulation index $k_L X = 1$ and an oscillating frequency $\omega_x/2\pi = 1$ MHz. The saturation parameter is kept constant by choosing a Rabi frequency $\Omega_1 = \gamma$, but we plot the spectrum for different values of the natural line-width: $\gamma = \omega_x/10$ (a), $\gamma = \omega_x/2$ (b) and $\gamma = 2\omega_x$ (c).

each band depends on the Bessel functions and the central band (ω_L) has an effective Rabi frequency $\Omega_1 \mathcal{J}_0(k_L X)$, the first sidebands ($\omega_L \pm \omega_x$) $\Omega_1 \mathcal{J}_1(k_L X)$, and the second sidebands ($\omega_L \pm 2\omega_x$) $\Omega_1 \mathcal{J}_2(k_L X)$. In the low saturation case where the atom response is proportional to the squared Rabi frequency, the excitation probability is the sum of the excitation induced by each line and

$$P_e(\delta) = \sum_{m=-\infty}^{m=+\infty} \frac{1}{2} \frac{\Omega_L^2 \mathcal{J}_m^2(k_L X)}{\Omega_L^2 \mathcal{J}_m^2(k_L X) + 2(\delta - m\omega_x)^2 + \gamma^2/2}. \tag{36}$$

Figure 3 shows different examples of spectra for different ratio γ/ω_x. The comparison of these spectra tells that for excitation on a broad transition ($\gamma > \omega_x$), the oscillating nature of the motion is not relevant to describe the spectrum as the motion sidebands are not resolved.

In this regime, where the broadband condition applies, called "weak binding regime", the ions can be treated as free (Figure 3(c)). On the contrary, for $\gamma < \omega_x$ (the "strong binding regime"), the motion sidebands are resolved. Each band is free from first-order Doppler broadening which is visible only in their envelope (Figures 3(a) and 3(b)). In this condition, is cooling required? As a rule of thumb, we can consider that the Bessel function $\mathcal{J}_m(k_L X)$ takes large values if $m \simeq k_L X$. As a consequence, if $k_L X \gg 1$, the coupling strength on the central band is very weak and it cannot be exploited for atom manipulation or spectroscopy. So, even with a resolved sideband spectra, it remains relevant to use Doppler cooling to reach the Lamb–Dicke regime for which $k_L X \ll 1$ and the central unshifted band is dominant. If the Doppler limit is assumed, the modulation index is

$\sqrt{2}k_L v_D/\omega_x$ and the smallest reachable value depends on the oscillation frequency. As an example, if the Ca^+ ion is considered as a two-level system, it takes $\omega_x/2\pi = 1$ MHz to have $k_L X = 1$ at the Doppler limit ($\lambda_L \simeq 400$ nm). Here, we touch an important issue concerning the trap requirement that must be taken into account when designing the trap. Reaching high oscillation frequency requires special cares that are dealt with in Chapter 1 (by Thompson) about Penning traps and Chapter 2 (by Knoop) about RF traps.

Observing resolved sidebands implies first that there is a transition in the strong binding regime. With the order of magnitude of 1 MHz for the oscillation frequency, optical dipole allowed transitions are ruled out because their width is in the 10 MHz range. Two different kinds of transition are commonly used, and they reduce the number of eligible atoms. The first solution is to choose a dipole forbidden transition. In several cases, it is an electric quadrupolar transition ($S \rightarrow D$), with natural line-width ≤ 1 Hz. It takes a heavy atom to have an appropriate D level. This is the case for Ca^+, Sr^+, Ba^+, Ra^+, Yb^+, Hg^+. Let's also mention experiments with In^+, making use of a hyperfine induced narrow electric dipolar transition. For other atoms, one can use Raman transitions in the optical domain between two sub-levels (Zeeman or hyperfine) of the ground state and a common excited state (for example Be^+, Mg^+, Zn^+, Cd^+). The effective line-width of the transition is then controlled by the two laser coupling parameters (Rabi frequency and detuning) and can be made as narrow as needed.

The laser(s) on the narrow transition may have a projection on several symmetry axis of the motion, which can include non-negligible micromotion and even excess micromotion. Then, the motion induced phase modulation has several terms:

$$\mathbf{k}_L.\mathbf{r} = k_x(X\cos\omega_x t + \epsilon_x)\left(1 + \frac{q_x}{2}\cos\Omega t\right) + k_z(Z\cos\omega_z t + \epsilon_z)\left(1 + \frac{q_z}{2}\cos\Omega t\right) \tag{37}$$

and the same spectral decomposition in Bessel functions can be done with several frequencies as long as these frequencies are not in a rational ratio.

4.2. *Quantum description of the motion*

For low temperature, this classical description of the motion is not sufficient to explain the observed spectrum and a quantum mechanical description is required. To this purpose, the atoms need to be treated like harmonic oscillator (HO) and the mechanical energy (kinetic + potential) has to be included in the Hamiltonian. The useful equations to play with HO are gathered in Appendix A.1. We can now think of the ion motion in terms of occupation of the vibrational energy level n. Doppler cooling results in a thermal distribution of n with an average,

$$\overline{n} = \frac{e^{-\hbar\omega_x/k_B T_D}}{1 - e^{-\hbar\omega_x/k_B T_D}} = \frac{e^{-2\omega_x/\gamma_a}}{1 - e^{-2\omega_x/\gamma_a}}, \tag{38}$$

where we now make a distinction between natural line-width γ_a for dipole allowed transition which gives access to strong coupling and γ_f for the narrow lines in the strong binding regime. In the case where $\omega_x < \gamma_a/2$, $\overline{n}$ is well approximated by $\gamma_a/2\omega_x$, with usual miniature trap designed to reach the Lamb–Dicke regime with single ions, Doppler cooling leads to $\overline{n} \simeq 5 - 15$. A quantum mechanical traitement of the motion is relevant when the population in the $n = 0$ vibrational state is non-negligible. This is not the case for large trap where ω_x is often limited to $\approx\gamma_a/50$.

To compute the time evolution of the internal DoF, it is easier to get rid of the free evolution and keep the evolution induced by atom–laser coupling by using the Interaction Picture (half-way between Schrödinger and Heisenberg, see Ref. [8]). Therefore, the interaction terms in the Hamiltonian are transformed through

$$\hat{V}^I = \hat{\mathcal{U}}_0^\dagger(t)\hat{V}\hat{\mathcal{U}}_0(t) \quad \text{with} \quad \hat{\mathcal{U}}_0(t) = \exp(-i\hat{H}_0 t/\hbar). \tag{39}$$

If only the internal DoF matters, $\hat{H}_0 = \hbar\omega_0(|e\rangle\langle e| - |g\rangle\langle g|)/2$ and

$$\hat{V}^I_{AL} = \frac{\hbar\Omega_1}{2}(|e\rangle\langle g|e^{-i\delta_L t}e^{i(k_L x+\psi)} + |g\rangle\langle e|e^{i\delta_L t}e^{-i(k_L x+\psi)}). \tag{40}$$

When the motion is also quantized, the self-Hamiltonian of the system is $\hat{H}_0 + \hat{H}_0^m$ (with eigenstates $|g,n\rangle, |e,m\rangle$):

$$\hat{V}^I_{AL} = \frac{\hbar\Omega_1}{2}(|e\rangle\langle g|e^{-i(\delta_L t-\psi)}e^{i\hat{H}_0^m t/\hbar}e^{ik_L\hat{x}}e^{-i\hat{H}_0^m t/\hbar} + \text{h.c.}), \tag{41}$$

where h.c. is the hermitian conjugate and a major difference between the two former equations is that $\hat{x}$ is now an operator and no more a simple parameter. By using the relations gathered in Appendix A.2, one can show that

$$\hat{V}^I_{AL} = \frac{\hbar\Omega_1}{2}(|e\rangle\langle g|e^{-i(\delta_L t-\psi)}\exp\left(i\eta\hat{a}^\dagger e^{i\omega_x t} + i\eta\hat{a}e^{-i\omega_x t}\right) + \text{h.c.}) \tag{42}$$

with $\eta = k_L x_0$, the Lamb–Dicke parameter (x_0 is the size of the ground vibrational state wave-packet).

This new form for the atom–laser coupling operator shows that motion and internal state are coupled in the transition. For each transition modifying the vibrational state from n to $n+p$, an effective Rabi frequency can be defined by

$$\Omega_{n,n+p} = \Omega_L |\langle n+p| e^{i\eta(\hat{a}+\hat{a}^\dagger)} |n\rangle|. \tag{43}$$

This expression was developed by Glauber in 1969, but we can gain insight by making a Taylor expansion of $\hat{V}^I_{AL}$ with η, which is sufficient for most practical cases. Up to the second order in η,

$$\begin{array}{ll} n \to n & \Omega n, n = \Omega_L(1-\eta^2 n), \\ n \to n+1 & \Omega n, n+1 = \Omega_L \eta \sqrt{n+1}, \\ n \to n-1 & \Omega n, n-1 = \Omega_L \eta \sqrt{n}, \\ n \to n+2 & \Omega n, n+2 = \Omega_L \eta^2/2\sqrt{(n+1)(n+2)}, \\ n \to n-2 & \Omega n, n-2 = \Omega_L \eta^2/2\sqrt{n(n-1)}. \end{array}$$

From these terms, we can extrapolate the p-sideband couplings scaling with $(\eta\sqrt{n})^p$ (it can also be demonstrated for general cases). It shows that for $\eta\sqrt{n} \ll 1$, only the first sidebands are excited. This is formally equivalent to the first-order expansion $\exp ikx \simeq 1 + ikx$ and is the formal condition for the **Lamb–Dicke** regime. The interaction term takes the simple form,

$$\hat{V}^I = \frac{\hbar\Omega_1}{2}|e\rangle\langle g|(\hat{1}e^{-i(\delta_L t-\psi)} + i\eta\hat{a}^\dagger e^{-i(\delta_L-\omega_x)t-\psi} + i\eta\hat{a}e^{-i(\delta_L+\omega_x)t-\psi} + \text{h.c.}), \tag{44}$$

which is very close to the Jaynes–Cummings Hamiltonian developed for photons in cavities (but here, there is an anti Jaynes–Cumming term!) Many experiments implying high-precision spectroscopy (QI, metrology,...) requires to reach this regime where the Doppler spectra is reduced to the main carrier (central) band and small first-order sideband. This is further developed in Schmidt's chapter about optical clocks and quantum logic spectroscopy (Chapter 18) and in an article by Roos about quantum information processing [9].

It takes $\eta \ll 1$ to be sure to reach the Lamb–Dicke regime once the Doppler cooling limit is reached. Once again, it has to be thought of when the trap is designed as it scales like

$$\eta = \sqrt{\omega'_{\text{rec}}/\omega_x} \tag{45}$$

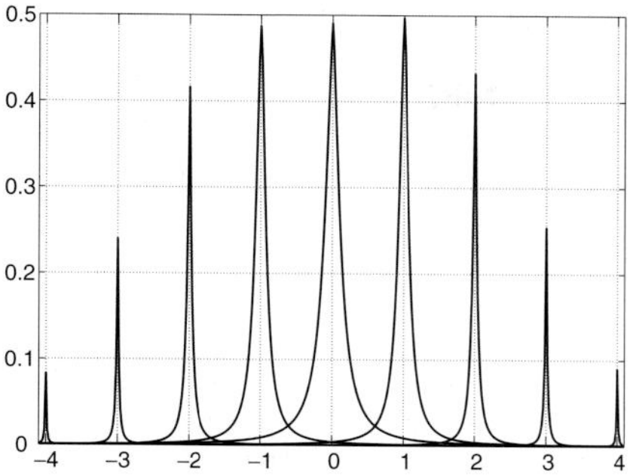

(a) $T = 2.5$ mK

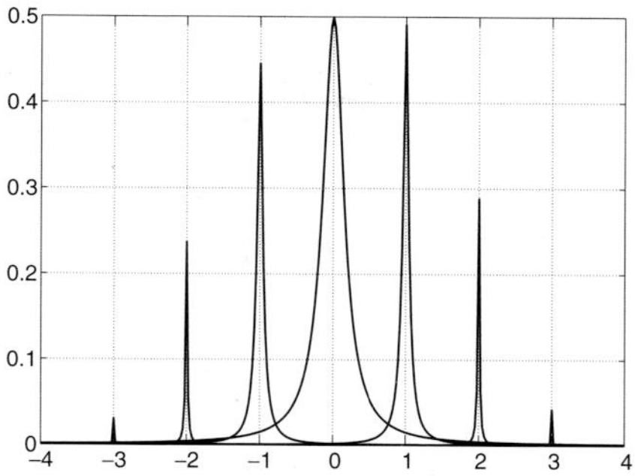

(b) $T = 0.5$ mK

Fig. 4. Calculated sideband spectra on the electric quadrupole transition of Ca^+ at $\lambda_L = 730$ nm with natural line-width of $1.1s^{-1}$. We assume a laser line-width of $\gamma_L/2\pi = 10$ kHz and a strong saturation of the line with $\Omega_1/2\pi = 1$ kHz. The oscillation frequency is $\omega/2\pi = 1$ MHz which leads a Lamb–Dicke parameter $\eta_0 = 0.094$. (a) The ion temperature is $T = 2.5$ mK which implies $\overline{n} = 51.6$. (b) $T = 0.5$ mK and $\overline{n} = 10$.

and ω_x needs to be large compared to the recoil frequency ω'_{rec} associated with the narrow line. Typical calculated sideband spectra are plotted an Figure 4 to illustrate the dependence of the laser coupling (visible on the power broadening) with the band index. For the colder case, the discrepancy between the ± 1 band illustrates the break down of the classical picture as it is due to the non-negligible occupation of the $n = 0$ vibrational state, which cannot be driven by a $n \to n-1$ transition. In his chapter, Roos shows how to use this discrepancy to measure $\overline{n}$ [9].

5. Resolved Sideband Cooling with Single Ions

The first experimental demonstration of resolved sideband cooling was in 1989 at NIST, on a single Hg^+ ion, by Wineland and coworkers. It takes advantage of the coupling between the internal and external DoF through the laser interaction to reduce the mechanical energy of the HO, namely by forcing $n \to n-1$ transition on the absorption. This is reached by choosing a laser detuning $\delta_L = -\omega_x$ to make resonant the last term in Equation (44), proportional to the annihilation operator $\hat{a}$. The net change in vibrational state is efficient if most spontaneous emission remains on the $n \to n$ line. This spontaneous emission rate, of the order of 1/s, is too low for experimental conditions which imply a different source of heating. To speed up the cooling cycle, the excited state lifetime γ_f^{-1} is shortened to γ_e^{-1} by coupling to a short-lived state by an extra laser.

The efficiency of resolved sideband cooling was analyzed by Stenholm in 1986 [10]. There, he assumes a low saturation of the transition and that the probability to be in the excited state is

$$P_e = \frac{\Omega^2}{\gamma_e^2}\frac{\gamma_e^2}{4\delta^2+\gamma_e^2} = \frac{\Omega^2}{\gamma_e^2}W(\delta), \tag{46}$$

where $W(\delta)$ is the Lorentzian profile. Excitation on the central band has the strength $\Omega = \Omega_1$ and $\Omega = \Omega_1\eta\sqrt{n}$ on the first red sideband. η is $(\mathbf{k}_L.\mathbf{x})x_0$ if we are interested in the cooling of the x-motion. The spontaneous scattering rate on $n \to n+1$ is included with an effective rate $\gamma_e\eta_e^2(n+1)$. η_e takes into account that only a fraction of the mean squared wave-vector corresponds to a recoil along Ox: $\langle k_x^2\rangle_{es} = \alpha\langle k_L^2\rangle$ and then $\eta_e^2 = \alpha(k_Lx_0)^2$ with $\alpha < 1$

$R^\pm$ is the rate for transition from $|g,n\rangle$ to $|g,n\pm1\rangle$. The first contribution represents $|g,n\rangle \to |e,n\rangle \to |g,n\pm1\rangle$, the second one is $|g,n\rangle \to |e,n\pm1\rangle \to |g,n\pm1\rangle$.

$$R^+ = W(\delta)\frac{\Omega_L^2}{\gamma_e^2} \times \gamma_e\eta_e^2(n+1) + W(\delta-\omega_x)\frac{\Omega_L^2\eta^2(n+1)}{\gamma_e^2} \times \gamma_e \tag{47}$$

$$= \frac{\Omega_L^2}{\gamma_e}\left(\eta_e^2W(\delta) + \eta^2W(\delta-\omega_x)\right)(n+1) = A^+(n+1), \tag{48}$$

$$R^- = \frac{\Omega_L^2}{\gamma_e}\left(\eta_e^2W(\delta) + \eta^2W(\delta+\omega_x)\right)n = A^-n. \tag{49}$$

The time evolution of the averaged vibrational number is

$$\frac{\mathrm{d}\overline{n}}{\mathrm{d}t} = R^+(+1) + R^-(-1) = (A^+ - A^-)\overline{n} + A^+. \tag{50}$$

If the detuning is tuned on the first red sideband $\delta = -\omega_x$ and if the line broadening remains small compared to the sideband splitting ($\omega_x^2 \gg \gamma_e^2$), then the averaged vibrational number is reduced and reach an equilibrium value,

$$\overline{n_f} \simeq \frac{A^+}{A^-} = \frac{\gamma_e^2}{4\omega_x^2}\left(\frac{1}{4} + \frac{\eta_e^2}{\eta^2}\right) \ll 1, \tag{51}$$

if no heating counteracts. This scaling is to be compared with the Doppler cooling one $n_D \simeq \gamma_a/2\omega_x$.

Here is a resume of the relevant orders of magnitude for laser cooling with trapped ions:

$$\begin{array}{ccccccc} \gamma_f & < & \omega_{\text{rec}}, \omega'_{\text{rec}} & < & \omega_{x,y,z} & < & \gamma_a \\ \simeq 1\text{ Hz} & & \simeq 10\text{ kHz} & & \simeq 1\text{ MHz} & & \simeq 10\text{ MHz}. \end{array}$$

Dipole allowed transitions of natural width γ_a are used for Doppler cooling, where the broad line approximation holds and the ions can be considered as free. There is nevertheless a major difference with neutral atoms: a single laser beam is sufficient to cool the three DoF as long as this laser beam has a projection on every symmetry axis of the trap or the sample is dense enough and expends in the three dimensions to make sure that Coulomb interactions couple the three DoF. This is the case for an ellipsoid shaped ion cloud but certainly not for a string of ions.

Dipole forbidden transitions or Raman transitions are used for resolved sideband cooling. Their effective width is tailored to increase the scattering rate. It is mandatory to have a projection of the laser beam on each direction of motion that needs to be cooled. As most of the time, the oscillation frequency is different for each direction, the three different sidebands have to be addressed sequentially to reach the vibrational ground state of the three orthogonal HO. The extrapolation of this method to more than one ion is limited as the number of vibrational eigenfrequencies to address increases with N. An alternative to resolved sideband cooling was developed to reach $\overline{n} < 1$ for a wide band of vibrational modes simultaneously. This method, based on the CPT process described in Section 2.4, is described in the following section.

6. EIT Cooling

As explained in Section 2.4, a Λ-scheme excitation gives rise to a trapping in a dark state when the two involved transitions share the same detuning. When in this dark state, the atoms do not absorb light and electromagnetically induced transparency (EIT) happens. Using this transparency to cancel absorption on the central band and enhance absorption on the first red sideband was proposed in 2000 by Morigi and coworkers [11] with the goal to cool motion with several eigenfrequencies simultaneously. The purpose of this section is to explain the concept of this method and to stress the experimental requirements for its efficiency, which are partly covered in Ref. [12] where the experimental realization of EIT cooling [13] is described.

6.1. *Concept of EIT cooling*

This method assumes that the atoms are already in the Lamb–Dicke regime and is based on coupling on the broad dipole transitions. The absorption on the central band ($n \to n$ transition) is canceled by choosing $\delta_c = \delta_p$. To enhance the $n \to n-1$ transitions, another feature associated with the Λ-scheme is used. The repumping transition $P \to D$ is strongly driven, whereas the cooling transition $S \to P$ is far under saturation (see Figure 2(a)), like in a pump-probe experiment. The eigenstate of the coupled dressed states {atom + repumping photons} are shifted in energy compared to the uncoupled ones by the light-shift δ_{LS}, which can be approximated by $\Omega_p^2/4\delta_p$ for large detuning. These eigenstates are linear combinations of dressed S and D states with a small mixing if the detuning is large compared to the Rabi frequency. In Figure 5, the narrow maxima in the excitation probability in the P state for $\delta_c = \delta_p + \delta_{\mathrm{LS}}$ corresponds to the laser coupling between the $|S\rangle$ and the $(|D\rangle + \epsilon|P\rangle)$ dressed states, where $\epsilon \ll 1$. The broad maxima corresponding to the other mixed state $|(P\rangle - \epsilon|D\rangle)$ is centered on $\delta_c = -\delta_{\mathrm{LS}}$, out of the range of the figure.

If now, the HO eigenenergy is incorporated in the dressed state energy, the $n \to n$ transitions are not shifted compared to transitions for stationary

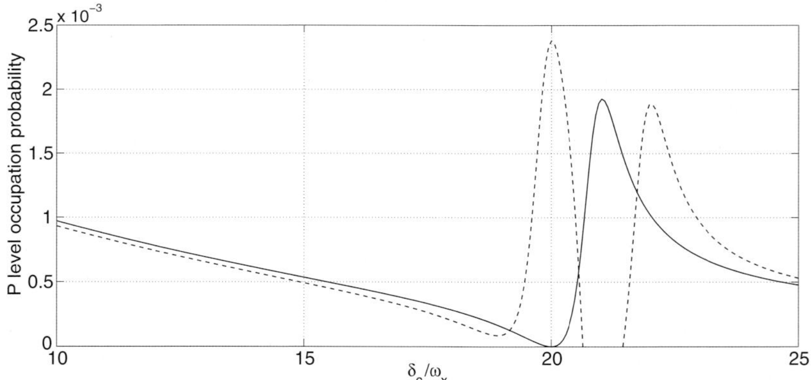

Fig. 5. Semi-classic calculation of the probability to populate the excited P state versus the cooling laser detuning δ_c in oscillation frequency scale ω_x, for a Λ-scheme atomic level. The calculation assumes an oscillating motion $X\cos(\omega_x t)$ along the laser propagation direction defined by $k_c X = 0.2$ but consider only ± 1 sidebands. $\delta_p = +20\omega_x$ and the dressing Rabi frequency is chosen to have a light-shift δ_{LS} matching ω_x. The full dark line plots the total probability of occupation, dominated by the central sideband excitation, whereas the dashed line the ± 1 sideband contribution expanded by a factor of 50.

ions. On the contrary, the $n \to n \pm 1$ transitions driven through the narrow dressed state ($|D\rangle + \epsilon|P\rangle$) are now centered on $\delta_c = \delta_p + \delta_{LS} \pm \omega_x$. By choosing the interaction parameters such that $\delta_{LS} = \omega_x$ (which requires $\delta_p > 0$), the $n \to n-1$ transition is on resonance for the CPT condition. In Figure 5, the $n \to n \pm 1$ contributions in the excitation probability are isolated from the $n \to n$ ones (and amplified) to illustrate this matching.

6.2. *Experimental constraints for EIT cooling*

This cooling process described above can still be efficient even if there is no perfect matching between the light-shift and ω_x, as long as the $n \to n-1$ transition remains a lot more probable than the $n \to n$ ones. This allows us to cool different HO DoF simultaneously, provided their eigenfrequencies are not too far apart and that the effective width of the transition can be adjusted by the pump coupling. The experimental results [12] report a simultaneous cooling of the motion of a single ion along two different directions with frequencies $\omega_x = 1.6$ and $\omega_z = 3.3$ MHz. Before EIT cooling, the averaged occupation numbers are measured to be $\overline{n}_z = 6.5(1.0)$ and $\overline{n}_x = 16(2)$. The cooling efficiency is quantified by the probability for the ion to occupy the vibrational ground state, which is $p_0 = 58\%$ for the x-HO and $p_0 = 74\%$ for the z-HO and set the ion deep in the Lamb–Dicke regime for the degrees of motion simultaneously.

The efficiency of this unresolved sideband cooling relies on a complete cancelation of the $n \to n$ transitions obtained by the dark line. In most experimental cases, the two-photon resonance condition results only in a grey line because of the relative phase drift of the two involved lasers. The need for a phase coherence between the two excitation lasers explains why the Λ-scheme chosen for the experimental demonstration of EIT cooling [13] is based on two Zeeman sub-levels of the ground state instead of two different electronic states (like S and D for Figure 2(a)). This choice allows one to produce the two radiations (dressing and cooling) from the same laser source by a modulation process (see Ref. [12] for details). As they share the same wavelengths (approximately), the two radiations are made different by their polarization, to address different Zeeman sub-levels. Any default in the polarization (which is very hard to cancel) drives the ions out of the designed Λ-scheme and may lead to an $n \to n$ or $n \to n+1$ transition, reducing the cooling efficiency. This may explain why, when a single degree of motion is cooled, the final state is limited to $p_0 = 84\%$ when ω_x is addressed and $p_0 = 90\%$ when ω_z is addressed, whereas the resolved sideband cooling allows the same group to reach $p_0 = 95\%$ for $\omega_x = 2$ MHz.

7. Conclusion

In this chapter, we have introduced two laser cooling techniques, the very basic and robust Doppler laser cooling which is the starting point of most cooling procedures, and the resolved sideband cooling, which takes small samples to lower temperature. Many other laser cooling techniques have been developed since the first proposals about Doppler laser cooling in 1975, but this sideband cooling seems very well suited for few trapped atoms. If your needs do not fit these specifications, there must be a better solution for you. Sisyphus cooling, CPT based techniques and many others may be more appropriate for you. You may not even be limited to atoms that can absorb light available on the laser market and take advantage of the sympathetic cooling allowed by the strong Coulomb interaction with another species that can be laser cooled efficiently. This method is one of the strategies used to cool molecules, like you can read about in Chapter 16 (by Wester).

8. Exercises

8.1. *Slowing an atomic beam*

Here, we want to use the radiation pressure to slow an atomic beam of sodium atoms with a counter-propagating laser beam.

(1) What is the recoil velocity v_{rec} induced by the absorption of one photon by a sodium atom? (atom: ^{23}Na, resonance transition wavelength: $\lambda = 589$ nm)
(2) The lifetime of the excited state τ is 16 ns, give an order of magnitude of the maximal force and acceleration of an atom in a resonant laser beam.
(3) The force on the atom induces a velocity change. Under which condition is it relevant to consider the atom velocity as a constant to compute this force? Is this condition fulfilled for sodium atom?
(4) What is the velocity v_T of atoms emitted by an oven with a temperature of 600 K? ($k_B = 1,38.10^{-23}$ J/K)
(5) $\omega_L/2\pi$ is the laser frequency in the lab frame. What is the laser frequency $\omega_{at}/2\pi$ in the atom frame when they escape the oven?
(6) v is the atom velocity in the lab frame. How to choose ω_L to be in resonance with the atomic transition defined by ω_0 for an atom at rest? How to choose the detuning $\delta = \omega_L - \omega_0$ to keep that laser tuned on the atomic resonance?

(7) Plot the magnitude of the force versus the atom velocity in case the laser is resonant for atoms with velocity v and in case of low saturation. What is the characteristic width of such a curve?

(8) Suppose $v = v_T$ to induce a force on atoms exiting the oven. What is the limit velocity reached by the atoms? Propose a solution to lower this limit.

(9) Assume that we are able to keep the laser tuned on the atomic transition all along the atom trajectory and that the acceleration is half of the maximum one, find the minimal distance required to bring the atom *"at rest"*.

Solution: the recoil velocity is 2.7 cm/s and at maximum, the atoms can scatter one photon every 2τ (or the scattering rate is $\gamma/2$), the acceleration is then $v_{\text{rec}}/(2\tau) = 8.7\times10^5$ m/s^2, which is huge compared to gravity! To consider the velocity as a constant in the force calculation, the system has to be in the broadband condition. Here, $\omega_{\text{rec}} = 1.4\times10^5\text{s}^{-1} \ll \gamma = 6.2\times10^7\text{s}^{-1}$, so the broadband condition is fulfilled.

In an atomic beam, the most probable velocity v_T is 1.22 times the thermal velocity $\sqrt{2k_BT/m}$ (to have more details on velocity in beams, see the book by Ramsey about molecular beams [14]). Here, v_T is 640 m/s. The laser frequency in the atom frame ω_L^{at} is shifted from $\omega_L/2\pi$ by the quantity $-\mathbf{k}_L.\mathbf{v}_T/2\pi = +v_T/\lambda = 1$ GHz. This shift is orders of magnitude larger than the natural line-width of the transition. To be resonant with the transition in the atom frame, the laser must be tuned such that $\omega_L^{at} = \omega_0$ if ω_0 is the frequency for an atom at rest. For a laser beam propagating against the atoms, it takes $\omega_L = \omega_0 - k_L v$.

The typical curve of the force is plotted in Figure 1 and its width is the capture range $\Delta v = \gamma/k_L$ which is 6 m/s for sodium atom. It means that if the laser is tuned to be resonant with atom exiting the oven, the atoms are out of resonant once their velocity reaches $v_T - v_c = 634$ m/s!

To lower this limit, one must find a way to keep the atomic transition and the laser frequency tuned while the atomic velocity is decreasing. One option is to shift the laser frequency, the other one consists in shifting the atomic transition frequency. The first option is called "chirp cooling" as the beam frequency interacting with the atoms must be chirped to stay tuned. The duration of this chirp is the time it takes to absorb $N = v_T/v_{\text{rec}}$ photons. If the tuning corresponds to half of the maximum acceleration, it takes $N4\tau = 1.5$ ms to sweep the frequency by 1 GHz, which can be done with electro-optics modulator or directly on the emitted light if the laser is based on semi-conductor. This choice implies a sequential cooling and a beam synchronized on the chirp as all the atoms in the beam experience the same laser frequency.

The other option circumvent this drawback by shifting the atomic resonance depending on the position of the atoms through a Zeeman effect proportional to the local magnetic field [15]. Depending on the Zeeman sub-level chosen m_J, the Zeeman shift can be written like $\mu(m_J)B/\hbar$ and it must compensate for $-k_L v$. For a constant deceleration, over trajectory of length L, the atom velocity behaves like $v_T\sqrt{1-z/L}$ and the required length L is $v_T^2/(2a)$. If the acceleration a is half the maximum, the length of the Zeeman slower or the trajectory inside the chirped beam is 47 cm for the assumed oven temperature.

8.2. *Increasing the brightness of an atomic beam*

Here, we want to use the radiation pressure to reduce the divergence of an atomic beam of Rubidium atoms ($\lambda = 780$ nm, $m = 85$ amu, $\tau_e = 27$ ns) with two sets of counter-propagating laser beams. The atoms leave the oven with a longitudinal velocity $v_z = 300$ m/s.

(1) What is the angular dispersion of the beam corresponding to the capture range of the Doppler laser cooling force (let's assume $\Delta_L = -\Gamma/2$)?
(2) For a saturation parameter of 1/10, how large must be the laser beams to make sure the lower achievable transverse temperature has been reached when the atoms exit the laser beam?
(3) What is the angular dispersion of the captured beam after this interaction?
(4) What is the gain in intensity for this part of the atomic beam?

Solution: if we assume for the capture range $\pm v_c = \pm\gamma/2k_L$ in the velocity space, it transfers into a divergence half-angle $\theta = v_c/v_z =$ 7.7 mrad. The time the atom spends in the laser beam is d/v_z if d is the beam diameter and this time must be larger than the Doppler cooling time τ_{DC} which reduces to $(2s_0\omega_{\mathrm{rec}})^{-1}$ for $\Delta_L = -\Gamma/2$. Here, the recoil frequency is $2,2\times10^4$ s^{-1} and τ_{DC} is 0.23 ms. The beam diameter must then be larger than 6.8 cm. If this size does not fit in your set-up, you can reduce and increase the laser intensity to reach a higher s_0. If the beam is large enough to reach the limit velocity, the final transverse velocity is the Doppler limit velocity $v_D = \sqrt{v_{\mathrm{rec}}v_c} = 0.11$ m/s which gives an angular divergence of 0.37 mrad. As the brightness scales with the surface of the beam, it is increased by v_c/v_{rec} which is 420 for Rubidium.

8.3. *Doppler laser cooling in case of extra sources of decoherence*

Here, we focus on the impact of extra sources of decoherence on the excitation efficiency and line profile. To that purpose, we go back to the OBE, but we now consider extra sources of decoherence like collision or excitation by a broadband laser. If we consider only elastic collisions, these processes do not force decay from the excited state and $\gamma_p = \gamma = 1/\tau$, but the coherence decays faster and all the decay rates must be added in $\gamma_d = \gamma/2 + \gamma_{coll} + \Gamma_L/2 + \cdots$ where Γ_L is the FWHM of the laser spectral profile. Use the following OBE equations to answer the questions:

$$\dot{u}(t) = \Delta_L v(t) - \gamma_d u(t), \tag{52}$$

$$\dot{v}(t) = -\Delta_L u(t) - \Omega_1 w(t) - \gamma_d v(t), \tag{53}$$

$$\dot{w}(t) = -\Omega_1 v(t) - \gamma_p (w(t) + 1/2). \tag{54}$$

(1) What is the stationary solution for the population inversion w_{st} or the probability for an atom be in the excited state $\rho_{ee} = w_{st} + 1/2$?
(2) By analogy with

$$\rho_{ee} = \frac{1}{2}\frac{s}{1+s}$$

and Equation (15), what is now the equivalent Rabi angular frequency driving the excitation and the relaxation rate it has to fight against?
(3) Derive the new expression for a saturation parameter s' compared to $s_0 = 2\Omega_1^2/\gamma^2$?
(4) What is now the FWHM of the transition the laser is exciting?
(5) What is now the condition for power broadening?

Solution: The steady state solution $\dot{u}(t), \dot{v}(t), \dot{w}(t) = 0$ of the OBE gives

$$\rho_{ee} = \frac{\Omega_1^2 \gamma_d/\gamma_p}{2(\Omega_1^2 \gamma_d/\gamma_p + \delta_L^2 + \gamma_d^2)}. \tag{55}$$

This equation is similar to Equation (15) with an effective coupling strength $\Omega_1^2/2$ replaced by $\Omega_1^2\gamma_d/\gamma_p$. Another saturation parameter s' can be defined by

$$s' = \frac{\Omega_1^2 \gamma_d/\gamma_p}{\delta_L^2 + \gamma_d^2}. \tag{56}$$

On resonance, this parameter reduces to $s_r' = s_0\gamma_p/(2\gamma_d) = \Omega_1^2/\gamma_p\gamma_d$. The ratio between γ_d and $\gamma_p/2$ reduces the laser coupling efficiency as it takes a larger laser intensity (in the ratio $2\gamma_d/\gamma_p$) to reach the saturation parameter that would be reached if $\gamma_d = \gamma_p/2$. Furthermore, these extra effects broaden the spectral line as the FWHM of the line is now $2\gamma_d\sqrt{1+s_r^{'}}$. Then, the smallest observable width is now $2\gamma_d = 1/\tau + 2\gamma_{coll} + \Gamma_L + \cdots$. Contrary to Doppler broadening, this is a homogeneous broadening as it is the same for all atoms.

Appendix

A.1. Summary of Useful Equations for HO

$$\hat{x} = \sqrt{\frac{\hbar}{2m\omega_x}}(\hat{a}^\dagger + \hat{a}) = x_0(\hat{a}^\dagger + \hat{a}),$$

$$\hat{p} = i\sqrt{\frac{m\hbar\omega_x}{2}}(\hat{a}^\dagger - \hat{a}), \tag{A.1}$$

$$\hat{N} = \hat{a}^\dagger\hat{a}, \tag{A.2}$$

$$\hat{H}_0^m = \frac{\hat{p}^2}{2m} + \frac{m\omega_x^2}{2}\hat{x}^2 = \hbar\omega_x\left(\hat{a}^\dagger\hat{a} + \frac{1}{2}\right), \tag{A.3}$$

$$[\hat{a}, \hat{a}^\dagger] = \hat{1}, \tag{A.4}$$

$$\hat{a}^\dagger|n\rangle = \sqrt{n+1}|n+1\rangle,$$

$$\hat{a}|n\rangle = \sqrt{n}|n-1\rangle. \tag{A.5}$$

A.2. Useful Commutation Relations with HO Operators

Using the property,

$$e^{\hat{A}+\hat{B}} = e^{\hat{A}}e^{\hat{B}}e^{-1/2[\hat{A},\hat{B}]} \quad \text{if} \quad [\hat{A},[\hat{A},\hat{B}]] = [\hat{B},[\hat{A},\hat{B}]] = 0 \tag{A.6}$$

and expressing the operator exponential $\exp(\hat{A}) = \hat{1} + \hat{A} + \hat{A}^2/2 + \hat{A}^3/6 + \cdots$, one can demonstrate these useful relations to move to the interaction picture:

$$\hat{a}^n e^{-i\omega t\hat{a}^\dagger\hat{a}} = e^{-i\omega t\hat{a}^\dagger\hat{a}}e^{-in\omega t}\hat{a}^n, \tag{A.7}$$

$$\hat{a}^{\dagger n} e^{-i\omega t\hat{a}^\dagger\hat{a}} = e^{-i\omega t\hat{a}^\dagger\hat{a}}e^{in\omega t}\hat{a}^{\dagger n}, \tag{A.8}$$

$$e^{i\eta(\hat{a}+\hat{a}^\dagger)} = e^{i\eta\hat{a}}e^{i\eta\hat{a}^\dagger}e^{-\eta/2}, \tag{A.9}$$

References

1. C. Cohen-Tannoudji *et al.*, *Photons and Atoms: Introduction to Quantum Electrodynamics*, pp. 169–199. New York, Wiley (1997).
2. G. Grynberg *et al.*, *Introduction to Quantum Optics*, pp. 45–104. Cambridge, Cambridge University Press (2010).
3. C. Foot, *Atomic Physics*, pp. 80–93 and pp. 178–201. Oxford, Oxford University Press (2005).
4. B. Bransden and C. Joachain, *Physics of atoms and molecules*, pp. 155–183. UK, Longman scientific and technical (1994).
5. P. Lett *et al.*, Optical molasses, *J. Opt. Soc. Am. B.* **6**(11), 2084 (1989).
6. C. Cohen-Tannoudji *et al.*, *Atom-Photon Interactions: Basic Processes and Applications*, pp. 400–450. Wiley (1997).
7. R. H. Dicke, The effect of collisions upon the doppler width of spectral lines, *Phys. Rev.* **89**, 472–473 (Jan, 1953). doi: 10.1103/PhysRev.89.472.
8. C. Cohen-Tannoudji *et al.*, *Quantum Mechanics*, pp. 300–320. New York, Wiley (2006).
9. C. Roos. Physics with Trapped Charged Particles: Lectures from the Les Houches Winter School. (*Eds. R. Thompson, M. Knoop, and N. Madsen*), *Quantum Information Processing with Trapped ions*, pp. 239–260. London, Imperial College Press (2013).
10. S. Stenholm, The semiclassical theory of laser cooling, *Rev. Mod. Phys.* **58**(3), 699–739 (1986).
11. G. Morigi *et al.*, Ground state laser cooling using electromagnetically induced transparency, *Phys. Rev. Lett.* **85**(21), 4458 (2000).
12. F. Schmidt-Kaler *et al.*, Laser cooling of trapped ions. In *Laser Physics at the limits*, pp. 243–260. Springer (2002).
13. C. Roos *et al.*, Experimental demonstration of ground state cooling with electromagnetically induced transparency, *Phys. Rev. Lett.* **85**(26), 5547 (2000).
14. N. Ramsey, *Molecular beams*, pp. 10–30. Oxford (1956).
15. W. Phillips *et al.*, Laser cooling and electromagnetic trapping of neutral atoms, *J. Opt. Soc. Am. B.* **2**(11), 1751 (1985).

CHAPTER SEVEN

NON-LASER COOLING TECHNIQUES

Laurent Hilico

Laboratoire Kastler Brossel, Université d'Evry Val d'Essonne, UPMC-Sorbonne Universités, CNRS, ENS-PSL Research University, Collège de France, 4 place Jussieu, 75005 Paris, France.
laurent.hilico@lkb.upmc.fr

We first review trapped ion radiative cooling and show that it is only efficient for high frequency oscillating particles in Penning traps. We then describe in detail resistive cooling and explain in the frame of an exercice why and how thermal equilibrium with the resistor is reached. We finally discuss buffer gas cooling in Paul traps.

1. Introduction

Cooling trapped ions is essential if one wishes to perform atomic or molecular spectroscopy with a high frequency resolution. Indeed, without cooling, the ion cloud temperature is of the order of the trap depth, i.e. from 0.1 eV per degree of freedom (DoF) ($\approx$1,200 K) to tens of eV (tens of 12,000 K) in Penning traps or in Radiofrequency (RF) Paul traps.[a] This temperature corresponds to high speed particles since the formula $\frac{1}{2}mv^2 = \frac{3}{2}k_BT$ leads to velocities $v \approx 1 \dots 3.1$ km/s for a molar mass of 20. The resulting first-order Doppler effect for a transition of wavelength λ is $v/\lambda \approx 1 \dots 3$ GHz, which is larger than most natural atomic or molecular line-widths. Even if one uses a Doppler-free spectroscopy technique such as a two-photon transitions with counter-propagating beams, the second-order Doppler effect shifts and broadens the lines. The relative effect is $\frac{\Delta\nu}{\nu} = -\frac{v^2}{2c^2} \approx 5.3 \times 10^{-11}$, e.g. 16 kHz for a transition at $\lambda = 1\mu$m. This is much larger than the state of the art transition frequency measurement.

[a]For a trapped ion with a harmonic motion, the total energy is $k_BT/2$ for the kinetic energy and $k_BT/2$ for the potential energy, i.e. k_BT per DoF.

The only way to perform high resolution spectroscopy of ions is to work with cold ions. The lowest temperatures are obtained using laser cooling when it is possible (see chapter 6 by Champenois in this book) i.e. when an efficient cooling transition is available and at the expense of rather complicated set-ups. Non-laser cooling techniques have been developed during the early age of ion traps. They allow cooling the ions down to about 4.2 K (liquid helium temperature), and find applications for ion manipulation, ion clocks or atomic and molecular spectroscopy. In this chapter, we will first review radiative cooling in Section 2, then resistive cooling in Section 3, and finally buffer gas cooling in Section 4. Many references can be found in Ref. [1] .

2. Radiative Cooling

The Larmor formula states that a charged particle of charge q undergoing an acceleration $\mathbf{a}$ looses energy with a rate given by Ref. [2]

$$\frac{dE}{dt} = -\frac{q^2}{6\pi\epsilon_0 c^3}\mathbf{a}^2. \tag{1}$$

We consider a particle oscillating in a trap with an amplitude $\mathbf{r_0}$ and a frequency ω. Assuming a low energy decay rate compared to ω, the trajectory, velocity, and acceleration are given by $\mathbf{r(t)} = \mathbf{r_0}\cos(\omega\mathbf{t} + \varphi)$, $\dot{\mathbf{r}}(t) = -\omega\mathbf{r_0}\sin(\omega\mathbf{t} + \varphi)$, and $\ddot{\mathbf{r}}(t) = -\omega^2\mathbf{r_0}\cos(\omega\mathbf{t} + \varphi)$ where φ is a phase factor depending on the initial conditions of the motion. The kinetic energy and the square of the acceleration are given by $E(t) = \frac{m\mathbf{r_0}^2\omega^2}{2}\sin^2(\omega t + \varphi)$ and $\ddot{\mathbf{r}}^2(t) = \mathbf{r_0}^2\omega^4\cos^2(\omega\mathbf{t} + \varphi)$. Taking the time average on a period of the oscillatory motion, the $\cos^2$ and $\sin^2$ lead to a factor 1/2, and we obtain $\langle E\rangle = m\mathbf{r_0}^2\omega^4/\mathbf{4}$ and $\langle\ddot{\mathbf{r}}^2\rangle = \mathbf{r_0}^2\omega^4/\mathbf{2} = \mathbf{2}\omega^2\langle\mathbf{E}\rangle/\mathbf{m}$. The time average of Equation (1) leads to

$$\frac{d\langle E\rangle}{dt} = -\frac{q^2\omega^2}{3\pi\epsilon_0 mc^3}\langle E\rangle = -\frac{\langle E\rangle}{\tau}. \tag{2}$$

The energy damping time constant,

$$\tau = \frac{3\pi\epsilon_0 mc^3}{q^2\omega^2} \tag{3}$$

can be evaluated for the cyclotron motion of an electron in a Penning trap using $\omega = \omega_c = qB/m$. Assuming a B field of 2 T, $m_e = 9.1\times10^{-31}$kg, $\omega_c \approx 56$ GHz, we have $\tau = 0.65$ s. The cyclotron frequency scales as $1/m$, so τ scales as m^3, so for any heavier charged species such as muons, protons, or

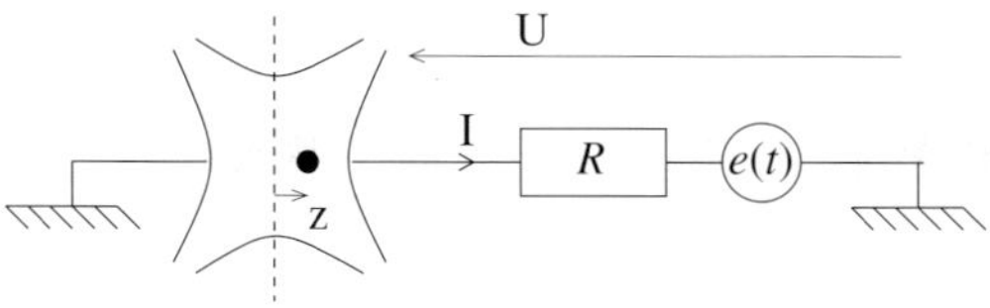

Fig. 1. Sketch of an ion trap where an electrode is connected to ground through a resistor R.

ions in a Penning trap, τ is increased by at least six orders of magnitude and is almost infinite. The axial and magnetron frequencies are smaller than the cyclotron frequency by some orders of magnitude leading to almost infinite time constants. In a Paul trap, the RF and secular frequencies are also much smaller than the electron cyclotron frequency, so radiative cooling can be neglected.

Actually, radiative cooling is only efficient for cyclotron motion damping of electrons or positrons in a Penning trap, leading to thermalization with local black-body radiation. This technique is currently applied in a number of experiments [1,3].

3. Resistive Cooling

An ion trap is made of metallic electrodes. By electrostatic influence, the charges confined in the trap influence the surrounding electrodes, creating *image charges*. An ion moving in front of an electrode creates an *image current*. The basic idea of resistive cooling is to connect a resistor to the electrode to dissipate energy through the Joule heating of the image current in the resistance as shown in Figure 1.

This process can be used to efficiently cool the cyclotron and radial motion in a Penning trap, as well as for the magnetron motion using sideband coupling. Resistive cooling has also been successfully used in an RF Paul trap [4]. In the following, we will focus on the axial motion damping in a Penning trap for a single ion. The detailed calculation of relaxation to equilibrium is studied in Problem 1; for cyclotron and magnetron resistive cooling, see Ref. [5].

3.1. *Image current in an electrode*

Figure 2(a) shows a parallel-plate capacitor of separation $2z_0$ containing a charge q_3 located at a distance z from the center of the electrodes and represented by a negligibly small spherical electrode. In order to determine the

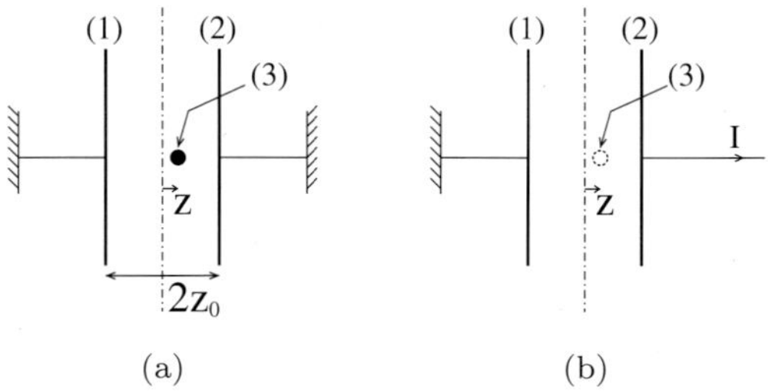

Fig. 2. Planar capacitor with two potentials and charge configurations. (a) ($V_1 = 0, q_1$), ($V_2 = 0, q_2$), and (V_3, q_3) (b) ($V_1' = 0, q_1'$), (V_2', q_2'), and ($V_3', q_3' = 0$).

relation between the q_3 charge velocity and the image current in electrode 2, we first have to determine the image charge q_2 of q_3. This can be done using the Gauss identity [2,6]. We consider a set of N electrodes and denote q_i the charges on the electrodes when the potentials V_i are applied to the electrodes and q_i' the charges when V_i' are applied. The Gauss identity states that

$$\sum_{i=1}^{N} q_i V_i' = \sum_{i=1}^{N} q_i' V_i. \tag{4}$$

Electrodes 1 and 2 are grounded, so $V_1 = V_2 = 0$, the potential of electrode 3 is V_3. Figure 2(b) shows the same set of electrodes with no charge on electrode 3, i.e. $q_3' = 0$. Electrode 1 is grounded and electrode 2 is at potential V_2', so the potential at electrode 3 is simply $V_3' = \frac{z+z0}{2z_0} V_2'$. The Gauss identity of Equation (4) writes $0 = q_2 V_2' + q_3 V_3'$ leading to $q_2 = -q_3 \frac{z+z0}{2z_0}$. Considering the orientation of the current I in Figure 2, the image current is given by

$$I = -\frac{dq_2}{dt} = \frac{q_3 \dot{z}}{2z_0}. \tag{5}$$

3.2. *Johnson–Nyquist noise in a resistor*

Following the fluctuation-dissipation theorem [7], the dissipative Joule effect in a resistor is associated with a voltage or current noise process. The equivalent circuit of a resistor at temperature T is shown in Figure 3 in the Thévenin or Norton representations. The voltage noise (and current noise) has zero mean values, i.e. $\langle e(t) \rangle = 0$ and $\langle i(t) \rangle = 0$ and symmetrized power spectral densities given by $S_e(\omega) = 4Rk_BT$ and $S_i(\omega) = \frac{4k_BT}{R}$. The dissipation in the resistor is responsible for the ion motion damping, whereas the voltage noise $e(t)$ explains the ion equilibrium temperature.

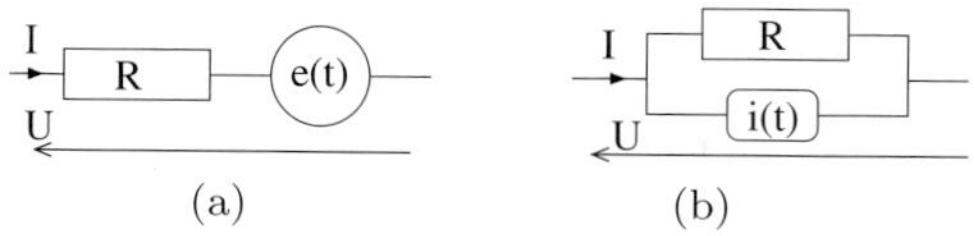

Fig. 3. Voltage noise (a) and current noise (b) equivalent circuit for a resistor R.

3.3. *Resistive cooling dynamics*

Resistive cooling of an ion in the trap depicted in Figure 1 is described by the four following equations:

$$
\begin{aligned}
V(z) &= \alpha \frac{z_0 + z}{2z_0} U(t), \\
E(z,t) &= -\alpha \frac{U(t)}{2z_0}, \\
I(t) &= \alpha \frac{q\dot{z}}{2z_0}, \\
U(t) &= RI(t) + e(t), \\
m\ddot{z} &= -m\omega_z^2 z + qE(z,t).
\end{aligned} \tag{6}
$$

The first equation is the electrostatic equation obtained in Section 3.1, the second one is obtained using the relation $E = -\frac{dV}{dz}$. The third equation is the image current expression of Equation (5), and the fourth one is the electrical equation of the circuit. The fifth one is the Newton's law applied to the ion including the trap restoring force $-m\omega_z^2 z$ and the electric force due to image charges $qE(z,t)$. Note that a geometrical factor α close to one has been added to take into account the fact that the trap is not a planar capacitor.

By eliminating I, U, and E in Equation (6), we obtain the evolution equation for the ion position $z(t)$ as

$$\ddot{z}(t) + \alpha \frac{q^2 R}{4mz_0} \dot{z}(t) + \omega_z^2 z(t) = -\alpha \frac{qe(t)}{2mz_0}. \tag{7}$$

This is a second-order differential equation describing a damped harmonic oscillator, which is driven by the Johnson–Nyquist noise of the resistor. The motion damping time constant τ_m and the kinetic energy damping time constant τ are linked by $\tau_m = 2\tau$, where $\tau = \frac{4mz_0^2}{\alpha q^2 R}$. For an electron in a trap with $z_0 = 1$ cm, $\alpha \approx 1$, and $R = 1\ \text{M}\Omega, \tau = 14$ ms; for a proton with $z_0 = 1$ mm, and $R = 1\ \text{M}\Omega, \tau = 260$ ms.

Resistive cooling is widely used in Penning traps. The expression of τ and those orders of magnitude show that resistive cooling is very efficient for light particles such as electrons and positrons even in rather large traps. It also works for much heavier ions in small traps and for highly charged ions taking advantage of the quadratic dependance of τ on q. Many details can be found in Refs. [8,9].

3.4. *Trapped ion equivalent circuit*

Eliminating U, E, z, and $\dot{z}$ in Equation (6), we obtain a relation between the image current $I(t)$ and the noise voltage $e(t)$ which can be written as

$$L_{\text{eff}}C_{\text{eff}}\frac{d^2I(t)}{dt^2} + RC_{\text{eff}}\frac{dI(t)}{dt} + I(t) = -C_{\text{eff}}\frac{de(t)}{dt}, \tag{8}$$

where the effective inductance and capacitance are given by $L_{\text{eff}} = \frac{4mz_0^2}{\alpha q^2} = \frac{R}{\tau}$ and $C_{\text{eff}} = \frac{1}{L_{\text{eff}}\omega_z^2}$. This means that the trapped ion behaves like a serial circuit $RL_{\text{eff}}C_{\text{eff}}$ with a resonance angular frequency ω_z. Note that the orders of magnitude of L_{eff} and C_{eff} are rather unphysical since for an electron in a trap with $z_0 = 1$ cm, $\omega_z = 2\pi \times 300$ kHz and $R = 1$ MΩ, one finds $L_{\text{eff}} = 14.2$ kH, $C_{\text{eff}} = 0.02$ fF. This corresponds to a very high quality factor $Q_{\text{eff}} = L_{\text{eff}}\omega_z/R = 26{,}800$. For a proton in a trap with $z_0 = 1$ mm, the same ω_z and R, we have $L_{\text{eff}} = 261$ kH, $C_{\text{eff}} = 0.001$ fF, and $Q = 4.9 \times 10^5$.

In most experimental set-ups, the electrode used for resistive cooling is connected to ground not only through a resistor R, but also through an RLC parallel circuit where C includes the electrode-to-ground capacitor and L is a real coil chosen such that $LC\omega_z^2 = 1$. The equivalent circuit is shown

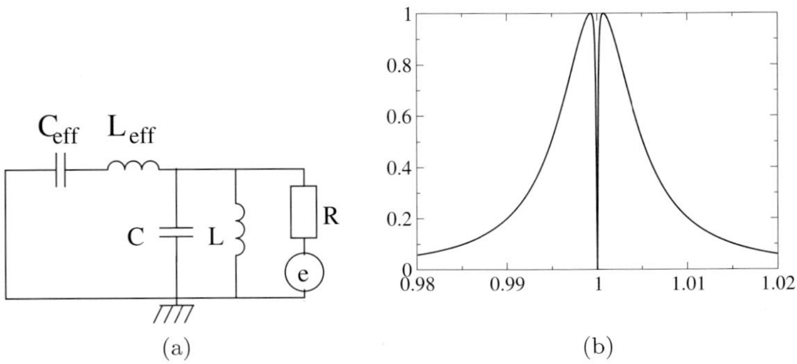

Fig. 4. (a) Equivalent circuit describing an ion in a trap connected to a resonant parallel LC circuit. (b) Transfer function $\frac{u(\omega)}{e(\omega)}$ for $Q = 100$ and $Q_{\text{eff}} = 5{,}000$.

in Figure 4(a). It can be seen as the combination of a parallel RLC circuit shortened by a narrower serial circuit $L_{\text{eff}}C_{\text{eff}}$. The transfer function — trap voltage to resistor noise voltage — is given by the divider bridge formula,

$$\frac{\underline{u}(\omega)}{\underline{e}(\omega)} = \frac{f(x)}{1+f(x)} \quad \text{with } f(x) = \frac{jQ_{\text{eff}}\,x(1-x^2)}{x^2 - Q(1-x^2)^2}, \tag{9}$$

where $x = \omega/\omega_z$ and where the parallel quality factor is $Q = R/L\omega_z$ and the serial quality factor is $Q_{\text{eff}} = L_{\text{eff}}\omega_z/R$. Figure 4(b) displays the transfer function $u(\omega)/e(\omega)$ versus ω/ω_z. It shows that the resistor voltage noise is filtered by the broad resonance of the parallel RLC circuit and shortened by the narrow series resonance. It nicely corresponds to the signal observed in Penning traps and used for accurate mass spectroscopy in Ref. [8].

3.5. *Resistive cooling of other modes*

Resistive cooling has been described for the axial motion in a Penning trap. The same idea can be applied to the cyclotron motion and, with more evolved techniques, to the magnetron motion.

The cyclotron motion takes place in a plane perpendicular to the trap axis. Image charge currents can be observed and used for cooling if the ring electrode is segmented into four segments as shown in Figure 5. The magnetron motion can also be cooled using sideband coupling to the axial motion. The underlying processes are beyond the scope of this tutorial and is described in detail in Ref. [5], see also Chapter 11 by Anderegg in this book. Note also that resistive cooling has also been demonstrated in an RF

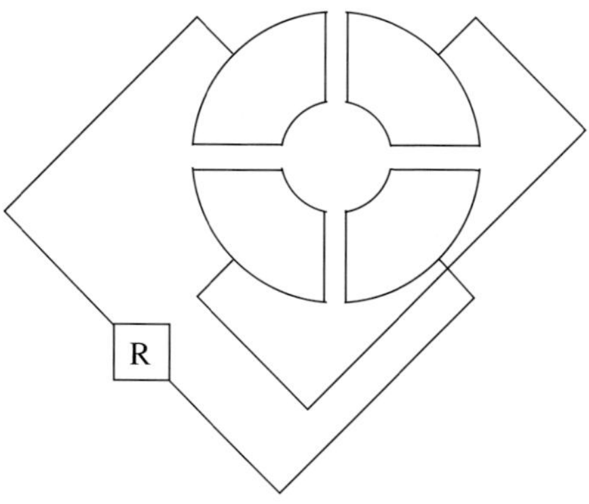

Fig. 5. Segmented ring electrode in a Penning trap and electrical connections used for resistive cooling.

Paul trap [4] with a room temperature resistor and a rather complicated resonant circuit design. Because of RF heating, the ion cloud temperature was only reduced by a factor of 3.3 from 3,000 K to 900 K, so this technique has not been further developed.

Problem 1. *Resistive cooling: route to thermal equilibrium.*
The coupling of an oscillating charged particle of mass m and charge q with the two electrodes of a parallel-plate capacitor is described by the mechanical and electrical Equation (6). $2z_0$ is the distance between the two electrodes of the trap. z is the position of the charged particle with respect to the center of the trap. ω_z is the oscillation frequency of the ion in the trap. $U(t)$ is the voltage across the two electrodes. $V(z)$ and $E(z)$ are the potential and electric field in the trap. α is a geometrical factor smaller than one. R is the resistance of the resistor. $e(t)$ represents the Johnson–Nyquist noise across the resistor; it is a random function with a zero average value and a symmetrized spectral noise density (defined for $\omega \geq 0$) given by $S_e(\omega) = 4Rk_BT$.

(1) *Show that the induced current $I(t)$ verifies the electrical circuit model given by*

$$L_{eff}C_{eff}\ddot{I}(t) + RC_{eff}\dot{I}(t) + I(t) + C_{eff}\dot{e}(t) = 0,$$

and give the expression of the effective inductance L_{eff} and capacitance C_{eff}.

(2) *Calculate L_{eff} and C_{eff} for $z_0 = 4\,mm$ and $^{12}C^{5+}$ with $q = 5q_e, m = 12 \times 1.67\ 10^{-27}$ kg and $\omega_z = 2\pi \times 300$ kHz.*

(3) *Using the complex impedance formalism, express $\underline{I}(\omega)$ with $\underline{e}(\omega), \omega, R, L_{eff}$, and C_{eff}. Show that*

$$\underline{\dot{z}}(\omega) = \frac{2z_0C_{eff}\omega_z}{q}\frac{j\omega/\omega_z\ \underline{e}(\omega)}{1-(\omega/\omega_z)^2+\frac{j}{Q}\omega/\omega_z},$$

and give the expression of Q.

(4) *The Wiener–Khintchine theorem states that the spectral density of a centered random function $h(t)$ is linked to the square modulus of its Fourier transform by $S_h(\omega) = |\underline{h}(\omega)|^2$. The variance is given by*

$$\langle h^2\rangle = \int_0^\infty S_h(\omega)d\omega/2\pi.$$

Use (3) and the relation between I and $\dot{z}$ to express the variance of the z-velocity distribution.

(5) *Show that the z-motion kinetic energy is given by $\langle\frac{m\dot{z}^2}{2}\rangle = \frac{k_BT}{2}$. Reminder: $\int_0^\infty u^2du/((1-u^2)^2+u^2/Q^2) \approx \pi Q/2$ for large Q.*

Solution. Route to equilibrium

(1) Insert $U(t) = RI(t) + e(t)$ into $E(z,t) = -\frac{U(t)}{2z_0}$ and $E(z,t)$ into $m\ddot{z} = -m\omega_z^2 z + qE(z,t)$, and use the relation between I and $\dot{z}$. One finds $L_{\text{eff}} = \frac{4mz_0^2}{q^2}$ and $C_{\text{eff}} = 1/(L\omega_z^2)$.
(2) $L_{\text{eff}} = 2 \times 10^8$ H, $C_{\text{eff}} = 1.4 \times 10^{-19}$ F.
(3) $\underline{I}(\omega) = \frac{jC_{\text{eff}}\omega\underline{e}(\omega)}{1-L_{\text{eff}}C_{\text{eff}}\omega^2+jRC_{\text{eff}}\omega}$ and $Q = \sqrt{L_{\text{eff}}/C_{\text{eff}}}/R$.
(4) $\langle \dot{z}^2 \rangle = \frac{1}{2\pi}\int_0^\infty \left|\underline{\dot{z}}(\omega)\right|^2 d\omega$

$\langle \dot{z}^2 \rangle = \frac{1}{2\pi}\frac{4z_0^2 C_{\text{eff}}\omega_z^2}{q^2}\int_0^\infty \frac{\left|\underline{e}(\omega)\right|^2(\omega/\omega_z)^2}{(1-(\omega/\omega_z)^2)^2+1/Q^2(\omega/\omega_z)^2}d\omega.$

(5) $\langle \frac{m\dot{z}^2}{2} \rangle = \frac{m}{2}\frac{1}{2\pi}\frac{4z_0^2 C_{\text{eff}}^2\omega_z^3}{q^2}4Rk_BT\int_0^\infty \frac{u^2}{(1-u^2)^2+u^2/Q^2}du$, setting $u = \omega/\omega_z$. Using the value of the integral and $QC_{\text{eff}}^2\omega_z^3 = \frac{1}{RL_{\text{eff}}}$, one gets the result.

4. Buffer Gas Cooling

The basic idea of trapped-ion buffer gas cooling is to utilize energy exchange during collisions with a neutral atomic or molecular gas to equilibrate the kinetic energy distributions of the ionic and neutral species to the vessel walls temperature. The main questions that arise are (i) the choice of the buffer gas, (ii) the cooling dynamics, and (iii) the final temperature that may be obtained. In this section, we will only address these questions for ions in an RF Paul trap and for elastic collisions. The effect of inelastic collisions is shortly addressed in paragraph 2.1.2 of Chapter 5 by Koelemeij and Knoop in this book. First, some orders of magnitude will be discussed.

- A typical collision cross-section is $\sigma = 10^{-20}\text{m}^2$ and the buffer gas pressure mostly used is $P = 10^{-8}\ldots 10^{-4}$mbar corresponding to a number density $n = 2.4 \times 10^8 \ldots 10^{12}\text{cm}^{-3}$, comparable or much larger than trapped ion densities. This leads to a mean free path $\lambda = k_BT/(\sqrt{2}\sigma P)$ between 3 km and 3 m, much longer than the usual trap length (with the notable exception of long storage rings). The collision rate is $Z = P\sigma\sqrt{8/(\pi k_BT\mu)}$ with μ the reduced mass of the collision partners. For He buffer gas, one finds Z between 0.04/s for low pressures and 400/s for high pressures. In both cases, the collision rates are much smaller than any oscillation frequency in an ion trap. These orders of magnitude justify the collision model used in numerical simulations (see Chapter 8 by Sillitoe and Hilico).
- A collision between an ion and a neutral particle is a short range event (sub-nm scale) that takes place at thermal energies with relative

velocities in the range above 100 m/s. The collision time is thus much smaller than the period of the axial or radial oscillation mode of the ions.

As a consequence, because collisions can be considered as low rate instantaneous events, a collision can be treated as a perturbation of the trapped-ion motion, and the buffer gas cooling dynamics can be obtained by averaging the effect of a large number of collisions on an ion.

4.1. *Buffer gas cooling in an RF Paul trap*

A simplified buffer gas cooling model in a Paul trap has been worked out by Moriwaki and co-authors and successfully compared to experiments [10, 11]. The oscillatory motion of an ion is described using the general expression of the x, y or z coordinate [12] (see also Chapter 2 by Knoop in this book)

$$u = A_u \sum_{j=-\infty}^{j=\infty} C_{2j,u} \cos\left(\frac{2\omega_u}{\Omega} + 2j\tau + \theta_u\right), \tag{10}$$

where ω is the trap RF angular frequency, $\tau = \Omega t/2$ the reduced time, ω_u is the secular frequency, and $C_{2j,u}$ relative coefficients of the different harmonics. Only A_u and θ_u depend on the initial conditions of the ion motion. The velocity of the ion is readily obtained by taking the time derivative of Equation (10).

The effect of an instantaneous collision is to modify the velocity of the ion without changing its position. In the model of Moriwaki, only direct head-on collisions are considered for simplicity, assuming that the ion and neutral velocities are colinear[b] (see Figure 6). For a head-on collision, the partner velocities before (v_1, v_2) and after (v_1', v_2') the collision can

Fig. 6. Head-on collisions of an ion and a neutral with velocities in the same (a) or opposite directions (b).

[b]This can be justified for a large ion cloud where most of the ions are far from the center of the trap and experience rather large micromotion, with an oscillatory velocity that exceeds the neutral root means square speed.

be deduced from energy and momentum conservation laws and one gets

$$v'1 = \frac{m_1 - m_2}{m_1 + m_2} v_1 + \frac{2m_2}{m_1 + m_2} v_2, \quad (11)$$

$$v'2 = \frac{2m_1}{m_1 + m_2} v_1 + \frac{m_2 - m_1}{m_1 + m_2} v_2. \quad (12)$$

The effect of the collision at time τ' of a neutral atom of mass m_n and velocity v_n on the trajectory of the ion is described by the equations,

$$u'(\tau') = u(\tau'), \quad (13)$$

$$\dot{u}'(\tau') = \frac{(m - m_n)u(\tau') + 2m_n v_n\ (2/\Omega)}{m + m_n}. \quad (14)$$

They can be solved in the form of Equation (10) with constants A'_u and θ'_u corresponding to the new initial conditions of the ion motion.

The end of the calculation is only outlined in the following, more details can be found in Moriwaki's papers [10,11]. The secular kinetic energy (SKE) of the ion motion in the direction u is defined by $\overline{W}_u = \frac{m}{2}\overline{\dot{u}}^2(\omega/2)^2$. By averaging the collision-induced kinetic energy variation on the collision time τ', the initial phase θ_u and on the neutral velocity distribution, the SKE mean-variation due to ion-neutral collisions is obtained. Using a similar approach, the mean-variation of the SKE due to Coulomb collision is also evaluated. Taking into account the ion-neutral and ion–ion collision rates, an SKE time-variation equation is obtained, with non-trivial dependance on the trapping (a, q) parameters and on the buffer gas properties (mass, pressure).

The predictions of this model are in good agreement with the measurements of ion cloud temperatures performed using Mg^+ ions in a hyperbolic ion trap and using He, H_2 or CH_4 as a buffer gas (see Ref. [11, Figure 1 or Figure 2]). The main conclusions are the following:

- There is a threshold for the buffer gas mass over which buffer gas cooling does not work. In practice, one has to use a very light buffer gas such as He or H_2. (Although H_2 leads to lower temperatures, it is not used because of possible chemical reactions with the trapped ions).
- The ion cloud temperature can be significantly larger than the buffer gas temperature, depending on the buffer gas pressure (the lower the pressure, the higher the temperature ratio) and on the trapping conditions (the higher the q parameter of the Paul trap, the higher the temperature ratio), both because of RF heating.

4.2. *Application examples*

(1) The first example is the microwave Hg^+ ion clock developed for space applications at Jet Propulsion Laboratory [13]. Although optical ion or neutral clocks are much more promising in terms of accuracy or stability, they usually require complex UV lasers that are not yet compatible with space environment. The Hg^+ microwave clock is operated on the ground state hyperfine transition at 40.5 GHz, corresponding to a wavelength of $\lambda = 7.4$ mm. Using a multipole RF trap with sub-cm radial dimensions allows trapping a large number of ions in the Doppler-free Lamb–Dicke regime. With uncooled ions, the clock resonance relative width and shift would be limited to

$$\frac{\Delta\nu}{\nu} = -\frac{v^2}{2c^2} = -\frac{3k_BT}{2mc^2} \tag{15}$$

due to the unavoidable second-order Doppler effect, which amounts to -4×10^{-12} at 3000 K. Using Buffer gas cooling with Ne at 300 K or He in a cryogenic environment at 4.2 K, the relative second-order Doppler effect is reduced to -4×10^{-13} or -5.6×10^{-15}, the latter being compatible with clock accuracies in the 10^{-16} range.

(2) The second example is an application to UV/IR photofragmentation spectroscopy of complex molecular ions such as protonated thyrosine [14] or many other ions (see for instance Ref. [15] or the work of Gerlich). Molecular ions have many vibrational and rotational levels that are excited at room or higher temperatures leading to very small populations of individual energy levels, and unresolved photofragmentation spectra. In this case, He buffer gas cooling not only cools the motional DoF but also cools the internal DoF, resulting in internal state resolved spectra that can be used as a fingerprint for molecular ion recognition.

(3) Very recently, He buffer gas cooling has been used for rotational cooling of sympathetically cooled MgH^+ ions [16], see also Chapter 15 by Drewsen in this book.

5. Conclusion

In this chapter, we have discussed non-laser cooling techniques that can be applied to trapped ions, among them, radiative cooling for fast oscillating light particles, resistive cooling, and buffer gas cooling. Other techniques have not been discussed, such as stochastic cooling or sympathetic cooling.

Acknowledgments

Thanks are due to D. Segal and C. Wunderlich for outlining the present chapter in the first PwTCP school.

References

1. M. Knoop *et al.*, *Physics with Trapped Charged Particles*, (*Eds D. Segal and C. Wunderlich*) World Scientific (2013).
2. J. D. Jackson, *Classical Electromagnetism*, New York, John Wiley (1999).
3. D. S. Hall, and G. Gabrielse, Electron Cooling of Protons in a Nested Penning Trap, *Phys. Rev. Lett.* **77**, 1962 (1997).
4. D. A. Church and H. G. Dehmelt, Radiative Cooling of an Electrodynamically Contained Proton Gas, *J. Appl. Phys.* **40**, 3421 (1969).
5. L. S. Brown and G. Gabrielse, Geonium theory: Physics of a single electron or ion in a Penning trap, *Rev. Mod. Phys.* **58**, 233 (1986).
6. C. Cohen Tannoudji, Cours du Collège de France 1984–1985. Available on: http://www. phys.ens.fr/~cct/college-de-france/.
7. P. Horowitz and W. Hill, *The Art of Electronics*, Chap. 7, pp 391–466. Cambridge, Cambridge University press (1996).
8. G. Werth *et al.*, Highly charged ions, quantum-electrodynamics, and the electron mass, *IJMS* **251**, 152 (2006).
9. H. Häffner *et al.*, Double Penning trap technique for precise g factor determinations in highly charged ions, *EPJD* **22**, 163 (2002).
10. Y. Moriwaki *et al.*, Collision Cooling of Ions Stored in Quadrupole Radio-Frequency Trap, *Jpn. J. App. Phys* **31**, L1640 (1992).
11. Y. Moriwaki *et al.*, Dependence of Temperature of Collision-Cooled Ions Stored in an RF Trap on Trapping Parameters, *Jpn. J. App. Phys* **35**, 757 (1996).
12. F. G. Major *et al.*, Eds, *Charged Particle Traps*, Chap 2, pp 17–46, Springer 2006.
13. J. D. Prestage *et al.*, *Mercury Ion Clock Based on Linear Multipole Ion Trap*, 2000 IEEE IFCS, Kansas City, Missouri, pp. 706710 (2000).
14. O. V. Boyarkin *et al.*, Electronic Spectroscopy of Cold, Protonated Tryptophan and Tyrosine, *JACS* **128**, 2816 (2006).
15. Juraj Jašík *et al.*, Probing Isomers of the Benzene Dication in a Low-Temperature Trap, *JACS* **136**, 2690–2692 (2014).
16. A. K. Hansen *et al.*, Efficient rotational cooling of Coulomb-crystallized molecular ions by a helium buffer gas, *Nature* **508**, 76 (2014).

CHAPTER EIGHT

NUMERICAL SIMULATIONS OF ION CLOUD DYNAMICS

Nicolas Sillitoe and Laurent Hilico*

Laboratoire Kastler Brossel,
Université d'Evry Val d'Essonne, UPMC-Sorbonne Universités,
CNRS, ENS-PSL Research University, Collège de France,
4 place Jussieu, 75005 Paris, France.
**laurent.hilico@lkb.upmc.fr*

We explain how to perform accurate numerical simulations of ion cloud dynamics by discussing the relevant orders of magnitude of the characteristic times and frequencies involved in the problem and the computer requirement with respect to the ion cloud size. We then discuss integration algorithms and Coulomb force parallelization. We finally explain how to take into account collisions, cooling laser interaction and chemical reactions in a Monte Carlo approach and discuss how to use random number generators to that end.

1. Introduction

Numerical simulations of trapped ions are a useful tool to prepare or accompany experiments. They can be performed in two rather different situations: (i) simulations of ion beam trajectories through an ion optical bench or (ii) simulations of trapped-ion cloud dynamics. In the first case (i), one usually has a complex arrangement of electrodes and/or magnets requiring an accurate modelization over a possibly large volume and the simulation time is very small (μs range) corresponding to a single flight through the apparatus. Commercial software allows to represent the ion optical bench and to fly ions through it including Coulomb repulsion, it is available at reasonable prices [1] . In the second case (ii), the trapped ions usually evolve in the reduced volume of the trapping region for long times from 1 to 100 ms or even more. During this time, the ions may interact with laser beams for laser cooling or photoexcitation or photodissociation, or undergo collisions with background gas leading to heating or chemical reactions. In this case, Coulomb repulsion plays an essential physical role and strongly dominates the computing time as soon as more than a few ions are taken into account. This is the domain of home-made optimized codes and the topic of this course.

In this chapter, we only address dynamics of a trapped ion cloud, and first present relevant orders of magnitude and hardware requirements in Sections 2 and 3. In Section 4, we discuss some integration algorithms and then the parallelization of Coulomb interaction in Section 5. Finally, Section 6 is devoted to the description of laser cooling, collisions, and chemical reactions.

2. Orders of Magnitude

The general scheme of ion beam or ion cloud simulations is the following:

(1) Represent the electric potential $V(\mathbf{r})$, the electric field $\mathbf{E}(\mathbf{r})$, and the magnetic field $\mathbf{B}(\mathbf{r})$ using either analytical formulae in simple cases or numerical representations.

(2) Represent the N charged particles by their mass m_i, charge q_i, position $\mathbf{r}_i$, velocity $\mathbf{v}_i$, and acceleration $\mathbf{a}_i$. A few boolean flags or integer variables may also be used to describe the internal state of the ion or any other peculiar properties.

(3) Evaluate the trapping force and the Coulomb force acting on each ion using the Lorentz law $q_i\mathbf{E}(\mathbf{r}_i, t) + q_i\mathbf{v}_i \times \mathbf{B}(\mathbf{r}_i, t)$ and the Coulomb law $\mathbf{F}_{i\leftarrow} = \sum_{j\neq i} \frac{q_i q_j}{4\pi\epsilon_0} \frac{\mathbf{r}_i - \mathbf{r}_j}{r_{ij}^3}$, and choose initial conditions.

(4) Integrate Newton's equations numerically taking into account laser interactions, collisions or chemical reactions at each time-step (see the detailed discussion in Section 6).

The last item raises the important questions of the integration algorithm, the time-step, the choice of a computing platform and of the programming language. They are addressed in the next paragraphs and sections.

The ion number of interest compatible with computation in reasonable times ranges from 1 to about 100,000.

2.1. *Choice of the integration time-step*

The trapped ion oscillation periods are summarized in Table 1. They typically vary from 0.01 to 200 μs. Collisions with low pressure neutral gas can be considered as instantaneous events that occur with rates from 100

Table 1. Characteristic oscillation times in Paul and Penning traps.

Trap	Motion	Period (μs)	Trap	Motion	Period (μs)
Paul	Radiofrequency (RF)	0.01 . . . 1	Penning	Cyclotron	0.01 . . . 0.1
	Secular	1 . . . 100		Axial	0.1 . . . 1
				Magnetron	10 . . . 200

to 10,000/s depending on the pressure (see Chapter 7 in this book). Laser interaction involves photon diffusion rates from 10^6 to 10^8/s, but only a large number of events lead to significant effect on an ion cloud. Characteristic ion cloud evolution times are then ms to hundred of ms. This shows that the physical problem involves both very short (10^{-8} s) and much longer (10 . . . 100 ms) times.

The evaluation of the characteristic time linked to Coulomb collisions deserves a special paragraph. We consider the head-on collision of two ions of mass m and charge q_1 and q_2. The collision energy can be evaluated from the minimal approach distance b or from the relative velocity v_{max} of the two ions at long distance $E_{\mathrm{coll}} = \frac{q_1 q_2}{4\pi\epsilon_0 b} = \frac{m v_{\mathrm{max}}^2}{2}$. For a safe integration of Newton's equations, the time-step must satisfy $v\delta t \ll b$. Taking into account the links between b and v_{max} through the expressions of E_{coll}, we obtain the criterion,

$$\delta t \ll \frac{q_1 q_2}{4\pi\epsilon_0} \frac{2}{m v_{\mathrm{max}}^3} = \frac{q_1 q_2}{4\pi\epsilon_0} \frac{\sqrt{m}}{\sqrt{2} E_{\mathrm{coll}}^{3/2}}. \tag{1}$$

Let's take an example: for an atomic mass of 20 amu, $v_{\mathrm{max}} = 1000\,\mathrm{m/s}$, we have $E_{\mathrm{coll}} = 100\,\mathrm{meV}$ and $\delta t \ll 1.3 \times 10^{-11}$ s. In case the integration time-step is too long, the spatial steps can be longer than the inter-ion distance and the ions may play leapfrog instead of repelling each other as shown in Figure 1.

In order to compare the prediction of Equation (1) with numerical simulations, we have systematically studied a head-on Coulomb collision between two identical ions in a 1D model. One ion is initially at rest and the second one is thrown on it with an energy E_{in}. Figure 2(a) shows the final energy E_{out} of the projectile ion (which is expected to be zero after the collision) versus the integration time-step for different values of E_{in}. For each energy, there is a threshold time-step below which the result is well converged. Figure 2(b) shows the threshold time-step versus E_{in}. The solid lines are fits with a $E_{\mathrm{coll}}^{-3/2}$ or $E_{\mathrm{coll}}^{-1.54}$ power law (red or green line). The fit agrees very well with the estimation of Equation (1).

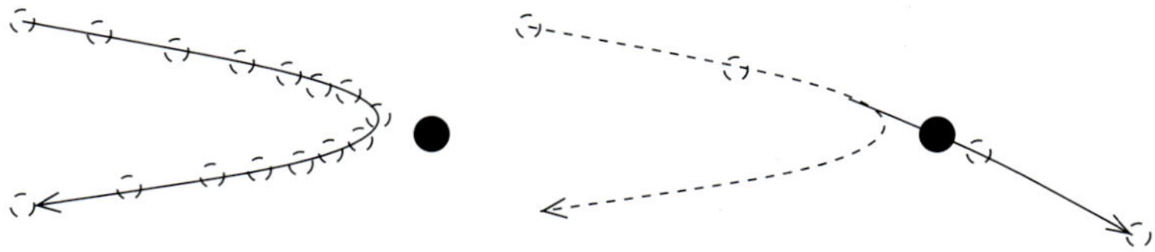

(a) (b)

Fig. 1. Numerical integration of Newton's equations for a Coulomb collision with a short enough time-step (a) and a too long time-step (b). Dashed circles: projectile ion positions in the frame of the target ion (solid circle).

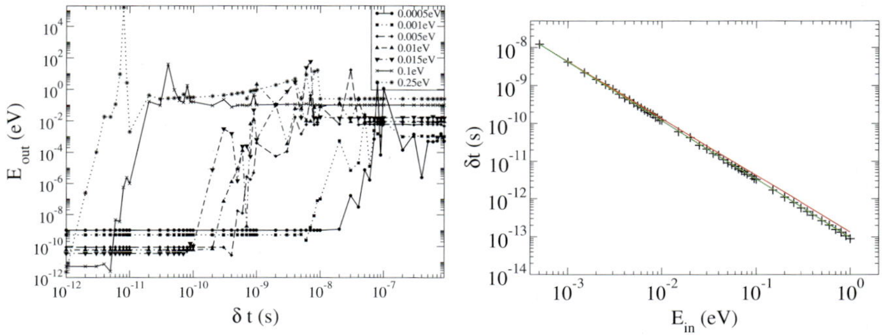

(a) (b)

Fig. 2. (a) Energy of the projectile ion after the collision. (b) Threshold time-step versus the collision energy. The red line is a fit by Equation (1) giving $1.35 \times 10^{-13}(E_{\text{in}}/\text{eV})^{3/2}$. The green line is the best fit given by $9.7 \times 10^{-14}(E_{\text{in}}/\text{eV})^{1.54}$. For both curves, $m_1 = m_2 = 1$.

From our tests, it would seem that $b > 0$ makes the criteria (1) looser, therefore it remains valid. As for $m_1 \neq m_2$, it seems that the time-step criteria becomes looser than Equation (1) using $m = \min(m_1, m_2)$. The condition states that δt must be much smaller than an upper bound. Our numerical tests showed that one tenth is a safe value.

2.2. *Coulomb force calculation*

An ion cloud containing up to 100,00 ions remains a mesoscopic system as can be seen in Figure 3. The detailed shape of the ion cloud is the result of the competition between the ion Coulomb repulsion and the trapping force that maintains the ions together. The dimensions of the ion cloud are not much larger than the typical inter-ion distance, and a non-negligible proportion of the ions belong to the outermost shell, so boundary conditions play

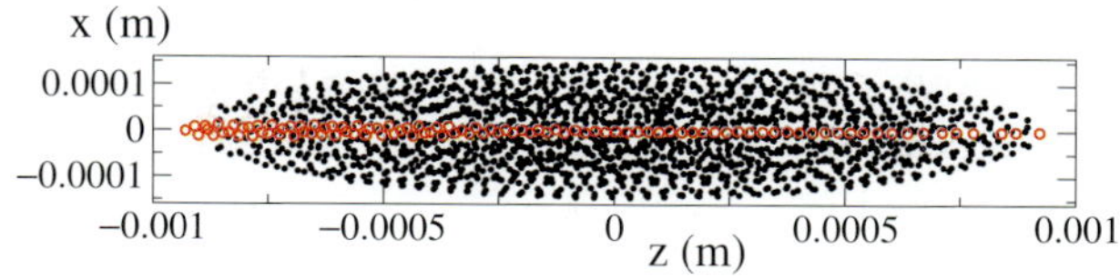

Fig. 3. Ion cloud confined in a Paul trap and containing 1,900 Be^+ ions (black solid circles) and 99 HD^+ ions. Trap characteristics: radius 3.5 mm, RF frequency 28 MHz, RF voltage amplitude 400 V and axial oscillation angular frequency $2\pi \times$ 67 kHz for Be^+. Laser cooling is applied on the axis from the right of the figure, on the Be^+ ions only with a beam waist of 1 mm, a detuning of $-\Gamma$, and an intensity equal to 1.5 saturation intensity (see Section 6). The sympathetically cooled HD^+ ions are pushed to the left of the ion cloud.

an important role. Hence, the ion cloud structure and dynamics can only be well simulated using the exact Coulomb force and any approximation would lead to non-reliable predictions.

2.3. *Conclusion*

The discussion of the orders of magnitude shows that a relevant numerical representation of a trapped ion cloud must be done using the exact Coulomb force and time dependent **E** or **B** fields, using time-steps no longer than 1 ns (and much smaller in case energetic events must be taken into account). Since the ion cloud evolution characteristic time exceeds tens of ms, a large number of steps is usually required (from 10^6 to 10^7 or even more). Because the Coulomb force calculation must be performed at each time-step with the unavoidable N^2 complexity, numerical simulation of ion clouds requires precise and intense computations with well-suited platform and algorithms.

3. Computer Requirements

3.1. *Memory (RAM) requirements*

In a computer, the representation of an integer needs 32 bits or 4 bytes, and 64 bits or 8 bytes for a double precision real number. Representing the ion positions, velocities, accelerations and internal states requires no more than 100 bytes per ion, which is less than 10 Mb for 10^5 ions that is negligible for present computers.

The representation of the **E** and **B** fields is negligible if analytical formulae (in an ideal trap) are used. It may rapidly become an issue if a numerical representation is used. Indeed, field discretization in a $1{,}000 \times 1{,}000 \times 1{,}000$ box requires 10^9 double precision numbers, i.e. 8 Gb per field component. One can easily saturate the amount of RAM if the discretization volume is not carefully optimized.

3.2. *Hard disk requirements*

Saving all the information on the computed trajectories (position, velocity, and acceleration) corresponds to nine double precision numbers, i.e. 72 bytes/step/ion. For a short simulation of 10^6 steps, this leads to 72 Mb/ion, and 72 Gb for 1,000 ions. For longer simulations involving more ions, one can very easily exceed several Terabytes per job. It is thus strongly recommended to only partially save data with a period much longer than the time-step, and to preprocess data of interest (energies, mean quantities, etc.) on the fly.

3.3. *Flops requirements*

Processor computational performance is expressed in Flop/s (Floating point operations per second). It depends on the processor clock frequency and hardware implementation. One can roughly consider that one addition (or one subtraction) and one multiplication take one clock period.[a] One division or one square root is more time consuming, taking about 10 clock periods. One integration step's Flop requirements can be split into a linear and a quadratic contribution with respect to the ion number. The linear part including **E** and **B** field evaluation, trap force evaluation, laser interaction and collisions represent less than 200 Flops. The quadratic part comes from the Coulomb force evaluation. It requires five additions or subtractions, eight multiplications, one division, and one square root corresponding to about 37 Flops. The amount of calculations scales as $37N_{\text{ion}}^2 + 200N_{\text{ion}}$. This estimation shows that the Coulomb interaction is the bottleneck as soon as $N_{\text{ion}} \geq 6$.

3.4. *CPU versus GPU*

Taking into account the amount of calculations that are required for a given simulation and the performances of Central Processing Unit (CPUs) and Graphics Processing Unit (GPUs), one can estimate the duration of a

[a]Modern processors can perform one addition and one multiplication at the same time.

Table 2. Computation time to simulate the dynamics of a cloud of N_{ions} ions with 10^8 time-steps. The computer performances are 100 GFlops for a 20 core CPU and 1.3 TFlops for the GPU.

N_{ions}	N_{op}/step	T for 10^8 steps 20 CPU	T for 10^8 steps GPU	6 GPU
100	370,000	6 min		
1,000	3.7×10^7	10 h20′		
10,000	3.7×10^9	43 days		
15,360	8.7×10^9	101 days	8 days	
86,016	2.7×10^11	≈ 9 years	243 days	41 days

calculation. The results are summarized in Table 2 for 20 CPU cores giving 100 GFlops, one GPU giving 1.3 TFlops and six parallelized GPUs. Here, the Flop Rates have been measured on a biprocessor system with two Intel Xeon ES-2680 v2 3.6 GHz and on a NVidia Titan Black GPU.

Parallelized CPU code is a good solution for ion clouds up to a few thousand ions. Above that, GPUs are much quicker while consuming much less energy.

4. Integration Algorithms

Newton's equations for N_{ion} ions are a set of three N_{ion} second-order coupled differential equations $\ddot{\mathbf{r}}_i = f(\ldots, \mathbf{r}_j, \ldots, \dot{\mathbf{r}}_j, \ldots, t)$ that can be written as a set of six N_{ion} first-order coupled differential equations in the form $(\mathbf{v}_i = \dot{\mathbf{r}}_i, \dot{\mathbf{v}}_i = f(\ldots, \mathbf{r}_j, \ldots, \dot{\mathbf{r}}_j, \ldots, t))$. They can be numerically solved using different algorithms. We analyze two of them. The simplest one, the Euler algorithm is shown to be intrinsically unstable for oscillatory problems and we will show in the following that it must be rejected since trapped ion motion is essentially oscillatory. The second one, the leapfrog [2] algorithm or Verlet-vitesse is show to be well suited for trapped ions.

4.1. *Euler algorithm*

For simplicity, we describe and analyze the Euler algorithm for a 1D problem. Newton's equation reads

$$\dot{x}(t) = v(t), \tag{2}$$

$$\dot{v}(t) = a(x(t), \dot{x}(t), t). \tag{3}$$

The idea of the Euler method is to determine the coordinates (x_{i+1}, v_{i+1}) at time $t_i + \delta t$ from the position x_i and velocity v_i at time t_i using a first-order expansion by using the algorithm,

$$(x_i, v_i) \rightarrow (x_{i+1} = x_i + v_i\delta t, v_{i+1} = v_i + a_i\delta t). \tag{4}$$

In the case of a harmonic oscillator of angular frequency ω, we have $a_i = -\omega^2 x_i$ so the algorithm writes

$$(x_i, v_i) \rightarrow (x_{i+1} = x_i + v_i\delta t, v_{i+1} = v_i - \omega^2 x_i\delta t). \tag{5}$$

The oscillator mechanical energy is given by $E = mv^2/2 + m\omega^2 x^2/2$. The mechanical energy at time t_{i+1} is given by $E_{i+1} = mv_{i+1}^2/2 + m\omega^2 x_{i+1}^2/2$. Replacing x_{i+1} and v_{i+1} by their expressions, we obtain

$$E_{i+1} = \left(1 + \omega^2\delta t^2\right) E_i. \tag{6}$$

This equation shows that with the Euler algorithm, the mechanical energy diverges (whereas it is physically preserved), and that the algorithm is never stable, even for very small time-steps.

4.2. *Leapfrog algorithm*

For the leapfrog algorithm, the discretized position velocities and acceleration are defined by $x_i = x(t_i)$, $v_i = v(t_i + \delta t/2)$, and $a_i = a(t_i)$ and an integration time-step is performed using the transformation,

$$\begin{cases} x_i \\ a_i \\ v_i \end{cases} \rightarrow \begin{cases} x_{i+1} = x_i + v_i\delta t + \frac{a_i\delta t^2}{2} \\ a_{i+1} = F(x_i, t_i) \\ v_{i+1} = v_i + \frac{a_i + a_{i+1}}{2} \end{cases}, \tag{7}$$

where $F(x_i, t_i)$ is the force at time t_i. For the stability analysis in the case of a 1D harmonic oscillator, we use $a_i = -\omega^2 x_i$ and set $\beta = \omega\delta t$. The transformation of Equation (7) can be recast into

$$\begin{pmatrix} \omega x_{i+1} \\ v_{i+1} \end{pmatrix} = \begin{pmatrix} 1 - \frac{\beta^2}{2} & \beta \\ -\frac{\beta}{2}(1-\beta^2) & 1 - \frac{\beta^2}{2} \end{pmatrix} \begin{pmatrix} \omega x_{i+1} \\ v_{i+1} \end{pmatrix}. \tag{8}$$

The mechanical energy is given by $E_i = \frac{m}{2}(v_i^2 + (\omega x_i)^2)$. The leap frog algorithm preserves energy of a 1D harmonic oscillator if at each time-step

$E_{i+1} = E_i$. This is the case if the matrix that appears in Equation (8) can be written

$$M(\beta) = \begin{pmatrix} \cos(\theta) & \sin(\theta) \\ -\sin(\theta) & \cos(\theta) \end{pmatrix} \tag{9}$$

with θ real. This is the case if $-1 \leq 1 - \frac{\beta}{2} \leq 1$, i.e. if $|\beta| = \omega\delta t \leq 1$, in other words, if the time-step is small enough with respect to the oscillation period.

The determinant of the matrix $M(\beta)$ is 1, so it is easy to check that $M(\beta)^{-1} = M(-\beta)$. This relation shows that the leap frog algorithm is time-reversible, and is a so-called *symplectic* algorithm.

4.3. *Discussion*

We have shown that the Euler algorithm has to be rejected because it is intrinsically unstable and also because it is a first-order method in δt. One can use more elaborate algorithms such as Runge–Kutta of order two or Runge–Kutta of order four that use a more accurate discretization scheme and can be found in libraries. The main drawback of those methods in the case of ion clouds is that they need two or four evaluations of the force per time-step, which is extremely time consuming.

The leap frog algorithm is a good trade-off between time consumption and performances because it is a second-order stable and time-reversible method requiring only one calculation of the force per time-step.

4.4. *Variable time-step methods*

We have seen that to perform relevant simulations, one has to carefully choose the integration time-step. A too short time-step leads to very long calculation times, and a too long one to possibly non-physical predictions.

A variable time-step can easily be implemented for algorithms that are local in time, i.e. for which the position and velocities at time $t + \delta t$ only depends on the positions and velocities at time t. This is the case for Euler, leapfrog and Runge–Kutta algorithms. Note that this is not the case for the Verlet algorithm (not described in this chapter) for which the position and velocities at time $t + \delta t$ depends on positions at time t and $t - \delta t$.

The constraints on the time-step come from the characteristic periods in the problem and from Coulomb collisions with high relative velocity, the latter possibly being more stringent. A variable time-step algorithm must then include a maximum time-step compatible with the typical periods of the ion oscillatory motions, as well as a "Coulomb collision analysis" at each time-step. In principle, this analysis should rely on the ion pair relative velocities, which scales as N_{ion}^2. Since the relative velocity of two particles is less than twice the maximum of the two velocities, the Coulomb collision analysis can rely on twice the maximum ion velocity (that can be evaluated with a linear complexity).

5. Coulomb Force Parallelization

At each time-step, the Coulomb force acting on each ion is evaluated from the position data set.

For a single CPU, the force on ion i can be simply written as a sum of the forces due to the other ions j with j varying from 1 to $i-1$ and from $i+1$ to N_{ion}. The pseudo-code looks like

```
do i=1,N_ion                            loop on i
 F_i=0                                  3D force initialization
 do j=1,i-1                             loop on j
  r_ij=r_i-r_j                          3D relative position
  r_ij2=r_ij.x^2+r_ij.y^2+r_ij.z^2      square of the distance
  r_ij1=sqrt(r_ij2)                     distance
  r_ij3=r_ij2*r_ij1                     cube of the distance
  F_i=F_i+q_j*r_ij/rij3                 Coulomb force of ion j on ion i
 enddo
 do j=i+1,N_ion
  .....                                 same as above
 enddo                                  end of loop on j
F_i=F_i*q_i*Coulombcoef                 final multiplication by q_i
enddo                                   end of loop on i
```

Note that one can save N_{ion} multiplications by doing the multiplication by q_i and by the Coulomb force coefficient $1/(4\pi\epsilon_0)$ at the end of the loops on j.

The Coulomb force parallelization can be implemented on a multicore CPU using the OPENMP library [3] on the outermost loop on i. The compiler directives are indicated as follows:

```
!$OMP parallel do private(j,Fi,r_ij,r_ij2,r_ij1,r_ij3)
do i = 1, N
  ...
enddo
!$OMP end parallel do
```

The loop on i is split into sub-loops executed by different cores. Note that some variables have to be defined locally in each thread; they are indicated in the private statement. The compilation is made using the `-openmp` option in `FORTRAN` or `-fopenmp` in `C`. Before execution, the number of threads and the size of the sub-loops are defined by the environment variables `OMP NUM THREADS` and `OMP SCHEDULE`. With a single CPU, the number of cores is limited to 12 and the number of threads to 24.

The Coulomb force calculation can also be implemented on multi-CPU platforms using the MPI [4] library. The calculation of the Coulomb force on a given ion requires an access to the position of all the other ions. This means that shared-memory platforms offering high data flow performance are preferable.

The Coulomb force calculation is performed independently for each ion using the same algorithm and the same position data set. This task perfectly matches the capabilities of GPU. These are *devices* that can be installed in a computer and that offer several thousands of threads. The specifics of GPU programming are out of the scope of this course. Nevertheless, here are a few examples of differences between CPU and GPU programming: (i) GPU's function in a host-device (master–slave) relationship with the host CPU; (ii) data need to be exchanged back and forth between CPU and GPU; (iii) for the sake of performance, it is important to efficiently use the hierarchy of different memories on the GPU. For the Coulomb force calculation, a useful reference is provided by Nvidia [5].

6. Laser Interaction, Collisions, and Chemical Reactions

We have shown in Section 1 that laser interaction, collisions with neutrals and possible chemical reactions can be considered as instantaneous processes with respect to the evolution times of the ion cloud, even if high velocity collisions are involved, that lead to a velocity kick on the ion undergoing the interaction. See Section 4 of Chapter 7, in this book for an evaluation of collision rates.

These interactions can be implemented numerically using a Monte Carlo approach as follows. At each time-step,

- randomly decide whether or not the interaction takes place,
- if the answer is positive, compute the velocity kick and add it to the ion velocity.

6.1. *Laser interaction*

We here restrict the analysis to Doppler laser cooling (see Chapter 6 by Champenois in this book for an analytical approach). The numerical implementation requires a variable describing the internal state of the laser cooled ions, denoted by $|g\rangle$ and $|e\rangle$ in the two-level model. An ion in the ground state $|g\rangle$ can only undergo a photon absorption with a probability $B_{12}\delta t$ and a velocity kick $\Delta\mathbf{v}_{\rm abs} = \hbar\mathbf{k}/m_{\rm lc}$ where $m_{\rm lc}$ is the laser cooled ion mass and $\mathbf{k}$ the photon wave-vector. An ion in the excited state $|e\rangle$ can undergo either spontaneous or stimulated emission with the probabilities $A_{21}\delta t$ and $B_{21}\delta t$ and with velocity kicks $\Delta\mathbf{v}_{\rm st} = \hbar\mathbf{k}'/m_{\rm lc}$ or $\Delta\mathbf{v}_{\rm sp} = -\hbar\mathbf{k}/m_{\rm lc}$, where $\mathbf{k}'$ is a wave vector with the same modulus as $\mathbf{k}$ and a random direction.

In the case of a two-level atom with a transition energy $\hbar\omega_0$ and width Γ, the elementary process probabilities during the interval δt are given by Ref. [6]

$$A_{21}\delta t = \Gamma\delta t, \tag{10}$$

$$B_{12}\delta t = \frac{I(\mathbf{r})}{I_{\rm sat}}\frac{1/2}{1+4\left(\frac{\omega_L+\mathbf{k}.\mathbf{v}-\omega_0}{\Gamma}\right)^2}, \tag{11}$$

$$B_{21}\delta t = B_{12}\delta t, \tag{12}$$

where ω_L is the laser angular frequency, $\mathbf{k}$ the wave vector, $\mathbf{v}$ the ion velocity, and $I(\mathbf{r})$ the laser intensity at the ion location and where the saturation intensity is given by $I_{\rm sat} = \frac{2\pi^2\hbar\Gamma}{3\lambda^3}$. For more complicated level structures, the energy level degeneracy has to be taken into account [7]. The cooling laser profile is usually Gaussian with a waist w_0 at a location $\mathbf{r}_{w_0}$, such that the laser intensity is given by

$$I(\mathbf{r}) = \left(\frac{w_0}{w(\zeta)}\right)^2 e^{-2r_\perp^2/w(\zeta)^2}, \tag{13}$$

where ζ is the projection of $\mathbf{r} - \mathbf{r}_{w_0}$ on the direction of $\mathbf{k}$, $r\perp$ the orthogonal projection, and $w(\zeta) = w_0\sqrt{1+(\frac{\lambda\zeta}{\pi w_0})^2}$[8], as defined in Figure 4.

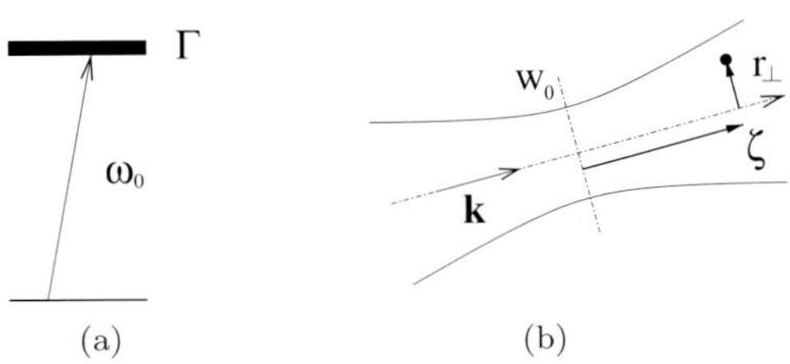

Fig. 4. (a) Two-level atom, transition angular frequency ω_0 and width Γ. (b) Gaussian laser cooling beam profile. The black circle is the ion location, ζ and $r\perp$ the axial and radial distances to the beam waist location.

Numerical implementation of laser cooling using a Monte Carlo approach can be done by deciding at each time-step whether or not one of the three processes occurs. The corresponding pseudo-code is as follows:

```
for each laser cooled ion
  evaluate the laser field at the ion location
  if ion_state=|g> then
    evaluate B12 dt
    uniformly choose a random number rn in [0,1]
    if rn < B12 dt
       then velocity kick = hbar k/m
       else no velocity kick
    endif
  if ion_state=|e> then
    evaluate A21 dt
    evaluate B21 dt
    uniformly choose a random number rn in [0,1]
    if rn < A21 dt
      then choose a random direction k'
           velocity kick = hbar k'/m
      else if A21 dt < rn < (A21+B21) dt
        then velocity kick = -hbar k/m
     endif
  endif
end loop on laser cooled ions
```

where dt, hbar, k, and k' represent δt, $\hbar$ and the vectors $\mathbf{k}$ and $\mathbf{k}'$, and where pseudo-random number generators with uniform and non-uniform distribution are used (see Section 7).

Laser-cooling damping can also be simulated using an effective drag force added to the trap and Coulomb forces. Nevertheless, in order to get physical equilibrium temperatures, it is essential to include the heating due to spontaneous emission in the form of random Langevin forces, which also need random numbers.

6.2. *Collisions, chemical reactions, and photodissociation*

Ion cloud trapping times are usually of the order of seconds to several minutes. Even if the vacuum conditions are extremely good, collisions heating the ions or chemical reactions changing the ion species or making it neutral may happen. In REMPD molecular ion spectroscopy experiments (resonance enhanced multiphoton dissociation), state selective photodissociation is used to detect transitions to excited states. For example, the energy released by the photodissociation $HD^+(v = 4 \cdots 9) + h\nu \rightarrow D^+ + H$ turns a HD^+ ion into a D^+ ion with a large initial velocity. This process can be described in terms of occurrence probability during δt depending either on the projectile gas flux or the photon flux and in terms of ion velocity kick events.

7. Pseudo-random Numbers

Most of the programming languages offer a uniform pseudo-random number generator in [0,1]. The pseudo-random series deterministically depends on the seed that initializes the generator; this is essential to be able to re-run a job with the same random numbers. Since two random series with different seeds are statistically independent, statistics on the simulations can simply be obtained by running the code with varied seeds.

For ion cloud simulations, non-uniform random series are required, e.g. Gaussian distributions to simulate thermalization to a temperature T. We first describe the *inverse sampling method* and then consider the case of a random direction distribution in 3D space needed for spontaneous emission or collision simulations.

7.1. *Inverse sampling method*

The question is to know how to get a random number series with a given distribution function $g(\nu)$ in the interval $[a, b]$. Since g is a probability distribution, it verifies $\int_a^b g(\nu)d\nu = 1$. Denoting G the primitive of g verifying $G(a) = 0$ and $G(b) = 1$, we have $\frac{dG(\nu)}{d\nu} = g(\nu)$. Using the change of variables $u = G(\nu)$, we have $du = \frac{dG}{d\nu}d\nu = g(\nu)d\nu$. This relation shows that if ν has a distribution function g, then u has a uniform distribution in [0,1]. Reciprocally, if u has a uniform distribution in [0,1], then $\nu = G^{-1}(u)$ has the distribution function $g(\nu)$. Consequently, the recipe to generate a random number series with distribution function $g(\nu)$ is the following: (i) generate a uniform random series u_k in [0,1] and (ii) compute $\nu_k = G^{-1}(u_k)$.

7.2. *Gaussian distribution*

The inverse sampling method can be used to obtain a centered Gaussian distribution $g(\nu) = \frac{1}{\sqrt{2\pi}\sigma}e^{-\nu^2/(2\sigma^2)}$, where σ is the RMS value. The primitive G satisfying $\lim_{\nu\rightarrow-\infty} G(\nu) = 0$ and $\lim_{\nu\rightarrow+\infty} G(\nu) = 1$ is linked to the

Gaussian error function erf by $G(\nu) = (1 + \text{erf}(\frac{\nu}{\sqrt{2}\sigma}))/2$. The main problem for the numerical implementation is to have the inverse of the erf function.

The Box–Muller method [9] offers a simple method to get two independent Gaussian distributions using standard functions only. This method is presented in Problem 1.

7.3. *Random direction in 3D space*

Choosing a uniformly random direction in a 3D space is equivalent to choosing a uniformly random position on a sphere of radius unity. Using spherical coordinate angles (θ, ϕ) with $0 \leq \theta \leq \pi$ and $0 \leq \phi \leq 2\pi$, the elementary solid angle $d\Omega = \sin(\theta) d\theta d\phi$ that can be rewritten:

$$\frac{d\Omega}{4\pi} = \frac{\sin(\theta) d\theta}{2} \frac{d\phi}{2\pi}. \tag{14}$$

A uniform solid angle distribution corresponds to a uniform distribution for ϕ in $[0, 2\pi]$ and to a distribution of density $g(\theta) = \frac{\sin(\theta)}{2}$ for θ. In the latter case, we have $G(\theta) = \frac{1-\cos(\theta)}{2}$. Following the inverse sampling method for θ and ϕ leads to the algorithm,

```
uniformly randomise u in [0,1]
uniformly randomise v in [0,1]
compute phi=2*pi*u
compute theta=arccos(1-2*u)
compute kappa_x=sinttheta) cos(phi)
        kappa_y=sin(theta) sin(phi)
        kappa_z=cos(theta)
```

to get a uniformly distributed unit vector κ in a 3D space.

Problem 1. *Random generator with a Gaussian distribution: Box–Muller method*

We consider u and v two uniformly distributed random variables in [0,1] and the random variables defined by $x = \sqrt{-2\ln u}\cos(2\pi v)$ *and* $y = \sqrt{-2\ln u}\sin(2\pi v)$. *We show that x and y are independent random variables with a normalized centered Gaussian distribution. To do so, we evaluate the mean value of a function* $f(x, y)$, *assuming that this mean is finite.*

(1) *Express the mean value* $\langle f \rangle$ *of* $f(x, y)$ *as a double integral on u and v.*
(2) *Use the changes of variable* $s = \sqrt{-2\ln u}$ *and* $\theta = 2\pi v$ *to express* $\langle f \rangle$ *as a double integral on s and* θ.

(3) *Use the change of variable* $(s, \theta) \to (x, y)$ *to obtain*

$$\langle f \rangle = \int_{-\infty}^{\infty} \int_{\infty}^{\infty} e^{-x^2/2} e^{-y^2/2} f(x, y) \frac{dx}{\sqrt{2\pi}} \frac{dy}{\sqrt{2\pi}}$$

and conclude.

(4) *Use the uniform random generator of your favourite software (Maple, Mathematica, Octave, . . .) or programming language (FORTRAN, C, C++, Cuda, Python, . . .) to generate a series of 1,000 numbers with a Gaussian distribution of standard deviation* σ. *Plot the histogram of the* x *and* y *values and compare with a Gaussian.*

Solution. Random generator with a Gaussian distribution: Box–Muller method

(1) $\langle f \rangle = \int_0^1 \int_0^1 f(\sqrt{-2\ln u}\cos(2\pi v), \sqrt{-2\ln u}\sin(2\pi v)) du dv$.
(2) $\langle f \rangle = \int_0^{2\pi} \frac{d\theta}{2\pi} \int_{-\infty}^{0} -f(s\cos(\theta), s\sin(\theta)) e^{-s^2/2} s ds$.
(3) The result is obtained by using $s^2 = x^2 + y^2$ and the polar to rectangular change of coordinate $(s, \theta) \to (x = s\cos(\theta), y = s\sin(\theta))$ with $s ds d\theta = dx dy$.

8. Conclusion

In this course, we have discussed trapped simulations of trapped ion clouds and shown that it is essential to accurately represent the trapping time-varying electromagnetic fields, and to use a short enough integration time-step to obtain reliable results. We propose a simple criterion to determine the upper bound of the integration time-step. We have discussed possible integration algorithms, the parallelization of the Coulomb force calculation, and the implementation of processes such as laser interaction for Doppler laser-cooling, collisions, and chemical reactions. Finally, we shortly discussed how to use the random number generator to get random number series with a given distribution.

Acknowledgments

Thanks are due to Pascal Monceau, Dominique Delande, Jofre Pedregosa, and Jean-Philippe Karr for the fruitful discussion on numerical simulations.

References

1. 12-21-2015 http://simion.com/, 12-21-2015 http://ibsimu.sourceforge.net/.
2. L. Verlet, Computer "experiments" on classical fluids, I. Thermodynamical properties of Lennard–Jones molecules, *Phys. Rev.* **159**, 98–103 (1967).
3. 12-21-2015, Available on: http://www.openmp.org/wp/.
4. See MPI internet links and tutorials.
5. 11-21-2015, GPU Gem3, Available on: http://http.developer.nvidia.com/GPUGems3/gpugems3_part01.html.
6. B. Cagnac, J.-C. Pebay-Peroula, Physique atomique tome 2, Annex VII.4, pp. 593–597, Dunod (1982).
7. R. C. Hilborn, Einstein coefficients, cross sections, f values, dipole moments, and all that, *Am. J. Phys.* **50**, 982–986 (1982) and *erratum* **51**, 471 (1983).
8. H. Kogelnik, and T. Lee, Laser beams and resonators, *App. Opt.*, **5**, 1550–1567 (1966).
9. G. E. P. Box and M. E. Muller, A note on the generation of random normal deviates, *Ann. Math. Stat.* **29**, 610–611, (1958).

CHAPTER NINE

PLASMAS IN PENNING TRAPS

D. H. E. Dubin
Dept of Physics UCSD, La Jolla CA 92093
ddubin@ucsd.edu

This chapter introduces the reader to the physics of plasmas in Penning traps. After a brief discussion of what constitutes a classical plasma, and a description of Debye shielding, the basic equilibrium properties of non-neutral plasmas in Penning traps are explained. Plasma rotation, the Brillouin limit, diamagnetic effects, the confined thermal equilibrium state, and constants of the motion are discussed.

1. Introduction: What is a Plasma?

A plasma is a state of matter with properties quite distinct from the solid, liquid, or gas phases that you are more familiar with from your physics classes. In fact, plasma is often referred to as the "fourth state of matter" [1, p. 2]. In the following two chapters, we will consider a few of the properties of the plasma state, particularly as they pertain to confined plasmas in Penning traps.

A plasma is a collection of charged particles moving freely under the influence of external force fields as well as self-generated electric and/or magnetic fields. In a plasma, these self-generated fields are sufficiently large to significantly affect the particle dynamics. Plasmas are often produced by heating a neutral gas until a significant fraction of the particles become ionized through collisional processes; however, low temperature plasmas also exist in both nature and the laboratory. In fact, plasma temperatures can be sufficiently low, and/or densities can be sufficiently high that quantum phenomena (such as Pauli exclusion [3] or quantized energies [4,5]) play an important role in the plasma equilibrium and dynamics. However, in these chapters, I will concentrate on those regimes where the plasma state is well described by classical mechanics. I will also neglect relativistic effects, assuming particle velocities are small compared to the speed of light (an excellent approximation in most Penning trap experiments).

Also, plasmas are not always charge-neutral — particularly in Penning trap experiments, the number of negative charges does not always balance the number of positive charges. Such plasmas are called "non-neutral" [6].

Below, I consider in more detail the requirements for a system to be in the plasma state.

1.1. *The Debye length*

The Debye length λ_D is a fundamental length scale in plasmas. It is the length over which static electric fields are "screened out" in an unmagnetized thermal classical plasma. To understand what this means, consider the following simple plasma configuration: a parallel plate capacitor is introduced into a neutral plasma consisting of electrons and singly-charged ions with equal densities n_0 and charges $-e$ and $+e$, respectively (Figure 1). I assume that this plasma has a well-defined temperature T, and I apply a potential V to the left capacitor electrode (at position $x = 0$) and ground the right electrode (which is at position $x = L$). If there were no plasma present, this would produce a potential between the electrodes given by

$$\phi(x) = V(1 - x/L), \tag{1}$$

which corresponds to a uniform electric field $E = V/L$ between the plates. However, the plasma *significantly affects* this potential, reducing the electric field to nearly zero after a "sheath" layer whose width is given by the Debye length. This is what is meant by "plasma screening". To analyze this screening phenomenon, I assume for simplicity that the plasma is in

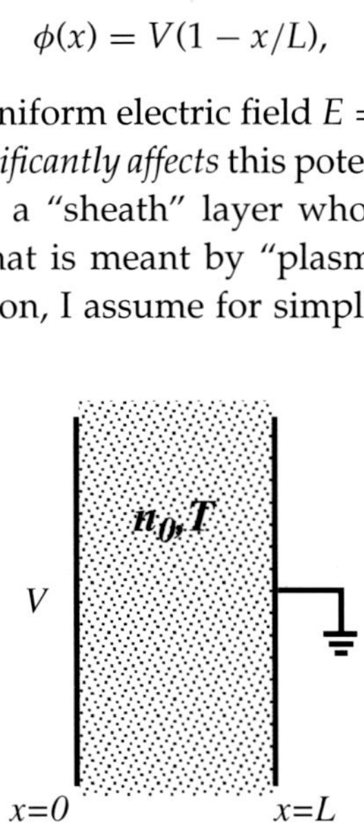

Fig. 1. A neutral plasma between the plates of a capacitor shields out the applied electric field.

a thermal equilibrium state at temperature T. (Here I should note in the interests of full disclosure that plasmas in contact with conducting plates as shown in the figure are typically not in thermal equilibrium because the plates draw current from the plasma, are not at the same temperature as the plasma, and may react chemically with the plasma, and consequently the plasma screening that occurs is much more complicated than the simple model put forward here. The conducting plates I am discussing are *magic plates* that can be heated to the same temperature as the plasma without vaporizing, and also somehow neither emit nor absorb electrons or ions.) The thermal equilibrium model implies that the electron and ion densities n_e and n_i are described by Boltzmann distributions [7]:

$$n_e(x) = n_0 \exp\left(e\phi(x)/T\right), \tag{2}$$

$$n_i(x) = n_0 \exp\left(-e\phi(x)/T\right). \tag{3}$$

That is, the electrons are attracted to the plate at positive potential, increasing their density there, while the ions are repelled from that region, and the zero of potential is defined to be in the region where the plasma achieves density n_0. (Note that in these chapters, temperature is regarded as having units of energy, and therefore, the Boltzmann constant k_B is unnecessary. Boltzmann, the founder of statistical mechanics and one of the great scientific innovators of the late 19th and early 20th centuries, deserves to have a better constant named after him!)

The charge distribution arising from Equations (2) and (3) has an appreciable effect on the electrostatic potential ϕ. The potential is determined from the Poisson equation,

$$\begin{aligned} \frac{d^2\phi}{dx^2} &= \frac{e}{\varepsilon_0}[n_e(x) - n_i(x)] \\ &= \frac{n_0 e}{\varepsilon_0}\left[\exp\left(e\phi/T\right) - \exp\left(-e\phi/T\right)\right]. \end{aligned} \tag{4}$$

Equation (4) can be solved subject to the boundary conditions that $\phi(0) = V$ and $\phi(L) = 0$. For simplicity, I will facilitate this solution by linearizing the equation in ϕ, assuming that $|e\phi/T| \ll 1$:

$$\frac{d^2\phi}{dx^2} = 2\frac{n_0 e^2}{\varepsilon_0 T}\phi. \tag{5}$$

The factor of two that appears on the right-hand side arises from the shielding effect of the two species considered here, i.e. electrons and singly-charged ions. If more species were added, with arbitrary charges, this factor would be modified [2].

The solution to Equation (5) that matches the required boundary conditions is

$$\phi(x) = V\frac{\exp\left(-\sqrt{2}x/\lambda_D\right) - \exp\left(\sqrt{2}(x-2L)/\lambda_D\right)}{1-\exp\left(-2\sqrt{2}L/\lambda_D\right)} \tag{6}$$

$$\simeq V\exp\left(-\sqrt{2}x/\lambda_D\right), \quad L \gg \lambda_D, \tag{7}$$

where the Debye length λ_D is defined in terms of the equilibrium density and temperature as

$$\lambda_D \equiv \sqrt{\frac{\varepsilon_0 T}{n_0 e^2}} \tag{8}$$

$$= 743\ \text{m}\sqrt{\frac{T(\text{eV})}{n_0(\text{m}^{-3})}}$$

Equation (7) implies that the electric field in the plasma is *exponentially suppressed*. The positively charged capacitor plate attracts plasma electrons and repels ions. After a sheath region which is a few Debye lengths thick, the electric field is nearly zero: it has been screened out by the plasma.

1.2. *Requirements for the plasma state*

These considerations lead us to our first requirement that a system be in the plasma state: in order for the plasma to significantly affect the potential, the Debye length must be small compared to the system size; otherwise, the screening effect of the plasma is negligible:

$$\lambda_D \ll L \text{ in the plasma state.} \tag{9}$$

If this requirement is not met and the Debye length is larger than L, one can see from Equation (6) that the potential returns to the vacuum form, Equation (1).

A second requirement follows from certain assumptions in the preceding analysis. In describing the ions and electron densities with Equations (2) and (3), I have implicitly treated them as continuous fluids. This is only a good approximation provided that the density varies slowly on the scale of the mean inter-particle spacing $a \equiv n_0^{-1/3}$. Since the density varies on the scale of the Debye length, it is necessary that $\lambda_D \gg n_0^{-1/3}$. This inequality is often rearranged to read

$$n_0 \lambda_D^3 \gg 1 \text{ in the plasma state.} \tag{10}$$

The dimensionless quantity $n_0 \lambda_D^3$, the number of charges in a "Debye-sphere", is called the plasma parameter [1, p. 11]. Some further intuition regarding this expression can be found by rewriting Equation (10) using Equation (8):

$$n_0 \lambda_D^3 = \left[\frac{T}{e^2/\varepsilon_0 a} \right]^{3/2}. \tag{11}$$

The quantity in the square brackets is the ratio of the mean kinetic energy of a particle, T, to the mean interaction potential energy $e^2/\varepsilon_0 a$ between nearest neighbors. This ratio must be large in the plasma state, so the plasma is a *nearly ideal gas* of weakly-interacting charges. However, this does not mean that one can ignore the *collective* interaction of many charges with one another, which gives rise to large potentials sufficient to screen out applied fields or produce plasma waves (as discussed in the next chapter).

Plasmas for which the plasma parameter is of order unity or even smaller than unity are referred to as non-ideal plasmas, or strongly-coupled plasmas [8]. Since the kinetic energy per particle is on the same order as, or even smaller than, the interaction energy, these plasmas might be better thought of as liquids or possibly even solids. The properties of non-ideal plasmas, and their study in Penning traps, will be the subject of other chapters in this course (for example, Chapters 12 and 15). Here, I will focus on "standard-issue" nearly-ideal plasmas.

Question (1a): If the capacitor plates are 1 cm apart and the plasma temperature is 10 eV, what density is required in order for there to be at least 10 Debye lengths between the plates?

Question (1b): The Orion Nebula is a roughly spherical mass of almost fully-ionized Hydrogen with a radius of about 20 light years and a mean charged particle density of roughly $n_0 = 10^8\,\text{m}^{-3}$. If it were in thermal equilibrium (it is not — portions of it are far from equilibrium!) with a temperature of $T = 100\,\text{eV}$, what would its Debye length be? Under these assumptions, would you classify the Orion Nebula as a plasma?

2. Non-neutral Plasmas in Penning Traps

A non-neutral plasma is a plasma in which the number of negative and positive charge species are unequal [6]. Most plasmas are at least slightly non-neutral; such plasmas are often referred to as "quasi-neutral". In this chapter, I will be concerned with fully-unneutralized plasmas consisting only of species with the same sign of charge. Many such plasmas that have been created and studied experimentally: pure electron plasmas [9], mixed electron and antiproton plasmas [10], mixed positron and positive ion plasmas [11], negative ion plasmas [12]. In these experiments, the plasmas can satisfy relations 9 and 10, and therefore exhibit strong Debye shielding of externally applied potentials.

These fully-unneutralized non-neutral plasmas are studied for a number of reasons. First and possibly foremost, they have exceptional confinement properties: they can be confined in a rotating thermal equilibrium state away from surrounding walls in an electromagnetic bottle called a Penning trap [13] that uses only static electric and magnetic fields [14]. (We will see that the same cannot be said of neutral plasmas!) The existence of a confined thermal equilibrium state implies that the plasmas are inherently low noise and reproducible since there is no free energy available to drive the kinds of instabilities that plague neutral plasma devices.

The range of densities that can be accessed by these non-neutral plasmas is smaller than for neutral plasmas, and it depends on the strength of the confining magnetic field. Densities are typically less than $10^{16}\,\mathrm{m}^{-3}$ for pure electron plasmas, and even less for ions. However, the temperatures in experiments can range over many orders of magnitude from 1 mK up to 10 eV or more, allowing a range of phenomena to be studied. For example, if a neutral plasma were cooled to 1 mK, it would immediately recombine to a neutral gas. However, in a fully-unneutralized plasma, there is no oppositely charged species with which to recombine. Furthermore, at such low temperatures, the plasma parameter is much smaller than unity and the plasma is strongly-coupled, exhibiting liquid and even crystalline phases. This interesting behavior will be discussed in, e.g. Chapters 12 and 15.

Here, I will first consider the confinement characteristics of a non-neutral plasma in a Penning trap.

2.1. *The Penning–Malmberg Trap*

Figure 2 shows a schematic of a Penning–Malmberg trap (a Penning trap with cylindrical electrodes [9]). Voltages are applied to the end electrodes in

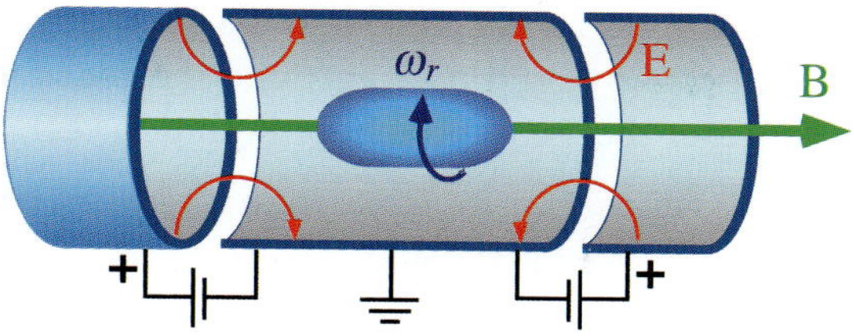

Fig. 2. Cutaway view of the cylindrical electrodes showing a positively-charged non-neutral plasma confined in a Penning–Malmberg trap.

order to produce a potential well in the axial direction that confines charges with a given sign of charge (assumed positive in the case of Figure 2). Confinement against radial plasma expansion is provided by the magnetic field $\mathbf{B} = B\hat{z}$, directed along the axis of symmetry of the trap. The plasma rotates around the axis of symmetry, and the rotational velocity provides an inward-directed $\mathbf{v} \times \mathbf{B}$ force that balances the outward-directed radial electric force from the unneutralized plasma charge.

To analyze this plasma configuration in more detail, I will apply fluid equations of motion. For a single-species plasma consisting of charges with mass m, charge q, and density n, the momentum equation for the plasma's fluid velocity $\mathbf{u}$ is (Section 3.3, [1,18])

$$mn\left(\frac{\partial \mathbf{u}}{\partial t} + \mathbf{u} \cdot \nabla \mathbf{u}\right) = qn\left(-\nabla\phi + \mathbf{u} \times \mathbf{B}\right) - \nabla p, \tag{12}$$

where p is the plasma's thermal pressure. In what follows, q is a signed quantity; it can be either positive or negative.

Throughout the rest of this chapter, I will also assume that the plasma has achieved a confined thermal equilibrium state. In this thermal equilibrium state, the plasma rotates, with a the time-independent fluid velocity given by the expression $\mathbf{u}(r) = -\omega_r r\widehat{\theta}$, where cylindrical coordinates are being employed, and ω_r is the rotation frequency (in radians per second). The negative sign in this expression reflects the fact that a positively charged plasma will rotate in the $-\widehat{\theta}$-direction; thus, for positive plasmas ω_r is a positive quantity; but for a negative plasma ω_r is less than zero.

In thermal equilibrium, the plasma rotation frequency is constant in time and uniform in space; if it were non-uniform, viscous effects would cause any such velocity shears to relax until the plasma rotates rigidly.

Also, in thermal equilibrium, the plasma pressure p is related to density and temperature T through the ideal gas law (since the plasma is a nearly ideal gas): $p = nT$, where T is time-independent and uniform in space (note that throughout the chapter I measure T in units of energy). If the temperatures were not uniform, it would relax through thermal conduction.

First, let us consider the z-component of Equation (12):

$$0 = -qn\frac{\partial \phi}{\partial z} - T\frac{\partial n}{\partial z}. \tag{13}$$

Consider first the "zero-temperature" limit (i.e. the regime where temperatures are small enough so that the second "pressure" term on the rhs can be neglected). In this limit, the equation implies that wherever the density is non-zero, the z-component of the electric field is zero. This is the Debye-shielding phenomenon discussed in the previous section, in the limit of zero Debye length. More generally, at finite T, the z-electric field is shielded out inside the plasma within a few Debye lengths of the plasma surface.

For finite T, Equation (13) can be integrated to yield the Boltzmann-like relation,

$$n(r,z) = N(r)\exp[-q\phi(r,z)/T], \tag{14}$$

for any function $N(r)$. This function is determined by the radial component of the momentum equation, which is given below:

$$-mn\omega_r^2 r = -qn\left(\frac{\partial \phi}{\partial r} + B\omega_r r\right) - T\frac{\partial n}{\partial r}. \tag{15}$$

The term on the lhs is the centripetal force density associated with rigid rotation arising from the $\mathbf{u}\cdot\nabla\mathbf{u}$ term in Equation (12). This force density must be in balance with the radial forces from the electric potential, rotation through the magnetic field, and pressure.

2.2. *Plasma density*

By substituting Equation (14) for the density into Equation (15), some cancelations occur and the result is a simple differential equation for $N(r)$:

$$T\frac{\partial N}{\partial r} = -m\omega_r(\Omega_c - \omega_r)r\,N, \tag{16}$$

where $\Omega_c = qB/m$ is the cyclotron frequency [a positive(negative) quantity for positive (negative) charges]. This equation can be integrated and the result combined with Equation (14) to yield the following expression for the plasma density in thermal equilibrium:

$$n(r,z) = C\exp\{-q[\phi(r,z) + \phi_{eff}(r)]/T\}, \tag{17}$$

where C is a constant of integration and where the *effective potential* ϕ_{eff} is defined as

$$q\phi_{eff}(r) \equiv \tfrac{1}{2}m\omega_r(\Omega_c - \omega_r)r^2. \tag{18}$$

This quadratic potential provides radial confinement due to rotation: provided that $\omega_r(\Omega_c - \omega_r) > 0$, the effective potential becomes large at large r, dominating over ϕ and forcing the density to become exponentially small (see Equation (17)). This inequality requires that $0 < \omega_r/\Omega_c < 1$ for confinement. If ω_r/Ω_c were greater than unity, the deconfining centrifugal force would win out over the confining $\mathbf{v} \times \mathbf{B}$ force.

In order to close the system and solve for the density, one must determine the potential $\phi(r, z)$. This is done solving the Poisson equation with boundary conditions given by the voltages on the cylindrical electrodes, and with density in terms of ϕ given by Equation (17):

$$\nabla^2\phi(r, z) = -qn(r, z)/\varepsilon_0. \tag{19}$$

2.3. *The uniform background charge, the Brillouin limit, and fluid drifts*

There is another useful way to think about the effective potential that aids in understanding the solution to Equation (19). A quadratic radial potential can also be produced by a cylinder of uniform density negative background charge. Using the Poisson equation, it is easy to show that the background density n_0 required to create an effective potential given by Equation (18) is

$$n_0 = 2\frac{m\varepsilon_0}{q^2}\omega_r(\Omega_c - \omega_r). \tag{20}$$

Thus, one can think of the plasma as being radially confined by this cylindrical neutralizing background charge rather than by rotation through a magnetic field; Equation (16) for the plasma density would be the same either way. Intuitively, one would then expect that, in equilibrium, the plasma matches its density to the background charge density, out to some surface of revolution (determined by the total number of particles, the uniform background density n_0, and the voltages applied to the electrodes) where the supply of plasma charge is exhausted and the density approaches zero. [15] In fact, this is just what the solutions to Equations (19) and (17) show. [17] At the plasma surface, the density falls from n_0 to zero on the scale of a few Debye lengths. Thus, within the plasma (i.e. several Debye lengths away from the edge) the density is uniform and given by Equation (20), provided that the plasma length and radius are both large compared to the Debye length.

Experiments with nearly-uniform density plasmas are often carried out in a regime where $\omega_r/\Omega_c \ll 1$. In this regime, one can easily solve Equation (20) for the rotation frequency in terms of the plasma density by approximating $\Omega_c - \omega_r \approx \Omega_c$ in Equation (20), yielding

$$\omega_r \approx \frac{q n_0}{2\varepsilon_0 B}. \tag{21}$$

This equation shows that, at low densities, increasing the density requires a higher rotation frequency in order to produce a larger $\mathbf{v} \times \mathbf{B}$ confining force that balances the larger electrostatic repulsion. However, Equation (20) shows that this balance only works up to a point: if the rotation rate is raised too high, centrifugal force begins to win out over the $\mathbf{v} \times \mathbf{B}$ force, and the density actually decreases as the rotation rate increases. For this reason, there is a maximum possible plasma density that can be confined in thermal equilibrium, called the *Brillouin limit*, [16]. The Brillouin limit follows from the form of Equation (20), which implies that as one varies ω_r the density reaches a maximum value n_B when $\omega_r = \Omega_c/2$, given by

$$\begin{aligned} n_B &= \frac{m\varepsilon_0 \Omega_c^2}{2q^2} \\ &= \frac{B^2}{2\mu_0 m c^2}, \end{aligned} \tag{22}$$

where I have used the identity $\varepsilon_0 \mu_0 = 1/c^2$. Equation (22) shows that the plasma's maximum rest energy density $n_B m c^2$ is equal to the magnetic energy $B^2/2\mu_0$. This implies a fairly low maximum density for magnetic fields currently available in the laboratory. For electrons in a 1 Tesla field, the density at the Brillouin limit is 4.8×10^{18} m^{-3}.

Another useful equation relating the plasma rotation frequency to the plasma density and potential is found by dividing Equation (15) by $mnr\Omega_c$ and rearranging terms so that the equation reads

$$\omega_r = -\frac{1}{Br}\frac{\partial \phi}{\partial r} - \frac{T}{qBrn}\frac{\partial n}{\partial r} + \frac{\omega_r^2}{\Omega_c}. \tag{23}$$

Thus, the uniform rotation frequency is a sum of three terms, which correspond to three different effects. The first term on the rhs of Equation (23) can be recognized as the rotation frequency arising from the $\mathbf{E} \times \mathbf{B}$ drift

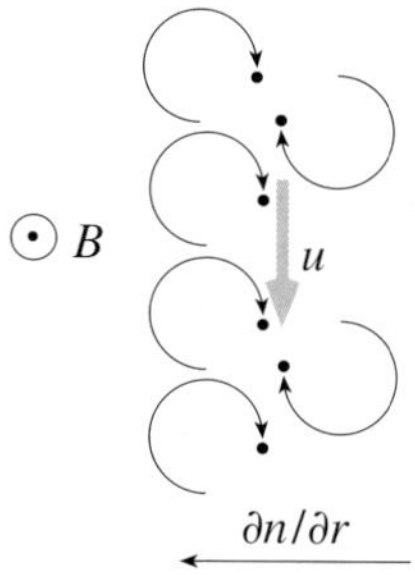

Fig. 3. The diamagnetic drift produces a contribution to the fluid velocity **u** at the plasma edge.

discussed in other chapters (see Chapter 3 for a derivation of this drift). At low rotation frequencies and in a cold plasma, this term dominates and is responsible for the rotation frequency given by Equation (21).

The last term in Equation (23) is a correction to the $\mathbf{E} \times \mathbf{B}$ drift caused by the centrifugal force from rotation, which produces an extra $\mathbf{F} \times \mathbf{B}$ drift. The middle term, proportional to the temperature, is a rotation of the plasma induced by the *diamagnetic drift*. This drift is caused by cyclotron motion in a non-uniform plasma. Figure 3 shows a close-up of a section of the plasma edge. The magnetic field is out of the page. In this figure, the $\mathbf{E} \times \mathbf{B}$ and centrifugal drifts are neglected, so charges simply undergo circular cyclotron motion. However, the existence of a density gradient implies that there are more particles on the left than on the right and consequently at any radius, the particle cyclotron motion causes a net fluid velocity downward (assuming positive charges), as depicted in the figure.

The diamagnetic fluid velocity is closely connected to the diamagnetic currents associated with diamagnetic materials. In these materials, an applied magnetic field induces magnetic dipole moments in particles making up the material, and these dipoles act to produce a surface current that creates a magnetic field opposed to the applied field. In the plasma, cyclotron motion due to the applied magnetic field produces current loops (see Figure 3) that also have magnetic moments, and there is therefore also a net surface current. Furthermore, one can show that this surface current creates a magnetic field that opposes the applied magnetic field; it is, truly, a *diamagnetic* current. This diamagnetic contribution to the magnetic field has been neglected (as have the contributions from the $\mathbf{E} \times \mathbf{B}$ and centrifugal drifts) because these self-generated fields are weak in most experiments (see Question 2 at the end of the chapter).

2.4. *The velocity distribution, canonical momentum, and the vortex frequency*

In thermal equilibrium, the full distribution function $f(\mathbf{r}, \mathbf{v})$ is a product of the equilibrium density given by Equation (17) and a Maxwellian velocity distribution, shifted by the fluid rotation velocity $\mathbf{u} = -\omega_r r\widehat{\theta}$:

$$f(\mathbf{r}, \mathbf{v}) = \frac{C}{(2\pi T/m)^{3/2}} e^{-q(\phi+\phi_{eff})/T} e^{-m(\mathbf{v}+\omega_r r\widehat{\theta})^2/2T} \tag{24}$$

$$= \frac{C}{(2\pi T/m)^{3/2}} e^{-H_r/T}, \tag{25}$$

where

$$H_r \equiv \frac{m}{2}(\mathbf{v} + \omega_r r\widehat{\theta})^2 + q\phi(r, z) + q\phi_{eff}(r). \tag{26}$$

The function H_r is the particle energy as seen in a frame rotating with the plasma: the particle velocity as seen in the rotating frame is $\mathbf{v} + \omega_r r\widehat{\theta}$, and the kinetic energy in this frame is proportional to the square of this apparent velocity. Also, this velocity is, on average, zero: the plasma is stationary when seen in the rotating frame (i.e. the mean fluid velocity is zero in this frame). The frame is not inertial and consequently there is an effective potential $e\phi_{eff}(r)$ due to centrifugal and Lorentz forces arising from rotation. When viewed in the rotating frame, the distribution function for this apparently stationary equilibrium plasma has the expected Boltzmann form, Equation (25) [14].

It is useful to rewrite the particle kinetic energy in terms of the *canonical momentum* $\mathbf{p} = m\mathbf{v} + q\mathbf{A}$, where $\mathbf{A}$ is the vector potential. For a uniform magnetic field $\mathbf{B} = B\hat{z}$, the vector potential can be expressed as $\mathbf{A} = Br\widehat{\theta}/2$. This implies one may write the particle velocity $\mathbf{v}$ in terms of $\mathbf{p}$ as

$$\mathbf{v} = \frac{\mathbf{p}}{m} - \frac{1}{2}\Omega_c r\widehat{\theta}.$$

Applying this expression for the velocity to Equation (26) yields

$$H_r = \frac{m}{2}(\mathbf{p} - m\Omega_v r\widehat{\theta}/2)^2 + q\phi(r, z) + q\phi_{eff}(r), \tag{27}$$

where I have introduced the vortex frequency Ω_v, defined as

$$\Omega_v \equiv \Omega_c - 2\omega_r. \tag{28}$$

The vortex frequency is the cyclotron frequency as seen in the rotating frame: one can recognize Equation (27) as the Hamiltonian of a charged particle as seen in this frame. The cyclotron frequency is shifted by coriolis force effects. It is well known that coriolis force caused by rotation has a form equivalent to the Lorentz $\mathbf{v} \times \mathbf{B}$ force, so it should not be too surprising that it acts to shift the cyclotron frequency.

Note that at the Brillouin limit, where the rotation frequency is half the cyclotron frequency, Equation (28) implies that the vortex frequency vanishes. At the Brillouin limit, particle motion as seen in the rotating frame is effectively unmagnetized.

2.5. *Total angular momentum*

Constants of the motion can be useful in understanding the dynamics of the plasma. Since the applied electromagnetic fields used to confine the plasma are (ideally) cylindrically-symmetric, the total canonical angular momentum P_θ is a conserved quantity. This quantity is a sum over the angular momentum of each particle:

$$P_\theta \equiv \sum_{i=1}^{N} \left(m v_{\theta i} r_i + \frac{qB}{2} r_i^2 \right). \tag{29}$$

The first term is the usual kinetic angular momentum, and the second term is the vector-potential contribution arising from the uniform magnetic field. In a strong magnetic field, this term dominates over the first term, and one may write

$$P_\theta \approx \sum_{i=1}^{N} \frac{qB}{2} r_i^2. \tag{30}$$

In other words, the angular momentum is proportional to the mean square radius of the plasma. Since the angular momentum is a conserved quantity, the plasma mean square radius cannot change over time, which greatly limits plasma loss in a Penning trap: if any plasma charge is lost to the electrodes surrounding the plasma, other charges must compensate by moving inward so that the mean square radius is unchanged.

Note also that in a neutral plasma, with both signs of charge present, angular momentum conservation does not aid confinement in this way: a positive and a negative charge can move outward together without changing P_θ. This is what makes neutral plasmas much more difficult to confine than non-neutral plasmas.

Finally, note that in real traps, slight torques on the plasma from asymmetries in the confinement fields, or from collisions with neutral gas, cause the angular momentum to change. These torques drag on the plasma, slowing its rotation. This makes the plasma expand radially (as well as heat) as the confining Lorentz force decreases. However, by operating in ultrahigh vacuum conditions, and by constructing the trap carefully so as to ensure a high degree of cylindrical symmetry in the electrodes, these torques can be minimized, allowing confinement times ranging from hours to even days. Also, a method known as the "rotating wall" has been used to counteract these effects and allow infinite-time confinement. The rotating wall method will be the subject of Chapter 11.

Question 2: Rotation of a long plasma column consisting of a single-species (say, positrons) with uniform density n_0 and radius r_p, produces a magnetic field. I neglected this magnetic field in this chapter. Evaluate this self-generated magnetic field, and explain why it is a good approximation to neglect it in typical Penning trap experiments. (*Hint*: In typical experiments, $\omega_r r_p \ll c$.) Does the induced field enhance or reduce the applied magnetic field $B\hat{z}$?

2.6. *Solutions to the exercises*

Question 1:

(a) Square both sides of the relation $L/\lambda_D = 10$ and substitute the definition of the Debye length, Equation (8), to obtain $L^2 e^2 n_0/(\epsilon_0 T) = 100$. Solve for n_0 using $T = 10\,\text{eV}$ and $L = 0.01$ m, to obtain $n_0 = 5.5 \times 10^{14}\ \text{m}^{-3}$.
(b) At the stated density and temperature, the Debye length is, according to Equation (8), $\lambda_D = 0.743\,\text{m}$. This is much smaller than the size of the system, meeting criterion (9). Also, the plasma parameter as given by Equation (11) is 4×10^7, which is much greater than unity, meeting criterion (10). At the given temperature and density, the Orion Nebula is a plasma.

Question 2: An electron column with uniform charge density $-en_0$, rotating rigidly with fluid velocity $\mathbf{u} = -\omega_r r\hat{\theta}$, will produce a current density $\mathbf{j} = en_0\omega_r r\hat{\theta}$ (where $\omega_r < 0$ for electrons). Such a current density produces a magnetic field $B_z(r)\hat{z}$. According to Ampere's law, this magnetic field satisfies the differential equation $\partial B_z/\partial r = -\mu_0 j_\theta(r)$. Solving this differential equation for $B_z(r)$ using the boundary condition that outside the plasma $B_z = B$ (where B is the constant externally-applied field) yields

$$B_z(r) = -\frac{\mu_0 e n_0 \omega_r}{2}(r^2 - r_p^2) + B, \quad r < r_p. \tag{31}$$

The total magnetic field is less than B inside the plasma (recall that for electrons, $\omega_r < 0$). The maximum change from B occurs at the origin, and is given by $B - B_z(0) = -\mu_0 e n_0 \omega_r r_p^2/2$. Using Equation (20), $\Omega_c = -eB/c$, and the identity $\mu_0 \epsilon_0 = 1/c^2$, this expression can be rewritten as

$$B - B_z(0) = B\frac{\omega_r^2 r_p^2}{c^2}\left(1 - \frac{\omega_r}{\Omega_c}\right). \tag{32}$$

Since $|\omega_r| r_p \ll c$ in typical experiments, this expression shows that the self-generated magnetic field is negligible compared to B.

References

1. F. Chen, *Introduction to Plasma Physics and Controlled Fusion*, 2nd. Ed. New York, Springer (2006).
2. S. Ichimaru, *Basic Principles of Plasma Physics*. MA, W. A. Benjamin, Reading (1973).
3. D. Pine and D. Bohm, A collective description of electron interactions: III. Coulomb interactions in a degenerate electron gas, *Phys. Rev.* **92**, 609–625 (1953).
4. W. J. De Haas and P. M. Van Alphen, The dependence of the susceptibility of diamagnetic metals, *Amsterdam Ac.* **33**, 1106–1118 (1930).
5. L. D. Landau, Paramagnetism of metals, *Z. Physik* **64**, 629–637 (1930).
6. R. Davidson, *Theory of Nonneutral Plasmas*. Benjamin, Reading MA (1974).
7. L. Boltzmann, Über die beziehung dem zweiten haubtsatze der mechanischen wärmetheorie und der wahrscheinlichkeitsrechnung respektive den sätzen über das wärmegleichgewicht, *Wiener Berichte*. **76**, 373–435 (1887).
8. S. Ichimaru, Strongly-coupled plasmas: high-density classical plasmas and degenerate electron liquids, *Rev. Mod. Phys.* **54**, 1017–1059 (1982).
9. J. H. Malmberg and J. S. deGrassie, Properties of nonneutral plasma, *Phys. Rev. Lett.* **35**, 577–580 (1975).
10. G. B. Andresen *et al.*, Centrifugal separation and equilibration dynamics in an electron-antiproton plasma, *Phys. Rev. Lett.* **106**, 145001 (2011).
11. B. M. Jelenkovic *et al.*, *Nuclear Instruments and Methods in Physics Research B* **192**, 117 (2002).
12. A. Kabantsev, *private communication*.
13. F. M. Penning, Die Glimmentladung bei niedrigem Druck zwischen koaxialen Zylindern in einem axialen Magnetfeld, *Physica (Amsterdam)* **3**, 873–894 (1936).
14. D. H. E. Dubin and T. M. O'Neil, Trapped nonneutral plasmas, liquids and crystals (the thermal equilibrium states), *Rev. Mod Phys.* **71**, 87–172 (1999).
15. J. H. Malmberg and T. M. O'Neil, Pure electron plasma, liquid, and crystal, *Phys. Rev. Lett.* **39**, 1333–1335 (1977).
16. L. Brillouin, A theorem of larmor and its importance for electrons in magnetic fields, *Phys. Rev.* **67**, 260–266 (1945).
17. S. A. Prasad and T. M. O'Neil, Finite length thermal equilibria of a pure electron plasma column, *Phys. Fluids* **22**, 278–281 (1979).
18. P. K. Kundu, *Fluid Mechanics*. San Diego, Academic Press (1990).

CHAPTER TEN

PLASMA MODES

D. H. E. Dubin

Dept of Physics UCSD, La Jolla, CA 92093
ddubin@ucsd.edu

This chapter explores several aspects of the linear electrostatic normal modes of oscillation for a single-species non-neutral plasma in a Penning trap. Linearized fluid equations of motion are developed, assuming the plasma is cold but collisionless, which allow derivation of the cold plasma dielectric tensor and the electrostatic wave equation. Upper hybrid and magnetized plasma waves in an infinite uniform plasma are described. The effect of the plasma surface in a bounded plasma system is considered, and the properties of surface plasma waves are characterized. The normal modes of a cylindrical plasma column are discussed, and finally, modes of spheroidal plasmas, and finite temperature effects on the modes, are briefly described.

1. Introduction: The Plasma Dielectric Tensor

When a single-species plasma trapped in a Penning trap is perturbed away from its equilibrium state, it rings at frequencies associated with normal modes of oscillation. These plasma modes are the subject of the following chapter. To describe the normal modes, I will use a fluid theory approach as in the previous chapter, but I will further simplify by assuming the plasma is cold, neglecting the thermal pressure in the equations of motion. Also, I will describe the modes in the rotating frame of the plasma, where in equilibrium it is stationary. I will also only consider small amplitude perturbations from equilibrium, oscillating in time with frequency ω (where ω is to be determined; note that this is the frequency as seen in the *rotating frame*, Doppler shifted with respect to the lab-frame frequency ω_{lab}).

Thus, within the plasma the density is $n(\mathbf{r}, t) = n_0 + \delta n(\mathbf{r})e^{-i\omega t}$, where δn is the density perturbation, and the equilibrium density n_0 is given by Equation (20). Also, the fluid velocity is $\mathbf{u}(\mathbf{r}, t) = \mathbf{0} + \delta\mathbf{u}(\mathbf{r})e^{-i\omega t}$, and the potential is $\phi(\mathbf{r}, t) = \phi_0(r, z) + \delta\phi(\mathbf{r})e^{-i\omega t}$, where ϕ_0 is the equilibrium potential (including the effective potential since we work in the rotating frame).

Then, to linear order in the perturbed quantities, the momentum equation, Equation (12) of the previous chapter, becomes

$$-i\omega\delta\mathbf{u} = -\frac{q}{m}\nabla\delta\phi + \Omega_v\delta\mathbf{u} \times \hat{z}. \tag{1}$$

The convective derivative $\mathbf{u} \cdot \nabla\mathbf{u}$ is dropped in Equation (12) because it is nonlinear in $\delta\mathbf{u}$, and the vortex frequency appears rather than the cyclotron frequency because we are working in the rotating frame (see Equation (28) of the previous chapter).

Equation (1) is linear in $\delta\mathbf{u}$ and can therefore be solved directly for $\delta\mathbf{u}$ (see Question 1). It is convenient to write this solution as

$$\delta\mathbf{u} = -\frac{\sigma \cdot \nabla\delta\phi}{qn_0}, \tag{2}$$

where σ is the conductivity tensor for the plasma, with components

$$\sigma = i\begin{pmatrix} \sigma_1 & i\sigma_2 & 0 \\ -i\sigma_2 & \sigma_1 & 0 \\ 0 & 0 & \sigma_3 \end{pmatrix}, \tag{3}$$

and where $\sigma_1 = \varepsilon_0\omega_p^2\omega/(\omega^2 - \Omega_v^2)$, $\sigma_2 = \varepsilon_0\omega_p^2\Omega_v/(\omega^2 - \Omega_v^2)$, and $\sigma_3 = \varepsilon_0\omega_p^2/\omega$. Here, I introduce the *plasma frequency* ω_p, defined in terms of the equilibrium density n_0 by

$$\omega_p \equiv \sqrt{q^2 n_0/\varepsilon_0 m}. \tag{4}$$

The plasma frequency is a natural frequency of oscillation in cold unmagnetized plasmas, as we will see.

The conductivity tensor σ expresses the linear relationship between the perturbed electric field $-\nabla\delta\phi$, and the perturbed current density $qn_0\delta\mathbf{u}$. The conductivity is a tensor rather than a scalar because an electric field in the x-direction produces a current in both the x- and y-directions (an effect caused by the magnetic field; see Question 1).

Question 1: Prove Equations (2) and (3) by solving Equation (1).

In order to obtain an equation for the mode frequencies, I will now combine Equation (2) with the continuity equation, describing the evolution of the particle density:

$$\frac{\partial n}{\partial t} + \nabla \cdot (n\mathbf{u}) = 0. \tag{5}$$

When this equation is linearized, one obtains

$$-i\omega\delta n + \nabla\cdot(n_0\delta\mathbf{u}) = 0. \tag{6}$$

Substituting for $\delta\mathbf{u}$ from Equation (2) and solving for δn yields

$$\delta n = -\frac{i}{q\omega}\nabla\cdot(\sigma \quad \cdot\nabla\delta\phi). \tag{7}$$

Finally, I combine this equation with the linearized Poisson equation, $\nabla^2\delta\phi = -\delta n/\varepsilon_0$, to obtain the following electrostatic wave equation:

$$\nabla\cdot\varepsilon\cdot\nabla\delta\phi = 0. \tag{8}$$

Here, $\varepsilon = \mathbf{1} + i\sigma/\omega\varepsilon_0$ is the frequency-dependent *plasma dielectric tensor* (where $\mathbf{1}$ is the unit tensor), with the following components:

$$\varepsilon = \begin{pmatrix} \varepsilon_1 & -i\varepsilon_2 & 0 \\ i\varepsilon_2 & \varepsilon_1 & 0 \\ 0 & 0 & \varepsilon_3 \end{pmatrix}, \tag{9}$$

and where the dielectric coefficients are

$$\begin{aligned} \varepsilon_1 &= 1 - \frac{\omega_p^2}{\omega^2 - \Omega_v^2}, \\ \varepsilon_2 &= \frac{\omega_p^2\Omega_v}{\omega(\omega^2 - \Omega_v^2)}, \\ \varepsilon_3 &= 1 - \frac{\omega_p^2}{\omega^2}. \end{aligned} \tag{10}$$

These coefficients follow from the components of the conductivity tensor given in Equation (3). For example, $\epsilon_2 = \sigma_2/(\epsilon_0\omega)$. The dielectric tensor is not isotropic because the applied magnetic field and plasma rotation break the isotropy. Note that if Ω_v is zero, the dielectric tensor takes the unmagnetized isotropic form $\varepsilon = \varepsilon_3\mathbf{1}$.

Equation (8) contains all the information about the electrostatic cold plasma modes of oscillation. This equation shows that one can think of the plasma as a dielectric medium; the motion of charges in a normal mode polarizes the dielectric producing an electric displacement $\mathbf{D} = -\varepsilon\cdot\nabla\delta\phi$ that satisfies the Poisson equation for dielectric media, $\nabla\cdot\mathbf{D} = 0$. The problem of finding the plasma normal modes is then reduced to finding non-trivial solutions to this equation.

2. Waves in an Unmagnetized Plasma

Within an unmagnetized uniform single-species plasma with $\Omega_v = 0$ (i.e. at the Brillouin limit), the dielectric is isotropic and Equation (8) can be written as

$$\varepsilon_3 \nabla^2 \delta\phi = 0, \tag{11}$$

where ε_3 is given by Equation (10). Thus, either $\nabla^2 \delta\phi = 0$ which by the Poisson equation implies there is no density perturbation (and hence no mode), or $\nabla^2 \delta\phi \neq 0$ and instead $\varepsilon_3 = 0$. By Equation (10), this condition requires that $\omega = \omega_p$. This is the frequency of plasma oscillations in a cold unmagnetized uniform single-species plasma. Interestingly, the spatial form of the plasma perturbation is unimportant; all such perturbations oscillate at the plasma frequency!

To understand why the plasma rings at this frequency, consider the simple perturbation sketched in Figure 1. A portion of the plasma in the shape of a slab is shifted slightly to the right by distance Δx. This increases the density to twice its original value in a narrow region of width Δx on the right side, and reduces it to zero in a narrow region of identical width on the left side. However, recall that there is a uniform neutralizing background that allows the unperturbed density to remain in equilibrium. Thus, the total charge density including the background in the narrow region on the right side is qn_0, and on the left side it is $-qn_0$. This configuration produces a uniform electric field E_x between the two sides:

$$E_x = -\frac{\Delta\sigma}{\varepsilon_0} = -\frac{qn_0\Delta x}{\varepsilon_0}, \tag{12}$$

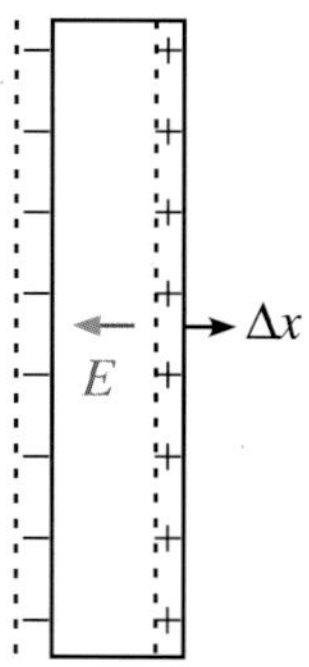

Fig. 1. A positively charged non-neutral plasma slab moves to the right by Δx, uncovering the neutralizing background charge on the left and overlapping the equilibrium plasma on the right.

where $\Delta\sigma$ is the charge per unit area in the narrow region on the right side. This electric field acts on the slab, pulling it back toward its equilibrium position where $\Delta x = 0$. According to Newton,

$$\Delta\ddot{x} = \frac{Q}{M}E_x = -\frac{qQn_0}{M\varepsilon_0}\Delta x, \tag{13}$$

where M and Q are the total mass and total charge of the slab respectively. However, since $Q/M = q/m$ in a single-species plasma, Equation (13) becomes $\Delta\ddot{x} = -\omega_p^2 \Delta x$ (see Equation (4)), a harmonic oscillator equation with frequency ω_p.

3. Waves in a Uniform Magnetized Plasma

If one neglects reflections from the plasma edges, assuming that the plasma is large, one can use a Fourier representation for wave solutions in the plasma of the form

$$\delta\phi(\mathbf{r}, t) = Ae^{i\mathbf{k}\cdot r - i\omega t}, \tag{14}$$

where ω and $\mathbf{k}$ are the frequency and wavenumber of a traveling wave within the plasma, and A is the wave amplitude. (Recall that for traveling waves moving in three dimensions, the wavenumber is a vector whose magnitude $k = |\mathbf{k}|$ yields the wavelength through the relation $\lambda = 2\pi/k$ and whose direction $\hat{k} = \mathbf{k}/k$ is the direction of propagation of the phase fronts of the wave.)

Waves of this form allow direct solution of Equation (8), since $\nabla\delta\phi = i\mathbf{k}\delta\phi$. Applying Equation (14) to Equation (8) then yields the dispersion relation for waves in a cold uniform magnetized plasma:

$$k_\perp^2 \varepsilon_1 + k_z^2 \varepsilon_3 = 0, \tag{15}$$

where k_z is the component of the wave-vector in the direction of the magnetic field (the z-direction) and $k_\perp$ is the magnitude of the component of the wave vector that is perpendicular to $\mathbf{B}$: $k_\perp^2 = k_x^2 + k_y^2$.

Substituting for the dielectric coefficients ε_1 and ε_3 from Equation (10) and rearranging terms yields a quadratic equation for ω^2. The two solutions of this quadratic correspond to two different types of propagating wave in the plasma. The frequencies of each wave can be expressed in the form

$$\omega^2 = \frac{\Omega_{uh}^2}{2} \pm \frac{\sqrt{k_\perp^2 \Omega_{uh}^4 + k_z^2(\Omega_v^2 - \omega_p^2)^2}}{2k}, \tag{16}$$

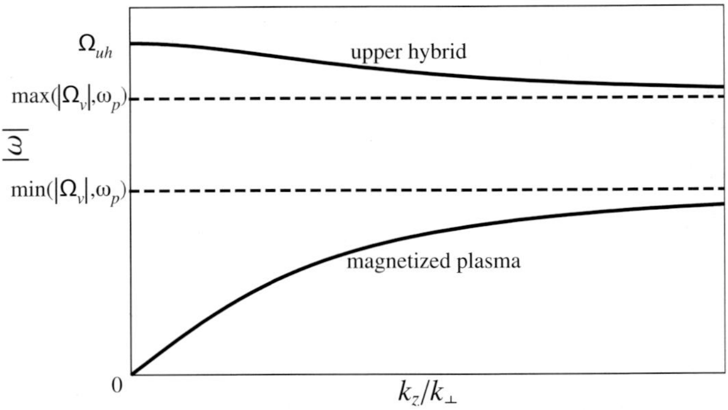

Fig. 2. Dispersion relation for upper hybrid and magnetized plasma waves in a uniform cold plasma.

where I have introduced the *upper hybrid frequency* Ω_{uh} (as seen in a rotating plasma) defined as

$$\Omega_{uh} = \sqrt{\Omega_v^2 + \omega_p^2}. \tag{17}$$

Waves with frequencies given by the upper sign in Equation (16) are generally referred to as *upper hybrid waves*, while waves with frequencies given by the lower sign are often called *magnetized plasma waves*. The dispersion relations for each wave are plotted in Figure 2. The frequency of each type of wave depends on the wavenumber only through its direction with respect to the magnetic field, parametrized in the figure by the ratio $k_z/k_\perp$. For waves propagating across the magnetic field, $k_z/k_\perp = 0$ and the wave frequencies for upper hybrid and magnetized plasma waves are Ω_{uh} and zero respectively. When the magnetic field vanishes, the upper hybrid waves become the unmagnetized plasma waves discussed in Section 2, and the magnetized plasma branch disappears. However, when the magnetic field is large so that $\Omega_v \gg \omega_p$, the dispersion relations for each branch simplify to

$$\omega^2 = \Omega_v^2 + \frac{k_\perp^2}{k^2}\omega_p^2, \quad \text{upper hybrid wave,} \tag{18}$$

$$\omega^2 = \frac{k_z^2}{k^2}\omega_p^2, \quad \text{magnetized plasma wave.} \tag{19}$$

In this regime, upper hybrid waves can be thought of as essentially a type of cyclotron motion with a frequency that is increased by the extra restoring force associated with the plasma response (see Question 2). The magnetized plasma waves are like unmagnetized plasma waves but with motion restricted to only the z-direction by the strong magnetic field.

Question 2: Recall that in Section 2, I analyzed unmagnetized plasma oscillations by considering a slab displaced in x by Δx. Redo this calculation but keep a magnetic field pointed in the z-direction, with cyclotron frequency Ω_v. Show that the plasma now rings at frequency Ω_{uh}. (*Hint*: The slab moves in both the x- and y-directions now.)

4. Modes in a Bounded Plasma

In a Penning trap, the plasma is not infinite and homogenous. This has several consequences. First, waves reflect from the plasma edges, setting up normal modes of oscillation. Most of these modes can be understood qualitatively by simply quantizing the possible values of k_z and $k_\perp$ in the previous dispersion relations obtained for homogeneous plasmas, such as Equation (16). For instance, for a long plasma column of length L, the modes have axial wavenumbers that roughly satisfy $k_z = m_z\pi/L$ for integer m_z. The lowest-order axial mode, $m_z = 0$, corresponds to a potential perturbation with no z-dependence within the plasma. The next axial mode, $(m_z = 1)$ has a single axial node in the center of the plasma, and so on. The possible quantized values of the perpendicular wavenumber $k_\perp$ for these modes are somewhat more difficult to categorize, requiring some algebra involving Bessel functions.

Another important finite plasma effect is the appearance of new modes associated with the plasma surface. The next subsection will analyze two types of surface plasma oscillations. For large magnetic fields they are referred to as a diocotron mode, with low frequency that scales as $1/B$, and a surface cyclotron mode, with a high frequency near the cyclotron frequency. (A third type of wave associated with the plasma surface(s), $\mathbf{E} \times \mathbf{B}$ modes, is discussed qualitatively at the end of the chapter.)

4.1. *Surface plasma waves*

Consider a plasma with density n_0 and a sharp edge at $x = 0$ as shown in Figure 3. As usual, there is a uniform magnetic field in the z-direction. Figure 3 could be thought of as a blow-up of a section of the plasma edge in a Penning trap plasma, with the x-direction the local direction of increasing plasma radius, and the y-direction in the direction of increasing θ. The

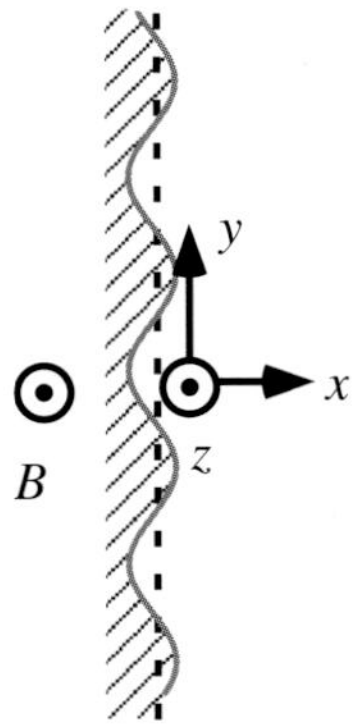

Fig. 3. A surface plasma wave perturbs the equilibrium surface (the dotted line) at $x = 0$.

plasma equilibrium is disturbed by a surface plasma wave. Such waves have potentials that are concentrated within a few wavelengths of the plasma surface. To simplify the analysis, I assume that the plasma radius and the distance to surrounding conducting walls are both large relative to the wavelength of the waves.

The waves propagate along the surface of the plasma, with a perturbed potential of the form

$$\delta\phi \propto e^{ik_y y + ik_z z - i\omega t}. \tag{20}$$

However, the x dependence of the potential is not so simple because of the plasma surface. Outside the plasma, where $x > 0$, the perturbed potential must satisfy the Laplace equation $\nabla^2 \delta\phi = 0$, which implies an exponential x dependence:

$$\delta\phi = e^{ik_y y + ik_z z - i\omega t}(Ae^{-kx} + Be^{kx}), \quad x > 0, \tag{21}$$

where A and B are undetermined constants, and $k = \sqrt{k_y^2 + k_z^2}$. Since the potential should not blow up at large x, one must set $B = 0$ in Equation (21).

On the other hand, inside the plasma, these surface waves satisfy Equation (8). Since the plasma is uniform, ε is a tensor with constant coefficients given by Equations (9) and (10). The equation then becomes

$$\varepsilon_1 \left(\frac{\partial^2 \delta\phi}{\partial x^2} + \frac{\partial^2 \delta\phi}{\partial y^2} \right) + \varepsilon_3 \frac{\partial^2 \delta\phi}{\partial z^2} = 0. \tag{22}$$

Substituting the assumed form for $\delta\phi$, Equation (20) implies that

$$\varepsilon_1 \frac{\partial^2 \delta\phi}{\partial x^2} = \left(k_y^2 \varepsilon_1 + k_z^2 \varepsilon_3\right) \delta\phi. \tag{23}$$

This differential equation has the general solution

$$\delta\phi = e^{ik_y y + ik_z z - i\omega t}(Ce^{-\kappa x} + De^{\kappa x}), \quad x < 0, \tag{24}$$

where $\kappa = \sqrt{k_y^2 + \varepsilon_3 k_z^2/\varepsilon_1}$. (For surface waves, κ is a real number, greater than zero.) The coefficient C must equal to zero in order to keep the solution from blowing up at large negative values of x.

The remaining coefficients A and D are related by matching the solution across the plasma boundary at $x = 0$. Continuity of the potential implies that $A = D$. However, the laws of electromagnetism also require that the normal component of the electric displacement $\mathbf{D} = -\varepsilon \cdot \nabla\phi$ be continuous across the boundary. When applied to Equations (21) and (24), and taking $A = D$ and $B = C = 0$, this requirement implies that

$$\hat{x} \cdot \varepsilon \cdot \nabla\, e^{\kappa x + ik_y y + ik_z z}|_{x=0} = -ke^{ik_y y + ik_z z}. \tag{25}$$

Applying Equation (9) and evaluating the LHS then yields

$$\kappa\varepsilon_1 + k_y \varepsilon_2 = -k. \tag{26}$$

This is the dispersion relation for surface plasma waves. Like the dispersion relation for waves in a uniform plasma, Equation (15), this dispersion relation depends on the direction of the wavenumber $\mathbf{k} = k_y\hat{y} + k_z\hat{z}$, but not its magnitude.

These surface waves propagate along the plasma surface, causing ripples in its shape, but their effect on the plasma falls off exponentially with distance from the surface, with length scale κ. The motion of the plasma surface can be understood in linear wave theory as causing a surface charge (charge per unit area) $\delta\sigma(y, z, t)$. Elementary electrostatics relates the surface charge to the jump in electric field across the surface:

$$\begin{aligned} \frac{\delta\sigma}{\epsilon_0} &= \frac{\partial\delta\phi}{\partial x}|_{x=0^-} - \frac{\partial\delta\phi}{\partial x}|_{x=0^+} \\ &= A(k+\kappa)e^{i(k_y y + k_z z - \omega t)}. \end{aligned} \tag{27}$$

The surface charge is due to a small change δx in the position of the surface as shown in Figure 3,

$$\delta\sigma = qn_0\delta x. \tag{28}$$

Combining Equations (27) and (28) gives the change in the position of the plasma surface due to the wave:

$$\delta x = A\frac{\epsilon_0}{qn_0}(k+\kappa)e^{i(k_y y + k_z z - \omega t)}. \tag{29}$$

There are two cases where the surface wave dispersion relation can be further simplified. First, for an ummagnetized plasma with $\Omega_v = 0$, Equation (10) implies that $\varepsilon_1 = \varepsilon_3 = 1 - \omega_p^2/\omega^2$ and $\varepsilon_2 = 0$, from which one may conclude that $\kappa = k$. Equation (26) then becomes

$$1 - \frac{\omega_p^2}{\omega^2} = -1,$$

which has the solution $\omega^2 = \omega_p^2/2$. This gives the frequency of unmagnetized surface plasma waves. Note that the frequency is the same for any wavenumber. These unmagnetized surface plasma waves do not just appear in Penning trap plasmas at the Brillouin limit. They are also observed propagating along the surface of metals, where they are usually called *surface plasmons* [1].

A second case that can be easily handled is when $k_z = 0$, i.e. propagation perpendicular to the magnetic field. In this case, $\kappa = k = k_y$ (assuming that k_y is positive), and Equation (26) becomes

$$\varepsilon_1 + \varepsilon_2 = -1. \tag{30}$$

Substituting for the dielectric coefficients from Equation (10) yields a quadratic equation for the wave frequency ω with the following two solutions:

$$\omega = -\frac{1}{2}\left(\Omega_v \pm \sqrt{\Omega_v^2 + 2\omega_p^2}\right). \tag{31}$$

Assuming that $\Omega_v > 0$, the upper sign gives the frequency of $k_z = 0$ *surface cyclotron waves*, and the lower sign yields the *diocotron wave* frequency. Although the waves have different frequencies, they both have the same value of $\kappa = k_y$ and hence the same functional form. When the vortex frequency is zero, Equation (31) returns to the unmagnetized surface plasma frequencies, but when $|\Omega_v| \gg \omega_p$, the two surface waves have the following approximate frequencies:

$$\omega \approx -\Omega_v - \frac{\omega_p^2}{2\Omega_v}, \quad \text{surface cyclotron wave,} \tag{32}$$

$$\omega \approx \frac{\omega_p^2}{2\Omega_v}, \quad \text{diocotron wave.} \tag{33}$$

The frequency of the diocotron wave in this large magnetic field regime scales as $1/B$ since in this regime, $\Omega_v \sim \Omega_c = qB/m$. Also, in this regime, the diocotron wave frequency (as seen in the frame rotating with the plasma) is the same as the plasma rotation rate itself (see Equation (21) in the previous chapter).

The sign of the frequency for these two surface waves has physical significance. Assuming $k_z = 0, k_y > 0$, and a positively-charged plasma, the surface cyclotron wave described by Equation (32) has negative frequency and a phase velocity in the $-y$ direction, while diocotron wave travels in the opposite $+y$ direction (as seen in the rotating frame where the equilibrium plasma is stationary). On a cylindrical plasma, the $-y$ direction corresponds to the $-\theta$-direction, so the surface cyclotron wave rotates around the plasma column in the same direction as the cyclotron motion of single particles. This is as opposed to the upper hybrid waves, which are in a similar frequency regime but can rotate in either direction on the plasma column.

Question 3: Show that in general there are two solutions to Equation (26) for the surface wave frequency *provided that* $\omega_p/|\Omega_v| \geq |k_z|/k$.

Question 4: Show that these solutions are

$$\omega = \frac{-k_y\Omega_v \pm \sqrt{2k^2\omega_p^2 + \Omega_v^2(k_y^2 + 2k_z^2)}}{2k}. \tag{34}$$

Question 5: Show that the values of κ for the two solutions are identical, for given values of the other parameters.

The dispersion curves given by Equation (34) are plotted in Figure 4 versus the direction of propagation of the waves as parametrized by k_z/k, and for three different magnetic field strengths, assuming $k_y \geq 0$ and a positively-charged plasma. In Figure 5, the value of κ/k is plotted. Note that in the large magnetic field limit, only $k_z = 0$ surface waves are allowed, but when $|\Omega_v|/\omega_p \leq 1$ waves may propagate along the surface in any direction. As $|\Omega_v|/\omega_p$ increases, the surface cyclotron frequency also increases in magnitude, following the (negative of) the cyclotron frequency, while the behavior of the diocotron branch is a bit more complicated: for small k_z/k the frequency decreases with increasing $|\Omega_v|$, as expected from Equation (31) or Equation (33), while for larger k_z/k the frequency can increase with increasing $|\Omega_v|$. For propagation parallel to **B** (which requires $|\Omega_v|/\omega_p < 1$), the two surface waves have equal but opposite frequencies, $\omega = \pm\Omega_{uh}/\sqrt{2}$. In this case, one might refer to the waves as surface upper hybrid waves.

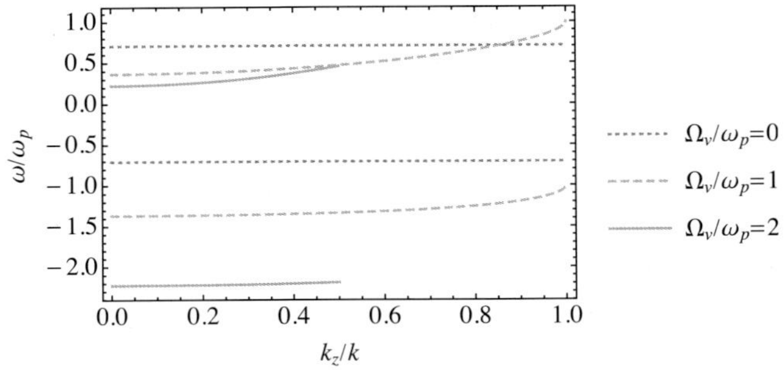

Fig. 4. Dispersion curves for the two surface plasma waves versus propagation direction, for three different magnetic field strengths.

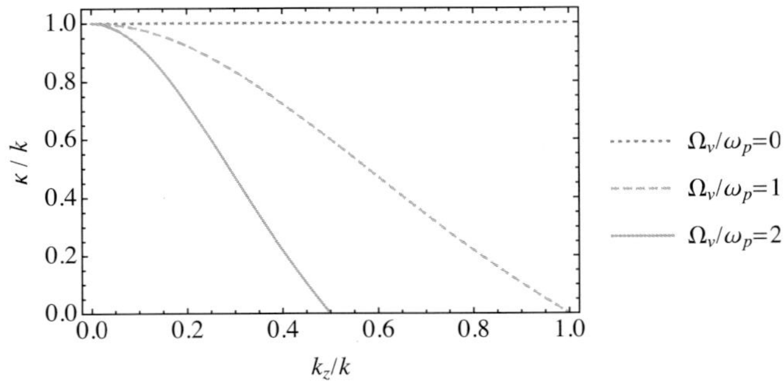

Fig. 5. Inverse decay length κ for surface plasma waves versus propagation direction, for three different magnetic field strengths.

4.2. *Cylindrical plasmas*

Plasma modes can be determined analytically in several other geometries of importance to Penning trap experiments. For a long uniform density plasma column of radius r_p and length L, running from $z = 0$ to $z = L$, and trapped along the axis of a hollow conducting cylinder of radius r_w, the dispersion relation involves Bessel function solutions of Equation (8), and is called the Trivelpiece–Gould (TG) dispersion relation [2]. The following remarks assume the reader's familiarity with basic properties of Bessel functions.

Within the plasma, where the tensor ϵ is uniform in space, Equation (8) can be expressed in cylindrical coordinates (r, θ, z) as

$$\varepsilon_1 \left(\frac{1}{r} \frac{\partial}{\partial r} r \frac{\partial \delta\phi}{\partial r} + \frac{1}{r^2} \frac{\partial^2 \delta\phi}{\partial \theta^2} \right) + \varepsilon_3 \frac{\partial^2 \delta\phi}{\partial z^2} = 0. \tag{35}$$

This differential equation is separable and the solution that is finite at the origin is

$$\delta\phi(\mathbf{r},t) = AJ_{m_\theta}(k_\perp r)\cos(k_z z)e^{im_\theta\theta - i\omega t}, \quad r < r_p, \tag{36}$$

where the non-negative integer m_θ is the azimuthal mode number, $k_z = m_z\pi/L$ where m_z is also a non-negative integer, and J_{m_θ} is a Bessel function of the first kind [19]. The transverse wavenumber $k_\perp$ is a separation constant that depends on k_z and ω through Equation (15):

$$k_\perp^2 = -k_z^2\epsilon_3/\epsilon_1. \tag{37}$$

The cosine form of the z dependence is chosen so that the axial electric field vanishes at the ends of the plasma column. For finite length plasma columns, this is a useful but rough approximation that improves as the length of the column increases [18,20].

Outside the plasma, the potential satisfies Laplace's equation (i.e. $\epsilon_1 = \epsilon_3 = 1$ in Equation (35)), and also vanishes at the conducting cylinder. The solution in this region is

$$\begin{aligned}\delta\phi(\mathbf{r},t) = B\left(I_{m_\theta}(k_z r)K_{m_\theta}(k_z r_w) - I_{m_\theta}(k_z r_w)K_{m_\theta}(k_z r)\right)\\ \times\cos(k_z z)e^{im_\theta\theta - i\omega t}, \quad r > r_p,\end{aligned} \tag{38}$$

where I_{m_θ} and K_{m_θ} are modified Bessel functions [19]. The coefficient B and the mode frequency ω are determined by matching the interior solution, Equation (36), to the above exterior solution. The potential must be continuous, implying that

$$AJ_{m_\theta}(k_\perp r_p) = B\left(I_{m_\theta}(k_z r_p)K_{m_\theta}(k_z r_w) - I_{m_\theta}(k_z r_w)K_{m_\theta}(k_z r_p)\right). \tag{39}$$

Also, integration of Equation (8) from $r = r_p^-$ to $r = r_p^+$ implies that

$$\hat{r}\cdot\epsilon\cdot\nabla\delta\phi|_{r_p^-} = \frac{\partial\delta\phi}{\partial r}|_{r_p^+}. \tag{40}$$

This result merely expresses the continuity of the normal component of the electric displacement $\mathbf{D} = \epsilon\cdot\nabla\delta\phi$ across the plasma surface, as discussed previously (see Equation (25)). Substituting for $\delta\phi$ from Equations (36) and (38) and using Equation (10) yields

$$\begin{aligned}&A\epsilon_1\frac{\partial}{\partial r_p}J_{m_\theta}(k_\perp r_p) + A\epsilon_2\frac{m_\theta}{r_p}J_{m_\theta}(k_\perp r_p)\\ &\quad = B\frac{\partial}{\partial r_p}\left(I_{m_\theta}(k_z r_p)K_{m_\theta}(k_z r_w) - I_{m_\theta}(k_z r_w)K_{m_\theta}(k_z r_p)\right).\end{aligned} \tag{41}$$

Substituting for A from Equation (39) yields the relation

$$\epsilon_1 \frac{\partial}{\partial r_p} J_{m_\theta}(k_\perp r_p) + \epsilon_2 \frac{m_\theta}{r_p} J_{m_\theta}(k_\perp r_p) = J_{m_\theta}(k_\perp r_p) \frac{\frac{\partial}{\partial r_p}\left(I_{m_\theta}(k_z r_p) K_{m_\theta}(k_z r_w) - I_{m_\theta}(k_z r_w) K_{m_\theta}(k_z r_p)\right)}{I_{m_\theta}(k_z r_p) K_{m_\theta}(k_z r_w) - I_{m_\theta}(k_z r_w) K_{m_\theta}(k_z r_p)}. \tag{42}$$

Equation (42) together with Equation (37) is the TG dispersion relation. In general, it yields real solutions for the mode frequency ω, but the solutions must be determined numerically. However, there are several limits where the dispersion relation can be simplified. For instance, when $k_z r_w \ll 1$, the rhs simplifies to yield

$$\epsilon_1 r_p \frac{\partial}{\partial r_p} J_{m_\theta}(k_\perp r_p) + \epsilon_2 m_\theta J_{m_\theta}(k_\perp r_p) = J_{m_\theta}(k_\perp r_p) \begin{cases} -m_\theta \frac{1+(r_p/r_w)^{2m_\theta}}{1-(r_p/r_w)^{2m_\theta}}, & m_\theta > 0, \\ -\frac{1}{\ln(r_w/r_p)}, & m_\theta = 0. \end{cases} \tag{43}$$

Several other simplifications can be made in various regimes, as described below.

The TG dispersion relation provides mode frequencies as seen in a frame rotating with the plasma. In the lab frame, there is a Doppler shift of the frequency caused by this rotation. The lab coordinate θ_{lab} is related to the rotating frame coordinate θ by a Galilean transformation, $\theta_{\text{lab}} = \theta - \omega_r t$. The factor $\exp[im_\theta\theta - i\omega t]$ in the mode potential can then be written in lab frame coordinates as $\exp[im_\theta\theta_{\text{lab}} - i(\omega - m_\theta\omega_r)t]$. This implies that the lab frame frequency is

$$\omega_{\text{lab}} = \omega - m_\theta\omega_r. \tag{44}$$

Figure 6 displays a sketch of the TG mode frequencies for a given value of $k_z \neq 0$ and $m_\theta \neq 0$, versus magnetic field. Also shown, as dashed lines, are the upper hybrid frequency and the vortex frequency. The plot for $m_\theta = 0$ has the appearance of the upper half of Figure 6 reflected about the x-axis into the lower half (i.e. the $m_\theta = 0$ modes come in $\pm\omega$ pairs).

The modes fall into three classes: upper hybrid modes, magnetized plasma modes, and two surface modes. The upper hybrid modes have frequencies in the range $\max(\omega_p^2, \Omega_v^2) < \omega^2 < \Omega_{uh}^2$. The magnetized plasma modes are in the range $\omega^2 < \min(\omega_p^2, \Omega_v^2)$. These ranges are the same as

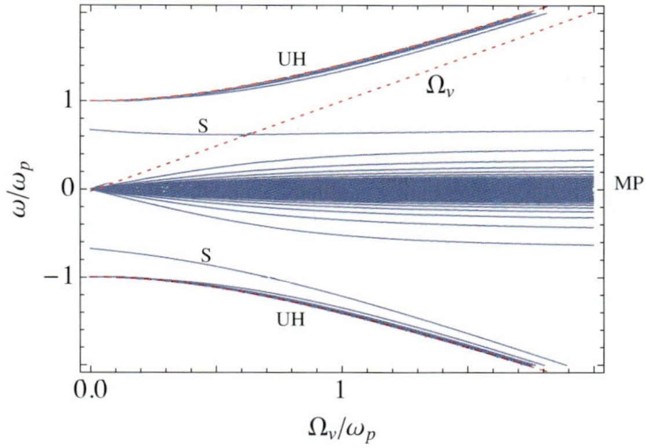

Fig. 6. A sketch of the frequencies of TG modes on a cylindrical plasma column versus the vortex frequency Ω_v for fixed values of $k_z > 0$ and $m_\theta > 0$. Dashed lines show the positive and negative upper hybrid frequencies and the vortex frequency. Modes labeled S, UH, and MP are surface modes, upper hybrid modes, and magnetized plasma modes respectively. The infinite set of upper hybrid modes are too close together to be distinguished in this sketch.

for a plasma with no boundaries; see Figure 2. The upper hybrid and magnetized plasma modes have an infinite number of possible branches with different values of $k_\perp$ for each, corresponding to different numbers of radial oscillations within the plasma column.

As Ω_v becomes large, and provided that $k_z \neq 0$, the positive frequency surface mode converts to a magnetized plasma mode with no radial nodes. For $k_z \neq 0$ and $m_\theta > 0$, the negative frequency surface mode joins the upper hybrid modes for large Ω_v; and for $m_\theta = 0$ this mode instead joins the magnetized plasma modes.

In the $k_z = 0$ limit discussed below, the two surface modes remain separate for all Ω_v; they are the diocotron and surface cyclotron modes. In this limit, all the upper hybrid branches are degenerate with $\omega = \pm\Omega_{uh}$ and the magnetized plasma modes all have $\omega = 0$, just as for an unbounded plasma (see Figure 2).

4.2.1. *TG magnetized plasma modes*

The TG plasma modes are finite k_z magnetized plasma oscillations on the cylindrical column, with a frequency of order the plasma frequency or less. For simplicity, I will consider the dispersion relation for these modes assuming that $k_z r_w \ll 1$ and taking the strong magnetic field limit where $\omega_p \ll \Omega_v$. One can then approximate $\epsilon_1 = 1$. The mode frequency then follows from Equation (37):

$$\omega^2 = \frac{\omega_p^2 k_z^2}{k_\perp^2 + k_z^2}. \tag{45}$$

This is the same as Equation (19) for a plasma with no boundaries. These TG modes are magnetized cold plasma waves with k_z and $k_\perp$ quantized by the finite plasma length and radius. The possible values of $k_\perp$ follow from Equation (43), taking $\epsilon_1 = 1$ and $\epsilon_2 = 0$ (the latter assumes that $k_z/k_\perp \gg \omega_p/|\Omega_v|$):

$$r_p \frac{\partial}{\partial r_p} J_{m_\theta}(k_\perp r_p) = J_{m_\theta}(k_\perp r_p) \begin{cases} -m_\theta \frac{1+(r_p/r_w)^{2m_\theta}}{1-(r_p/r_w)^{2m_\theta}}, & m_\theta > 0, \\ -\frac{1}{\ln(r_w/r_p)}, & m_\theta = 0. \end{cases} \tag{46}$$

There are multiple solutions to Equation (46) corresponding to waves with different numbers of radial nodes within the plasma column. For example, for $m_\theta = 0$ there is a solution with no radial nodes that roughly satisfies

$$k_\perp r_p = \sqrt{\frac{2}{\ln(r_w/r_p)}}, \tag{47}$$

assuming that $r_w \gg r_p$. (This follows by Taylor expansion of the $m_\theta = 0$ Bessel functions in Equation (46) around $k_\perp r_p = 0$, assuming that $k_\perp r_p \ll 1$.) The solutions with more nodes roughly satisfy $J_1(k_\perp r_p) = 0$, so that

$$k_\perp = j_{1,n}/r_p, \quad n = 1, 2, 3, \ldots, \tag{48}$$

where $j_{m_\theta,n}$ is the n'th zero of the Bessel function $J_{m_\theta,n}(x)$, counting out from, but not including, the origin.

For $m_\theta > 0$, and again assuming $r_w \gg r_p$, the rhs of Equation (46) can be approximated as $-m_\theta J_{m_\theta}$. Then a Bessel function identity [19] allows one to write the equation as $k_p r_p J_{m_\theta - 1}(k_\perp r_p) = 0$, so that the solutions for $k_\perp$ are

$$k_\perp = j_{m_\theta-1,n}/r_p, \; n = 1, 2, 3, \ldots. \tag{49}$$

These solutions correspond to a potential with $n-1$ radial nodes. The $n = 1$ case with no radial nodes and with positive frequency (for $\Omega_v > 0$) connects to the positive frequency surface mode; see Figure 6.

The formulae in this section, while useful in their regimes of validity, are only approximate. The frequencies found by solving the full TG dispersion relation can differ from these formulae, sometimes substantially, depending on the circumstances. Two examples are shown in Figure 7. The solid curves

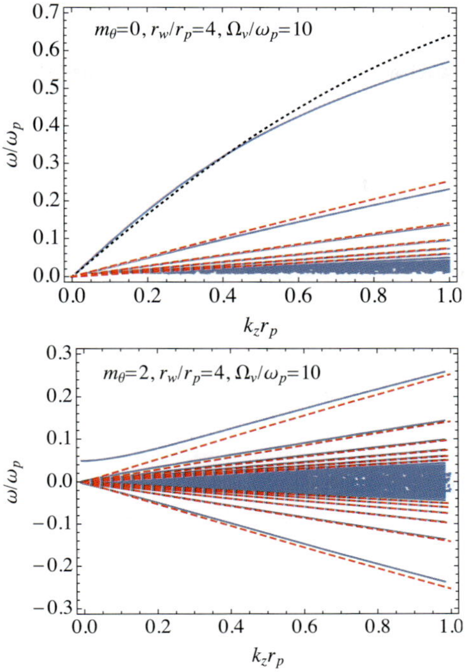

Fig. 7. Frequency versus wavenumber for TG modes with $|\omega| < \omega_p$. Solid curves are solutions of the full TG dispersion relation, Equation (42). Dotted and dashed curves are approximate analytic dispersion relations described in the text. Only the first six approximate dispersion curves are shown, corresponding to waves with between zero and five radial nodes.

are frequencies versus wavenumber k_z, obtained from the full dispersion relation for a plasma with $r_w/r_p = 4$, $\Omega_v/\omega_p = 10$ and $m_\theta = 0$ in (a) and $m_\theta = 2$ in (b). The dotted curve in (a) is Equation (47), and the dashed curves are Equation (48), both combined with Equation (45). In Figure 7(b), the dashed curves are Equations (49) and (45). The approximate dispersion relations are just that, approximate, particularly for small $k_z r_p$ in the $m_\theta = 2$ example, where the assumption that $k_z/k_\perp \gg \omega_p/\Omega_v$ is breaking down and the ϵ_2 term in the TG dispersion relation cannot be neglected. Here the upper TG mode is becoming a surface mode, poorly described by Equation (45), and the other modes are not well-described by Equation (49). [In fact, one can show [18] that for $k_z/k_\perp < \omega_p/\Omega_v$ and $m_\theta \neq 0$ the TG modes (other than the surface mode) are better-described by $k_\perp = j_{m_\theta,n}/r_p$ rather than Equation (49).]

4.2.2. *Upper hybrid modes*

In the large magnetic field regime $|\Omega_v| \gg \omega_p$, there is also a set of upper hybrid modes whose frequencies have a magnitude close to that of the vortex frequency $|\Omega_v|$. For these modes, one can set $\epsilon_3 = 1$, which implies through Equation (37) that $\epsilon_1 = -k_z^2/k_\perp^2$. Using Equation (10), this equation can be rewritten as

$$\omega^2 = \Omega_v^2 + \frac{k_\perp^2}{k_\perp^2 + k_z^2}\omega_p^2, \tag{50}$$

the upper hybrid dispersion relation in the strong magnetic field regime. This dispersion relation is the same as Equation (18), except that now k_z and $k_\perp$ are quantized. The possible values of $k_\perp$ follow from Equation (42), or Equation (43) if $k_z r_w \ll 1$ (I will assume this here for simplicity). In the large magnetic field regime with $\omega \sim \pm\Omega_v$, one may set $\epsilon_1 = -k_z^2/k_\perp^2$ and $\epsilon_2 = \pm(1-\epsilon_1) = \pm(1 + k_z^2/k_\perp^2)$, so that Equation (43) becomes

$$\begin{aligned} -k_z^2 r_p \frac{\partial}{\partial r_p} J_{m_\theta}(k_\perp r_p) &\pm (k_\perp^2 + k_z^2) m_\theta J_{m_\theta}(k_\perp r_p) \\ &= k_\perp^2 J_{m_\theta}(k_\perp r_p) \begin{cases} -m_\theta \frac{1+(r_p/r_w)^{2m_\theta}}{1-(r_p/r_w)^{2m_\theta}}, & m_\theta > 0, \\ -\frac{1}{\ln(r_w/r_p)}, & m_\theta = 0, \end{cases} \end{aligned} \tag{51}$$

where the $\pm$ sign in the equation corresponds to $\omega \sim \pm\Omega_v$. Upper hybrid modes with positive ω and m_θ have a positive azimuthal phase velocity, and generally do not have the same $k_\perp$ as modes which rotate on the column in the negative azimuthal direction because the magnetic field breaks the reflection symmetry normally associated with these two directions.

There are multiple solutions to Equation (51) for $k_\perp$, corresponding to upper hybrid modes with different numbers of radial nodes. One simple case is $k_z = 0$ (i.e. $m_z = 0$), where the solutions are $k_\perp = j_{m_\theta,n}/r_p$, $n = 1, 2, 3, \ldots$. These solutions correspond to a z-independent potential that vanishes outside the plasma. These upper hybrid modes are internal waves with n radial nodes (not counting the node at $r = 0$ for $m_\theta \neq 0$), one of which is at the plasma edge. These modes have no effect outside the plasma, and hence cannot be observed or excited using external electrodes. All of these waves have the same frequency (as seen in the rotating frame), the upper hybrid frequency $\pm\Omega_{uh}$.

Another simple case is $\omega < 0$, $m_\theta > 0$, and $(r_p/r_w)^{2m_\theta} \ll 1$, so that the rhs in Equation (51) can be approximated as $-m_\theta k_\perp^2 J_{m_\theta}$. Then for the lower sign in the equation corresponding to $\omega < 0$, a Bessel function identity [19] allows one to rewrite Equation (51) as $-k_z^2 k_\perp r_p J_{m_\theta - 1}(k_\perp r_p) = 0$. Thus, in this case, the solutions for $k_\perp$ are

$$k_\perp = j_{m_\theta - 1, n}/r_p, \quad n = 1, 2, 3, \ldots . \tag{52}$$

These solutions have a potential with $n - 1$ radial nodes within the plasma column (again, not counting the node at $r = 0$). The $n = 1$ case has no radial nodes and connects to a surface mode; see Figure 6.

In using these formulae, remember that the same caveat with respect to their approximate nature holds as for the magnetized plasma modes discussed in the previous section.

4.2.3. *Surface modes for an unmagnetized cylindrical plasma*

At the Brillouin limit where $\Omega_v = 0$, the plasma is unmagnetized when seen in the rotating frame, and the TG mode dispersion relation simplifies. In this limit, $\epsilon_2 = 0$ and $\epsilon_1 = \epsilon_3$ so Equation (37) implies $k_\perp^2 = -k_z^2$; i.e. $k_\perp$ is imaginary. In this case, the Bessel functions of the first kind convert to modified Bessel functions through the identity $J_{m_\theta}(ix) = i^{m_\theta} I_{m_\theta}(x)$. These modified Bessel functions are exponentially large for large argument, implying that the modes are surface modes concentrated at $r = r_p$. The frequency of these modes follows from Equation (42):

$$\begin{aligned} \epsilon_3 &= 1 - \omega_p^2/\omega^2 \\ &= \frac{I_{m_\theta}(k_z r_p)}{\frac{\partial}{\partial r_p} I_{m_\theta}(k_z r_p)} \frac{\frac{\partial}{\partial r_p}\left(I_{m_\theta}(k_z r_p) K_{m_\theta}(k_z r_w) - I_{m_\theta}(k_z r_w) K_{m_\theta}(k_z r_p)\right)}{I_{m_\theta}(k_z r_p) K_{m_\theta}(k_z r_w) - I_{m_\theta}(k_z r_w) K_{m_\theta}(k_z r_p)}, \end{aligned} \tag{53}$$

which can be easily solved for ω^2. In the limit of large m_θ or large k_z, the rhs simplifies to -1, yielding $\omega^2 = \omega_p^2/2$, giving the surface plasma frequency familiar from the slab geometry case considered previously.

As the magnetic field increases from zero, eventually ϵ_1/ϵ_3 changes sign, $k_\perp$ becomes real, and (for $k_z \neq 0$) the two surface modes join the magnetized plasma and (for $m_\theta \neq 0$) upper hybrid branches, as discussed in relation to Figure 6.

4.2.4. *Diocotron modes and surface cyclotron modes*

Another simplifying limit of the TG dispersion relation is when $k_z \to 0$ and $m_\theta \neq 0$. In this limit, Equation (37) implies $k_\perp \to 0$ as well, provided that $\epsilon_1 \neq 0$ so that we avoid the upper hybrid modes discussed previously. Taylor expansion of Equation (43) in $k_\perp$ then yields

$$m_\theta(\epsilon_1 + \epsilon_2) = -m_\theta \frac{1 + (r_p/r_w)^{2m_\theta}}{1 - (r_p/r_w)^{2m_\theta}}. \tag{54}$$

This is the dispersion relation for $k_z = 0$ surface waves on the cylindrical plasma column. Compared to Equation (30), Equation (54) differs from the previous slab-geometry result only through the terms involving $(r_p/r_w)^{2m_\theta}$. These terms encode the effect on the mode of image charges in the cylindrical electrodes, which were neglected in the slab-geometry discussion of surface waves. The slab geometry result is approached when m_θ is large or when $r_p/r_w \to 0$, so that $(r_p/r_w)^{2m_\theta} \to 0$, i.e. when image charge effects are negligible.

Equation (54) can be solved for ω to yield two roots:

$$\omega = -\frac{\Omega_v}{2} \pm \sqrt{\frac{\Omega_v^2}{4} + \omega_p^2 \frac{1 - (r_p/r_w)^{2m_\theta}}{2}}. \tag{55}$$

When $\Omega_v = 0$, the roots are equal and opposite and correspond to the surface plasma waves discussed in the previous section, shifted in frequency by image charge effects. For large Ω_v, these roots correspond to a high frequency surface cyclotron mode and a low frequency diocotron mode. For $\Omega_v^2 \gg \omega_p^2$ the low frequency solution is

$$\omega = \frac{\omega_p^2}{2\Omega_v}\left[1 - \left(\frac{r_p}{r_w}\right)^{2m_\theta}\right], \tag{56}$$

the *diocotron frequency* (as seen in the rotating frame). The surface cyclotron frequency (as seen in the rotating frame) is given by $\Omega_v - \omega$, where ω is the diocotron frequency. Equation (56) is identical to the slab geometry diocotron wave frequency in the large magnetic field limit, Equation (33), except for a frequency shift caused by the effect of image charges in the conducting wall.

The functional form of the diocotron and surface cyclotron mode potential inside and outside the plasma is given by Equations (36) and (38), taking $k_\perp \to 0$ and using Taylor expansions for the Bessel functions:

$$\delta\phi(\mathbf{r}, t) = Ce^{i(m_\theta\theta - \omega t)} \begin{cases} r^{m_\theta}, & r < r_p, \\ \frac{r^{m_\theta} - (r_w^2/r)^{m_\theta}}{1 - (r_w/r_p)^{2m_\theta}}, & r > r_p. \end{cases} \tag{57}$$

This potential corresponds to a z-independent distortion of the shape of the plasma, producing a travelling wave on the plasma surface that propagates in the θ-direction. The radial change $\delta r(\theta, t)$ in the position of the plasma surface due to the mode can be obtained using an argument similar to that which led to Equation (29), and is left as an exercise (see below). For instance, the $m_\theta = 1$ mode is a displacement of the entire column off of the axis of symmetry of the conducting cylinder. The off-axis plasma is attracted to its image in the conducting walls and this force, for the diocotron mode, causes the entire plasma to $\mathbf{E} \times \mathbf{B}$ drift around the cylinder. The $m_\theta = 1$ surface cyclotron mode has the same distortion, except that its motion is at higher frequency: it is essentially cyclotron motion of the entire column, with a frequency slightly shifted by image charge forces. Both modes rotate in the same direction as seen in the lab frame: the direction of the cyclotron motion (i.e. the negative $\hat{\theta}$-direction for positive charges).

Question 6: Using Equation (57) show that the radial change δr in the position of the plasma surface produced in a surface cyclotron or diocotron mode is given by

$$\delta r = C \frac{2\epsilon_0 m_\theta r_p^{m_\theta - 1}}{q n_0 \left[1 - (r_p/r_w)^{2m_\theta}\right]} e^{i(m_\theta \theta - \omega t)}. \tag{58}$$

4.3. *Other geometries;* E × B *modes; finite temperature effects*

Plasma modes can be determined analytically in a few other geometries of importance to Penning trap experiments. For instance, for spheroidal plasmas of small size compared to the distance to the electrodes, the dispersion relation has been worked out in terms of Legendre functions [3,9]. The functional form of this dispersion relation will not be discussed further here; the interested reader is referred to the references.

The modes of a spheroid consist of upper hybrid waves, magnetized plasma waves, and surface waves, each with quantized wavenumbers, just as for the TG dispersion relation. However, in the strong magnetic field regime there is also an extra set of modes: modes with low frequencies of order $1/B$, that consist of vortical $\mathbf{E} \times \mathbf{B}$ motions in the x–y plane [4]. These modes differ from the diocotron surface mode (which also has frequency of order $1/B$) in that they have finite frequency due only to the varying axial length of the spheroid as a function of cylindrical radius. As an axial rod of plasma is convected radially by $\mathbf{E} \times \mathbf{B}$ motion, it feels a restoring force due to the varying length of the plasma during the motion, which compresses (or expands) the rod [5]. In a cylindrical plasma column with flat ends, such motions would merely rearrange the fluid elements within the column without changing the density or potential; there would be no linear restoring force and the motions would be inherently nonlinear. These "zero-frequency" nonlinear motions are referred to as *convective cells*, and are important in the study of plasma turbulence [6]. Variation of the equilibrium length of the plasma column with radius breaks the degeneracy of the convective cells, giving them a range of low but finite frequencies.

An analogy has also been drawn between these $\mathbf{E} \times \mathbf{B}$ modes and certain low-frequency oceanic and atmospheric disturbances called *Rossby waves* [7]. Radial variation of the plasma length can be thought of as analogous to the longitudinal variation in coriolis force that drives these waves in the ocean and the atmosphere [8]. This analogy could allow simulation of geophysical phenomena in a non-neutral plasma.

Within the plasma spheroid these finite-length $\mathbf{E} \times \mathbf{B}$ modes are nearly z-independent, and as $|\Omega_v|/\omega_p$is reduced below unity they convert to magnetized plasma modes with small axial wavenumbers and hence low frequencies, approaching zero frequency as $\Omega_v \to 0$ (see Figure 2).

For simplicity, the theory of plasma waves considered in this chapter neglected effects associated with finite temperature. Finite temperature effects on magnetized plasma modes [10,11] and diocotron modes [12] have been observed and studied theoretically; rather less is known concerning these effects on surface cyclotron and upper hybrid modes although work is ongoing [13,14]. For example, the magnetized plasma mode frequencies are shifted upward by finite temperature as plasma pressure increases the wave restoring force. These shifts are sufficiently well understood to be used as a plasma thermometer in some experiments [15–17].

Furthermore, finite temperature effects can produce mode damping through the process called *Landau damping* [21], in which charged particles moving with nearly the same velocity as the wave phase velocity (due to the particle's thermal speed) are resonantly accelerated by the wave potential and hence remove energy from the wave.

In addition, a new set of temperature-dependent modes with frequencies near multiples of the cyclotron frequency is predicted to occur at finite temperature [13, 22]. These "Bernstein modes" have been observed in recent experiments on non-neutral plasmas [14, 22], but more work is needed to fully understand their dispersion and damping in such plasmas.

4.4. *Solutions to the exercises*

Question 1

Equation (1) has three components,

$$-i\omega\delta u_x = -\frac{q}{m}\frac{\partial\delta\phi}{\partial x} + \Omega_v \delta u_y,$$

$$-i\omega\delta u_y = -\frac{q}{m}\frac{\partial\delta\phi}{\partial y} - \Omega_v \delta u_x,$$

$$-i\omega\delta u_z = -\frac{q}{m}\frac{\partial\delta\phi}{\partial z}.$$

The last equation implies $\delta u_z = -iq/(m\omega)\partial\delta\phi/\partial z$. The first two equations are coupled, but can be easily solved to yield

$$\delta u_x = -\frac{iq}{m}\frac{\omega\partial\delta\phi/\partial x + i\Omega_v\partial\delta\phi/\partial y}{\omega^2 - \Omega_v^2},$$

$$\delta u_y = -\frac{iq}{m}\frac{\omega\partial\delta\phi/\partial y - i\Omega_v\partial\delta\phi/\partial x}{\omega^2 - \Omega_v^2}.$$

This solution can be written in matrix form as shown in Equations (2) and (3).

Question 2

Referring to Figure 1, there is now a magnetic field out of the page (in the z-direction). The magnetic field modifies the equations of motion of the plasma slab, so that Equation (13) is replaced by the coupled equations

$$\Delta\ddot{x} = -\omega_p^2\Delta x + \Delta\dot{y}\Omega_v,$$

$$\Delta\ddot{y} = -\Delta\dot{x}\Omega_v.$$

Integrating the second equation to obtain $\Delta\dot{y} = -\Delta x\Omega_v$, and substituting this into the first equation, yields $\Delta\ddot{x} = -(\omega_p^2 + \Omega_v^2)\Delta x$. This harmonic oscillator equation implies that position of the slab oscillates at the upper hybrid frequency.

Questions 3 and 4

Write Equation (26) as $\kappa\epsilon_1 = -k - k_y\epsilon_2$, square both sides, and substitute $\kappa^2 = k_y^2 + \epsilon_3 k_z^2/\epsilon_1$. This yields $k^2 + 2kk_y\epsilon_2 + k_y^2\epsilon_2^2 = k_y^2\epsilon_1^2 + k_z^2\epsilon_3\epsilon_1$. Using the definitions of ϵ_1, ϵ_2, and ϵ_3, this equation can be expressed as

$$\frac{2k^2\omega^2 + 2kk_y\omega\Omega_v - k^2\omega_p^2 - k_z^2\Omega_v^2}{\omega^2\left(\omega^2 - \Omega_v^2\right)} = 0.$$

The numerator is a quadratic function of ω, whose solution is given by Equation (34). However, this solution arises from squaring both sides of the original equation, so there is an extra requirement: $\kappa\epsilon_1$ must have the same sign as $-k - k_y\epsilon_2$. Assuming that κ is real (see the solution to Question 5), the sign of ϵ_1 must be the same as $-k - k_y\epsilon_2$. We have already shown this to be the case at $k_z = 0$, where $\epsilon_1 = -1 - \epsilon_2$ (and $k = k_y$), so as k_z/k increases from zero the sign changes only where $-k - k_y\epsilon_2$ passes through zero. This expression can be written as

$$\frac{k\omega\Omega_v^2 - k\omega^3 - k_y\Omega_v\omega_p^2}{\omega(\omega^2 - \Omega_v^2)}.$$

However, using Equation (34) this becomes

$$\frac{k^2\omega_p^2 - k_z^2\Omega_v^2}{2k(\omega^2 - \Omega_v^2)},$$

which changes sign when $k_z^2/k^2 = \omega_p^2/\Omega_v^2$.

Question 5

Substitute Equation (34) into $\kappa^2 = k_y^2 + \epsilon_3 k_z^2/\epsilon_1$. After some algebra, one obtains the expression

$$\kappa^2 = k^2\left(\frac{k^2\omega_p^2 - k_z^2\Omega_v^2}{k^2\omega_p^2 + k_z^2\Omega_v^2}\right)^2, \tag{59}$$

independent of the sign of the square root in Equation (34). This expression also shows that κ is real.

Question 6

The change in radial position δr of the plasma surface is related to a surface charge $\delta\sigma$ through $\delta r = \delta\sigma/(qn_0)$. The surface charge is related to the jump in radial electric field across the surface (see Equation (27)): $\delta\sigma/\epsilon_0 = \frac{\partial\delta\phi}{\partial r}|_{r=r_p^-} - \frac{\partial\delta\phi}{\partial r}|_{r=r_p^+}$. Substituting for $\delta\phi$ from Equation (57) leads directly to Equation (58).

References

1. R. H. Ritchie, Plasma losses by fast electrons in thin films, *Phys. Rev.* **106**, 874–881 (1957).
2. A. W. Trivelpiece and R. W. Gould, Space charge waves in cylindrical plasma columns, *J. Appl. Phys.* **30**, 1784–1793 (1959).
3. D. H. E. Dubin, Theory of electrostatic fluid modes in a cold spheroidal non-neutral plasma, *Phys. Rev. Lett.* **66**, 2076–2079 (1991).
4. D. H. E. Dubin, Effect of correlations on the thermal equilibrium and normal modes of a non-neutral plasma, *Phys. Rev. E* **53**, 5268–5290 (1996).
5. T. J. Hilsabeck and T. M. O'Neil, Finite length dicotron modes, *Phys. Plasmas* **8**, 407–422 (2001).
   J. A. Krommes, Statistical Descriptions and Plasma Physics
6. J. A. Krommes, *Statistical Descriptions and Plasma Physics* (*Eds M. Rosenbluth and R. Sagdeev*) Chapter 5.5 Handbook of Plasma Physics, vol. II, p. 183.North-Holland, Amsterdam (1984).
7. C. G. Rossby, Relation between variations in the intensity of the zonal circulation of the atmosphere and the displacements of the semi-permanent centres of action, *J. Mar. Res.* **2**, 38–55 (1939).
8. J. M. Finn *et al.*, Compressional effects in nonneutral plasmas, a shallow water analogy and the m = 1 instability, *Phys. Plasmas* **6**, 3744–3758 (1999).
9. J. J. Bollinger *et al.*, Electrostatic modes of ion trap plasmas, *Phys. Rev. A* **48**, 525–545 (1993).
10. F. Anderegg *et al.*, Thermally excited modes in a pure electron plasma, *Phys. Rev. Lett.* **90**, 115001 (2003).
11. M. D. Tinkle *et al.*, Low-order modes as diagnostics of spheroidal non-neutral plasmas, *Phys. Rev. Lett.* **72**, 352–355 (1994).
12. K. S. Fine and C. F. Driscoll, The finite-length diocotron mode, *Phys. Plasmas* **5**, 601–607 (1998).
13. D. H. E. Dubin, Cyclotron waves in a non-neutral plasma column, *Phys. Plasmas* **20**, 042120 (2013).
14. M. Affolter *et al.*, Cyclotron mode frequency shifts in multi-species ion plasmas, *Phys. Lett. A* **378**, 2406–2409 (2014).
15. M. Amoretti *et al.*, Complete nondestructive diagnostic of nonneutral plasmas based on the detection of electrostatic modes, *Phys. Plasmas* **10**, 3056–3064 (2003).
16. H. Higaki *et al.*, Electron cooling of high-energy protons in a multiring trap with a tank circuit monitoring the electron-plasma oscillations, *Phys. Rev. E* **65**, 046410 (2002).
17. A. Speck *et al.*, Density and geometry of single-species plasmas, *Phys. Lett. B* **650**, 119–123 (2007).
18. S. A. Prasad and T. M. O'Neil, Waves in a cold pure electron plasma of finite length, *Phy. Fluids* **26**, 665–672 (1983).
19. G. N. Watson, *A Treatise on the Theory of Bessel Functions*. Cambridge, Cambridge University Press, (1995).

20. J. K. Jennings *et al.*, Numerical calculation of axisymmetric electrostatic modes for cold finitelength nonneutral plasmas, *Phys. Plasmas* **2**, 2630–2639 (1995).
21. L. Landau, On the vibrations of the electronic plasma, *JETP* **16**, 574–579 (1946).
22. R. W. Gould, Theory of cyclotron resonance in a cylindrical nonneutral plasma, *Phys. Plasmas* **2**, 1404–1411 (1995).

CHAPTER ELEVEN

ROTATING WALL TECHNIQUE AND CENTRIFUGAL SEPARATION

François Anderegg

University of California San Diego, Physics Dept. 0319, La Jolla CA 92093, USA

fanderegg@UCSD.edu

This chapter describes the "rotating wall" technique which enables essentially unlimited confinement time of 10^9–10^{10} charged particles in a Penning trap. The applied rotating wall electric field provides a positive torque that counteracts background drags, resulting in radial compression or steady-state confinement in near-thermal equilibrium states.

The last part of the chapter discusses centrifugal separation in a rotating multi-species non-neutral plasma. Separation occurs when the centrifugal energy is larger than the mixing due to thermal energy.

1. Introduction

Let us consider a non-neutral plasma contained in a Penning–Malmberg trap as shown in Figure 1. The trap consists of a series of cylindrical electrodes carefully aligned with the magnetic field $\boldsymbol{B} = -B\hat{z}$. Longitudinal confinement is produced by potentials V applied to the end electrodes, and radial confinement is produced by the magnetic field. For simplicity, let us assume that the plasma consists of positive charges, so our choice of $\boldsymbol{B}$-direction will make all rotation frequencies and velocities positive.

The charges produce a radial electric field pointing to the wall, creating an azimuthal $\boldsymbol{E} \times \boldsymbol{B}$ drift of the particles $v_\theta = E_r/B$, resulting in a rotation frequency:

$$f_E = \frac{v_\theta}{2\pi r} = \frac{E_r}{B2\pi r}. \tag{1}$$

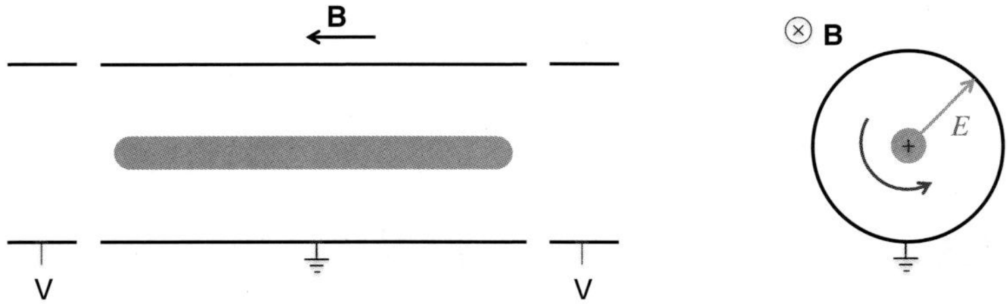

Fig. 1. Penning–Malmberg trap.

The electric field satisfies Gauss' law:

$$\nabla \cdot E = \frac{nq}{\epsilon_0}, \tag{2}$$

and in cylindrical coordinates, the radial component is:

$$\frac{1}{r}\frac{\partial}{\partial r}(rE_r) = \frac{nq}{\epsilon_0}. \tag{3}$$

Multiplying by r and integrating gives:

$$rE_r = \frac{q}{\epsilon_0}\int_0^r n(r')r'dr'. \tag{4}$$

For a radially uniform density:

$$E_r = \frac{q}{\epsilon_0 r} = \frac{1}{2}r^2 n = \frac{rnq}{2\epsilon_0}, \tag{5}$$

therefore,

$$f_E = \frac{nq}{4\pi\epsilon_0 B}. \tag{6}$$

One sees that for a uniform density plasma the rotation is constant out to the plasma edge r_p; that is, the plasma is rotating as a rigid rotor, at a rate proportional to the density n.

Non-neutral plasma has extraordinary confinement properties [1], in particular, in an azimuthally symmetric system the plasma angular momentum P_θ is conserved

$$P_\theta = \sum_j (mv_{\theta j} + qA_\theta r_j), \tag{7}$$

with $A_\theta = Br/2$ for a uniform magnetic field. The first term is the mechanical angular momentum and the second is the canonical angular momentum.

For large magnetic field, the canonical angular momentum term dominates and

$$P_\theta \cong \sum_j \frac{qBr_j^2}{2}, \tag{8a}$$

$$P_\theta^T \cong \sum_j \frac{qB}{2}\left(r_j^2 - R_W^2\right), \tag{8b}$$

where the sum on j is overall the particles in the trap. The P_θ^T of Equation (8b) explicitly includes both the plasma charges and an equal number of image charges located at R_W and may be seen as more intuitive. Note that Equation (8b) is valid for a cylindrical trap with a uniform wall radius, and reflects the fact that the magnitude of the total angular momentum is minimum when all particles have been lost at the wall.

Therefore, if one particle moves outward increasing its r_j, other particles have to move inwards. Consequently in theory, non-neutral plasmas relax towards a confined thermal equilibrium state as viewed in a frame rotating at rate f_E.

In reality, perfect symmetry is never realized in the laboratory. Residual gas, magnetic field asymmetries, and electrode imperfections create drags on the rotating plasma, reducing its rotation rate and therefore decreasing its density and angular momentum.

There are several methods to add angular momentum to the particles of a Penning trap:

- In the single particle regime, a sideband technique known as *"axialization"* couples the magnetron motion to the "other" motion in the trap (either cyclotron or axial). The "other" motion is damped, either by laser cooling or by a resonant circuit, resulting in a radial compression of the particle density. The axialization technique works in the single particle regime, but not in the plasma regime where the Debye length λ_D is smaller than the plasma radius r_p. This axialization technique has been presented in detail during the winter school and Chapter 1 written by R. Thompson in this volume covers the subject.
- The radiation pressure of a laser has been successfully used to torque on the plasma and increase its density [2].
- In principle, rotating the entire trap at the plasma rotation frequency f_E would alleviate the drag on the plasma, but this is rather impractical since non-neutral plasmas typically rotate at $1\,\text{kHz} \leqslant f_E \leqslant 100\,\text{MHz}$.

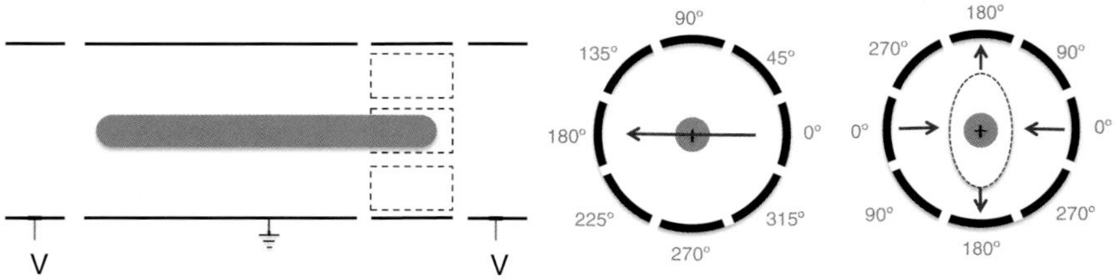

Fig. 2. Segmented electrode to apply "rotating wall" perturbation with dipole $m_\theta = 1$ and quadrupole drive $m_\theta = 2$.

No macroscopic objects can rotate at these rates due to the limitation of material strength. A more practical solution is to apply a time-varying potential to azimuthally sectored electrode, at frequencies f_{RW}.

Figure 2 shows schematically an azimuthally segmented electrode for applying a "rotating wall" perturbation. The time dependent potential applied to each azimuthal sector is:

$$\begin{aligned} \phi_j(\theta, t) &= A_{\mathrm{RW}} \cos\left[m_\theta \left(\theta_j - 2\pi f_{\mathrm{RW}} t\right)\right], \\ \theta_j - \frac{\Delta\theta}{2} &< \theta < \theta_j + \frac{\Delta\theta}{2}; \end{aligned} \tag{9}$$

here $m_\theta = 1$ represents a dipole drive and $m_\theta = 2$ a quadrupole drive. The signal applied to each sector is a sine wave with a phase shifted by θ_j. Inside the trap, a charged particle "*sees*" a rotating electric field.

The fundamental concept of a rotating electric field is simple but due to the finite size of sectored electrodes, unwanted spatial harmonics can be significant. An extreme example is applying a quadrupole drive with only four electrodes, where the amplitude of the backward rotating electric field ($m_\theta = -2$) is as large as the forward one ($A_{m_\theta=-2}/A_{m_\theta=2} = 1$). One should note that the plasma may still couple to one direction preferentially, since the rotating perturbation is Doppler shifted in the plasma rotating frame. Using eight sectors significantly improves the quality of the drive. Here, the strongest backward rotating component is $m_\theta = -6$, ($A_{m_\theta=-6}/A_{m_\theta=2} \cong 2/3$), that is, the useful $m_\theta = 2$ component is about 60% of the signal compared to about 40% of $m_\theta = -6$ rotating backward.

1.1. *Torque balance*

The plasma is in equilibrium when the sum of all the torques applied to the plasma equals zero. Ambient, lab-frame effects such as collisions with residual gas particles or an asymmetric $\boldsymbol{B}$ field will exert a "drag" on the rotating plasma. In contrast, a rotating wall with $f_{\mathrm{RW}} > f_{\mathrm{E}}$ will "spin-up" the plasma. A drag decreases the magnitude of P_θ^T and increases $\langle r_j^2 \rangle$, whereas spinning-up increases the magnitude of P_θ^T and decreases $\langle r_j^2 \rangle$. This can be proven formally using thermodynamic arguments [3].

Steady state is achieved when

$$|\tau_{\mathrm{RW}}| = |\tau_{\mathrm{ambient}}|, \tag{10}$$

and the compression of the plasma happens when

$$|\tau_{\mathrm{RW}}| > |\tau_{\mathrm{ambient}}|. \tag{11}$$

In principle, any electric field rotating faster than the plasma will exert a torque on the plasma and compress it; but Debye shielding may render the rotating wall torque too small to be useful. The rotating wall field can be greatly enhanced by a plasma wave resonance, and working in the vicinity of azimuthally rotating plasma modes has generally been successful. It is often easier to couple to these rotating modes from the end of the plasma column.

Any radially expanding plasma is necessarily releasing electrostatic energy, resulting in plasma heating. The minimum heating that the plasma will have in the presence of an *"ideal"* rotating wall balancing ambient torques will be:

$$2\pi f_{RW}\tau_{RW} = 2\pi f_E \tau_{\mathrm{ambient}}. \tag{12}$$

In general, the heating will be larger due to the presence of unwanted spatial harmonics and imperfection in the rotating wall drive. Typically, the unwanted spatial harmonics are reduced by increasing the number of azimuthal sectors, but no systematic experiments have been performed yet.

At high temperatures, plasma modes are damped and plasma is less collisional; both effects are reducing coupling to the rotating wall electric field. Therefore, to successfully implement the rotating wall technique, a cooling sufficient to balance the unwanted heating is necessary.

1.2. *Typical form of cooling used for rotating wall*

1.2.1. *Cyclotron radiation*

An accelerated charge q radiates energy at a rate given by the Larmor formula:

$$\frac{dE}{dt} = \frac{q^2 a^2}{6\pi\epsilon_0 c^3}. \tag{13}$$

For a charged particle gyrating in a magnetic field, the acceleration is $a_\perp = \Omega_c v_\perp$ and energy is $E_\perp = \frac{1}{2}mv_\perp^2$ resulting in:

$$\frac{dE_\perp}{dt} = \frac{q^2\Omega_c^2 E_\perp}{3\pi\epsilon_0 mc^3}. \tag{14}$$

Averaging the above equation over a Maxwellian distribution yields [4,5]:

$$\frac{dT_\perp}{dt} = \frac{-3T_\perp}{2\tau_r}, \tag{15}$$

with radiation time τ_r given by

$$\tau_r = \frac{-3T_\perp}{2\dot{T}_\perp} = \frac{3}{2}\frac{T_\perp 3\pi\epsilon_0 mc^3}{q^2\Omega_c^2 T_\perp} = \frac{9}{2}\frac{\pi\epsilon_0 m^3c^3}{q^4B^2}. \tag{16}$$

One sees that the radiation time is short for light particles in a large magnetic field; for electrons (or positrons):

$$\tau_r = \frac{3.86 \text{ s}}{B_{\text{T}}^2}. \tag{17}$$

In contrast, ions are too massive to be cooled by cyclotron radiation in any practical trap magnetic field.

1.2.2. *Collisions with residual gas particles*

Effective ion cooling can be achieved from collisions with residual gas particles at rate ν_{iN}. The gas is at temperature T_N and the cooling rate is:

$$\dot{T} \cong \nu_{iN}(T - T_N). \tag{18}$$

One sees that if the difference of temperature in between the gas and the plasma is large, then collisions with background gas is effective. The ion-neutral collision rate ν_{iN} is typically of the order of $10^{-2}\,\text{s}^{-1}$. For example, magnesium ions colliding with H_2 through dipole interactions, one obtains:

$$\nu_{iN} \cong 0.019\ \text{s}^{-1}\left(\frac{P_N}{10^{-9}\ \text{mbar}}\right) \quad (\text{Mg}^+ \text{on H}_2). \tag{19}$$

Succesful cooling of positron has also been achieved using vibrational modes of large gas molecules [6].

1.2.3. *Laser cooling*

This technique has been presented in detail during the winter school and Chapter 6 written by Champenois in this volume covers the subject. Laser cooling is effective to cool ions, but only a few kind of ions can be laser cooled since a closed two-level system is preferred.

Sympathetic cooling has been successfully used to cool other ions through collisions with laser cooled ions [7], or to cool antiprotons with electrons that are cooled by cyclotron radiation [8].

2. Results from Various Experiments

The rotating wall technique has been implemented on numerous experiments. Here, I will briefly review results from three experiments. The first one is the original demonstration of the rotating wall technique, demonstrating the importance of plasma modes in the coupling. The second shows the "strong drive regime", and the third experiment demonstrates that a crystallized plasma can phase-locked its rotation to the rotating wall drive.

2.1. *Rotating wall coupled through plasma modes*

Experiments in Penning–Malmberg traps containing about 10^9 magnesium ions or 3×10^9 electrons have demonstrated that a rotation wall perturbation can control the plasma density and radius; and that the confinement time of the particles is essentially "infinite" (weeks) [9]. For electron experiments with a magnetic field of 4 T, cyclotron cooling is rapid with cooling time $\tau_r \sim 0.24\,\mathrm{s}$. For the data presented in this section, ion plasmas are cooled by weak collisions with residual gas particles giving cooling time $\tau \sim 20\,\mathrm{s}$.

Both dipole ($m_\theta = 1$) and quadrupole ($m_\theta = 2$) rotating wall drive produce significant plasma compression for both electrons and ions. The experimental arrangement used a rotating wall perturbation applied to the end of the plasma column as shown in Figure 2. Density profiles for both electron and ion plasmas are shown in Figure 3(a). The electron density is measured with a destructive plasma dump on a moveable collimator plate with a small hole. The charge passing through the small hole is measured by a Faraday cup resulting in a line integrated density. The density is obtained by dividing the line integrated density by the plasma length.

A low density plasma (A) is compressed by sweeping up the rotating wall frequency slowly into profiles (B) and (C). The ion density profiles measured with Laser Induced Fluorescence are shown on the upper frame.

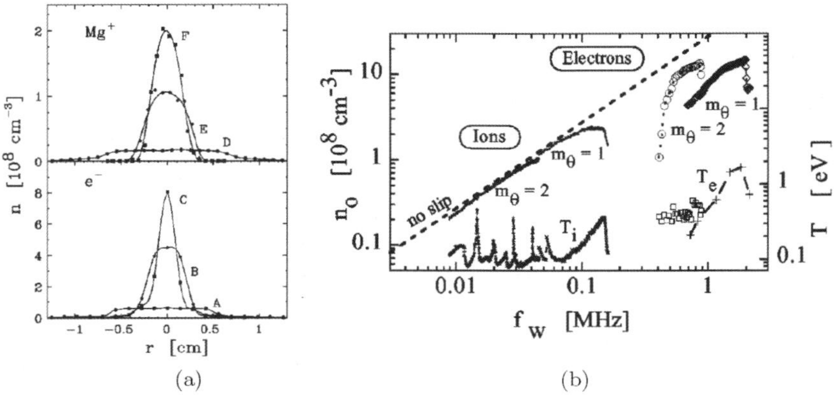

Fig. 3. (a) Electron and ion density profiles. (b) Density and temperature during rotating wall frequency sweep.

These profiles are steady state and confined for periods of weeks. One should note that ion plasmas that are confined for a long time exhibit slow chemical reactions even at ultrahigh vacuum, with residual background gas (mainly H_2) converting metallic ions into metal hydride ions.

Figure 3(b) shows the central plasma density plotted versus the rotating wall frequency. As the frequency is ramped up, the plasma density increases and the rotation frequency f_E of Equation (6) increases. The plasma rotation frequency is always lower than the rotating wall frequency ($f_{RW} > f_E$) and therefore some "slip" is present. The maximum ion density achieved in this experiment was 13% of the Brillouin density (i.e. maximum stable density in a Penning trap). As the density increases, the background drag increases as $\sim n_0^2$ while the rotating wall torque remains constant, so the slip increases. More heating is generated and the rotating wall coupling decreases, leading to an abrupt reduction of the density in the trap.

Also, the plasma temperature shows spikes each time the rotating wall driven imperfections excite a longitudinal plasma mode. Here, the longitudinal plasma modes are detrimental to the rotating wall coupling. Care should be taken to rapidly change the rotating wall frequency when one such mode is encountered, otherwise the control of the plasma density may be lost since the coupling decreases as the temperature increase.

Figure 4 demonstrates that the coupling of the rotating wall to the plasma is much larger in the vicinity of azimuthal (rotating) plasma modes, for both $m_\theta = 1$ and $m_\theta = 2$. Here, the electron plasma profile B of

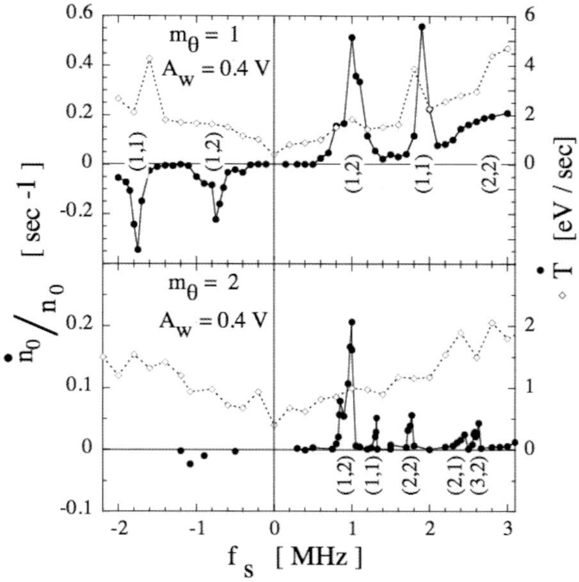

Fig. 4. Compression rate versus rotating wall frequency for $m_\theta = 1$ and $m_\theta = 2$ drives.

Figure 3(a) is in equilibrium with the rotating wall at $f_{\rm RW} = 0.5$ MHz, then $f_{\rm RW}$ is changed and the compression rate is measured at $r = 0$. When the rotating wall frequency is close to an azimuthal plasma mode characterized by (m_z, m_r), the compression rate is significantly larger. When the rotating wall is phased so as to rotate backwards (labeled as negative frequencies in Figure 4, rapid expansion is observed in the vicinity of backward traveling modes).

Compression peaks are broadened and their amplitude is reduced due to Landau damping when the temperature gets too high. Depending on the plasma geometry and particles masses, compression peaks due to plasma modes can be very broad and appear continuous.

In Figure 4, one sees that the heating rate increases as $f_{\rm RW}$ increases due to increased slip rate.

2.2. *Strong drive regime*

This technique relies on a large amplitude drive and seems to be less sensitive to plasma modes, when the cooling rate is large enough and the background drag small enough. The geometry of this experiment is similar to

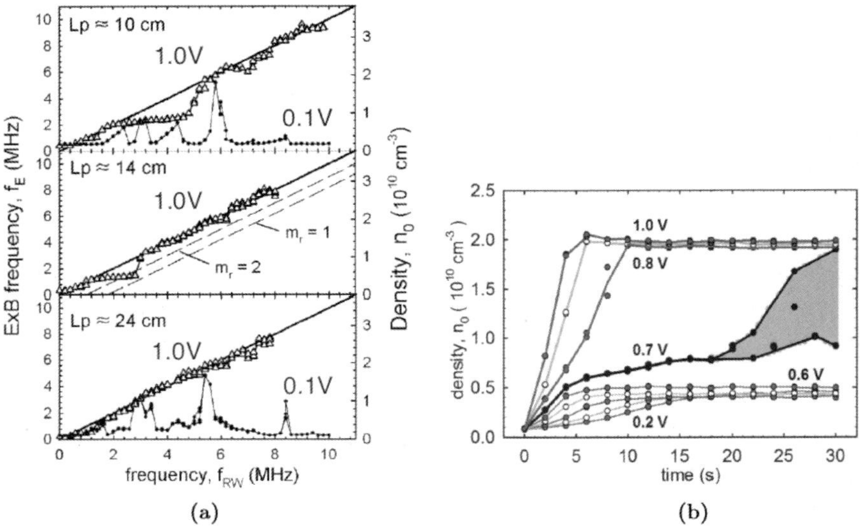

Fig. 5. (a) Weak (0.1 V) and strong drive (1.0 V), and (b) Density below and above critical amplitude (0.7 V).

the canonical Penning–Malmberg trap, with a rotating wall applied at the end of the plasma column as shown in Figure 2. Typically, $\sim 10^9$ electrons are confined in a magnetic field of $B = 5$ T resulting in strong cyclotron radiation with a cooling time $\tau_r = 0.15$ s. A dipole ($m_\theta = 1$) drive is applied at a fixed frequency [10].

Two distinct plasma responses are observed depending on the strength of the rotating wall drive. At low amplitude (0.1 V), compression is observed only at discrete rotating wall frequencies as shown in Figure 5(a), due to plasma mode couplings. At large amplitude (1.0 V), compression is observed over a wide range of frequencies and no significant slip is observed. In this experiment, the rotation frequency is inferred from a density measurement, and no direct rotation frequency measurement is performed. At large amplitude, the central frame of Figure 5(a) suggests that the plasma is rotating faster than the rotating mode frequencies indicted by dashed lines.

Also, a bifurcation behavior is observed as the amplitude of the drive exceeds a critical strength of 0.7 V as shown in Figure 5(b), the plasma density rapidly reaches $n = 2 \times 10^{10}\,\mathrm{cm}^{-3}$.

Here, the increased cyclotron cooling and the low background transport is what allows this new regime to be observed.

2.3. *Phased-locked rotating crystal*

Beryllium ions contained in a Penning trap are laser cooled to $T < 10\,\mathrm{mK}$ ($\sim 10^{-6}$ eV). The plasma consists of $10^2 < N < 10^6$ ions, and is strongly coupled, since the potential energy between neighboring ions is larger that the ion thermal energy. The rotating wall perturbation is applied uniformly across the axial extend of the plasma with two sets of azimuthally segmented electrodes (the compensation electrodes). Plasma compression is observed with both $m_\theta = 1$ and $m_\theta = 2$ drives [11].

Theoretically, the dipole field ($m_\theta = 1$) cannot control the plasma rotation of a single-species plasma in a quadratic trap. This is because it only causes a center-of-mass orbital motion about the trap axis and is thus decoupled from the internal plasma rotation. Experimentally, the dipole field ($m_\theta = 1$) works in the presence of impurity ions, while the quadrupole field ($m_\theta = 2$) always works. The NIST trap is shown schematically in Figure 6(a).

Figure 6(b) shows the plasma rotation frequency inferred from the measured plasma aspect ratio. The plasma rotation frequency increases linearly with the applied rotating wall frequency in both weakly and strongly coupled plasmas.

For a more accurate determination of the rotation rate, the time dependance of Bragg-scattered light from the rotating crystal has been detected

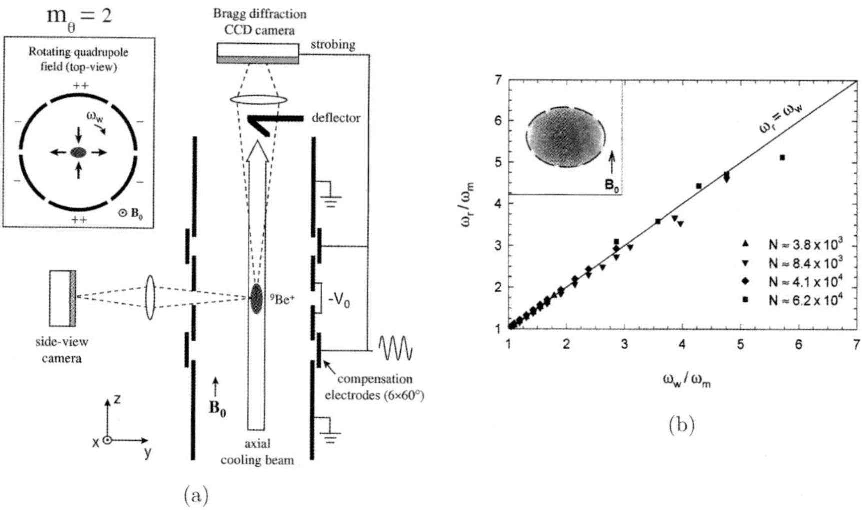

Fig. 6. (a) NIST trap for ion crystal. (b) Plasma rotation controlled with rotating wall frequency.

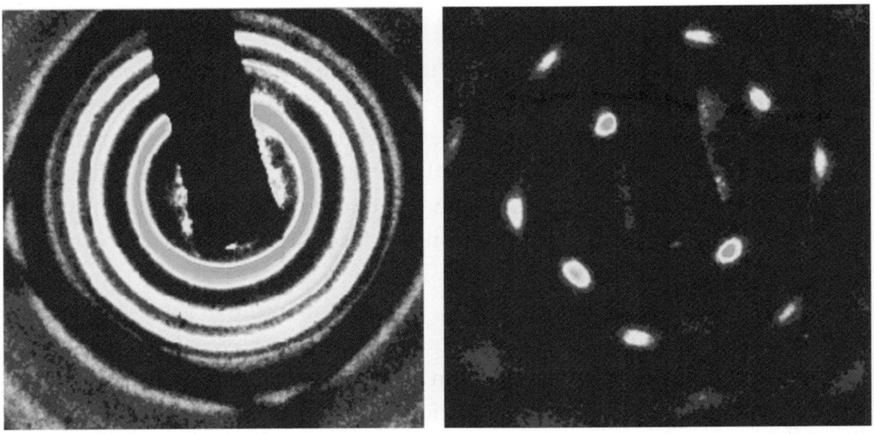

(a) (b)

Fig. 7. (a) Time averaged diffraction pattern and (b) strobed diffraction pattern.

by strobing the camera. Without strobing, Figure 7(a) shows the time averaged diffraction pattern of concentric ring because of the plasma rotation about the axial laser beam. With strobing, Figure 7(b) shows a time-resolved pattern accumulated over 10^6 rotations. The well-defined rectangular dot pattern demonstrates that the crystal is phase-locked to the rotating field that is ($f_E = f_{RW}$).

Here, the rotating wall electric field changes the trap potential in the rotating frame, the plasma boundary is slightly deformed to a tri-axial ellipsoid, and the shear force in the crystal transmits the torque to the interior. The plasma shape deformation has been measured and is typically less than 1%, but it generates sufficient torque to phase-lock the plasma rotation.

The NIST group demonstrated that the rotating wall technique works in the strongly coupled regime, and that the plasma rotation is phased-locked to the rotating wall drive for a long period of time.

2.3.1. *Rotating wall summary*

The rotating wall is a very successful technique, allowing essentially unlimited confinement of non-neutral plasmas. The frequency of the rotating wall controls the plasma density. The coupling of the rotating perturbation to the plasma is well understood for crystallized plasma, but in the "plasma" regime many plasma distortions (such as waves) can contribute.

3. Centrifugal Separation

The bulk rotation of a multi-species ion plasma tends to produce centrifugal separation of its component species. To understand the mechanism, let us write the radial force balance of a small piece of plasma located at radius r.

$$0 = n_a(r)\left[qE(r) - qB\omega_{ra}r + m\omega_{ra}^2 r\right] - \frac{\partial p_a}{\partial r}, \tag{20}$$

where $p_a = n_a k_B T_a$ is the thermal pressure of species a. With $B > 0$ and $B = -B\hat{z}$ here, all frequencies (ω_{ra}, ω_E) are positive and $\omega_r \equiv \dot{\theta}$. [Other conventions chose $B = B\hat{z}$, and define a *"rotation frequency"* $\tilde{\omega}_r \equiv -\dot{\theta}$ so as to make $\tilde{\omega}_r > 0$].

Equation (20) can be rewritten in terms of rotation ω_E and cyclotron Ω_{ca} "frequencies":

$$\omega_E(r) = \frac{E(r)}{Br} \quad \text{and} \quad \Omega_{ca} = \frac{qB}{m_a}, \tag{21}$$

giving:

$$\omega_{ra} = \omega_E(r) - \frac{1}{qBn_a(r)r}\frac{\partial p_a}{\partial r} + \frac{\omega_{ra}^2}{\Omega_{ca}}. \tag{22}$$

The last term is the centrifugal correction to the rotation rate; it is generally small but it causes centrifugal separation. Before reaching thermal equilibrium, each species rotates at a different rate, and the collisional drag between species causes torques which drive one species out and the other in. Consider a drag force for species a of the form

$$F_{\theta a} = -\sum_b \nu_{ab}\, m_a r(\omega_{ra} - \omega_{rb}), \tag{23}$$

where ν_{ab} is the collision rate between species a and b. This drag θ-force produces a $F_\theta \times B$ drift in the radial direction that causes centrifugal separation. The resulting radial flux Γ_{ra} of species a is simply the charge density times the drift velocity. Combining the last two equations, one gets:

$$\Gamma_{ra} = n_q\frac{F_{\theta a}}{qB} = \sum_b \frac{D_{ab}}{k_B T_a}\left[\frac{\partial p_a}{\partial r} - \frac{n_a}{n_b}\frac{\partial p_b}{\partial r} + n_a\left(m_b\omega_{rb}^2 - m_a\omega_{ra}^2\right)r\right], \tag{24}$$

where $D_{ab} = \nu_{ab}\, r_{ca}^2$ is a diffusion coefficient and $r_{ca} = \sqrt{k_B T_a}/\Omega_{ca}$ is the thermal cyclotron radius of species a. The first two terms are diffusive fluxes, which tend to mix the species, while the last term is a mobility term separating the species due to centrifugal force acting on each species. Note that the flux Γ_{ra} vanishes when $T_a(r) = T_b(r) = T, \omega_{ra}(r) = \omega_{rb}(r) = \omega_r$ and the densities satisfy thermal equilibrium.

In thermal equilibrium, each species density can be written as [3]:

$$n_a(r) = n_a(0) \exp\left[\frac{-q_a}{k_B T}\left(\phi(r) - \frac{m_a}{q_a}\frac{\omega_r^2 r^2}{2} - \frac{B\omega_r r^2}{2}\right)\right]. \tag{25}$$

Note that the only difference between species comes from the ω_r^2 term, and for the separation to be significant, this term must be large compared to the thermal energy $k_B T$. More precisely for the simple two species case, the following has to be satisfied:

$$q\left|\frac{m_1}{q_1} - \frac{m_2}{q_2}\right| \omega_r^2 R_p^2 > k_B T. \tag{26}$$

The separation length is defined as:

$$l_{sep} \equiv \frac{k_B T}{|m_1 - m_2|\,\omega_r^2 R_p}. \tag{27}$$

When $l_{sep} < R_p$ separation occurs in the plasma, and when $l_{sep} \ll \lambda_D$ then complete separation takes place, with species arranged in separate concentric rings.

For two species carrying the same charge, Equation (25) leads to:

$$\frac{n_a(r)}{n_b(r)} = C_{ab} \exp\left[\frac{1}{2k_B T}(m_a - m_b)\,\omega_r^2 r^2\right], \tag{28}$$

where C_{ab} is a constant determined by the overall fraction of each species.

The measured density profiles for a warm plasma with negligible separation and for a cold plasma with strong separation [12] are shown in Figure 8. The symbols represent LIF-measured densities of magnesium ion isotopes. The solid flat line is the total density n_0 obtained from the rotation frequency. The curves are predictions of Equation (28), here the theory prediction has been convoluted with the finite size probe laser beam σ_l so they can be compared directly with the experimental measurements. At $T = 4.8 \times 10^{-3}$ eV, the species are uniformly mixed. Note that the sum of the Mg^+ isotopes is 25% lower than to the total plasmas density due to the presence of impurity ions H_3O^+ and O_2^+ not detected by the LIF diagnostic. As the plasma is laser cooled down to $T = 7.1 \times 10^{-5}$ eV, the species centrifugally separate and concentrate into radial annuli. The central hole observed in the Mg^+ density is the result of the lighter impurity species H_3O^+.

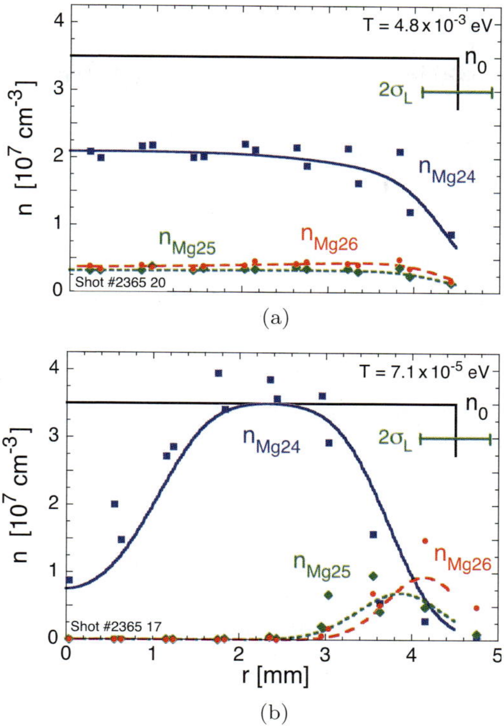

Fig. 8. Radial density profile of multi-species plasma showing warm un-separated plasma (a), and cold separated plasma (b).

More dramatic separation is routinely observed in electron–antiproton plasmas [13].

The rate $\mathcal{R}$ at which the centrifugal separation occurs can be easily estimated if the mobility flux is smaller or equal to the diffusive flux. This rate is then roughly the rate required for particles to diffuse across the plasma radius r_p.

$$\mathcal{R} \sim \frac{D_{ab}}{r_p^2} \sim 0.1 s^{-1} \left(\frac{n_0}{10^7 \mathrm{cm}^{-3}}\right) \sqrt{\frac{\mu(\mathrm{amu})}{T}} \left(\frac{1}{B(\mathrm{Tesla}) R_p(\mathrm{cm})}\right)^2. \tag{29}$$

The re-mixing rate of previously separated magnesium ion isotopes is shown in Figure 9. The plasma is abruptly heated with a burst of cyclotron heating, changing from $T \sim 5 \times 10^{-5}$ eV to $T \sim 10^{-3}$ eV. The squares are LIF measurements of the normalized density ratio $\mathrm{Mg}_{25}/\mathrm{Mg}_{24}$. The solid

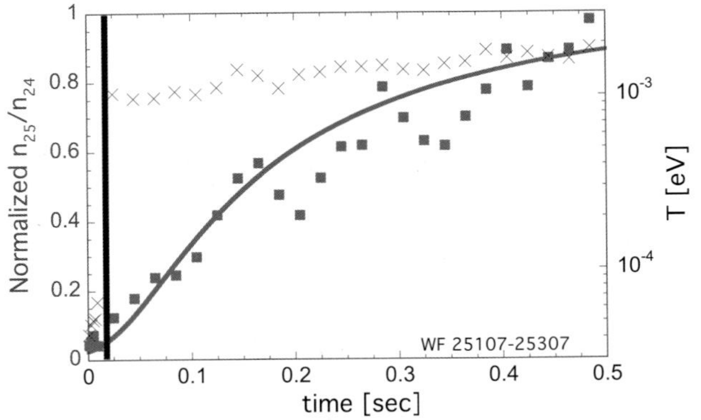

Fig. 9. Re-mixing of magnesium isotopes after a burst of heat (black vertical bar). $\times$ represents temperature and squares are concentration of Mg_{25}.

line is the result of a calculation of the flux Γ_{ra} from Equation (24) starting from the initially measured density profiles and measured $T(t)$.

3.1. *Centrifugal separation summary*

We have seen that multi-species plasmas are centrifugally separated when the centrifugal energy is larger than the thermal energy (Equation (26)) and that the separation is complete when the separation length is smaller than the Debye screening length (Equation (27)). For plasma close to thermal equilibrium, the radial densities distribution and the separation-remixing rate are correctly described by a drag force due to collision between species.

4. Simple Tutorial Problems

4.1. *Problem* 1

Calculate the $\boldsymbol{E} \times \boldsymbol{B}$ rotation frequency of a single-species, uniform plasma, of density 10^7 cm^{-3} in a 3 T magnetic field.

(a) Consider an electron plasma.
(b) Consider a Magnesium ion plasma.

As we have seen in the first section of this chapter, $\boldsymbol{E} \times \boldsymbol{B}$ rotation rate of a constant density plasma is:

$$f_E = \frac{nq}{4\pi\epsilon_0 B} \cong \frac{10^{13} \cdot 1.6 \times 10^{-19}}{4\pi \cdot 8.8 \times 10^{-12} \cdot 3} \cong 4.8\,\text{kHz}.$$

Note that here we are assuming that the density is low compared to the maximum density achievable in a Penning trap ("*Brillouin density*"). For most plasmas in Penning traps, this assumption is satisfied (i.e. $2\omega_r \ll \Omega_c$). Here, the cyclotron frequency of a singly ionized magnesium ion is $\Omega_c^{Mg_{24}}/2\pi \cong 1.9\,\text{MHz}$, clearly within our approximation. For plasmas approaching the Brillouin limit, a rigorous description is given by Dubin in Chapter 9 on Plasmas in Penning trap.

$E \times B$ drifts are independent of the mass of the trapped charged particles, but dependent on the charge q. Therefore, ions and electrons rotate in opposite direction. Figure 1 of this chapter show the (positive) rotation direction for positive charges in $\boldsymbol{B} = -B\hat{z}$.

4.2. *Problem 2*

Estimate the minimum rotation frequency necessary to observe centrifugal separation of magnesium 24 from magnesium 25 for a temperature of 10 K and a plasma radius of 5 mm.

Assuming thermal equilibrium, we have seen that for singly ionized ion the separation occurs when:

$$|m_1 - m_2|\,(2\pi f_E R_p)^2 > k_B T.$$

Therefore,

$$\begin{aligned} f_E &> \frac{1}{2\pi R_p}\sqrt{\frac{k_B T}{|m_1 - m_2|}}, \\ &> \frac{1}{2\pi \cdot 5 \times 10^{-3}}\sqrt{\frac{1.38 \times 10^{-23} \cdot 10}{|25 - 24| \cdot 1.67 \times 10^{-27}}}, \\ &> 9.15\,\text{kHz}. \end{aligned}$$

Acknowledgments

This work was supported by National Science Foundation Grant PHY-1414570, Department of Energy Grant DE-SC0002451and Department of Energy High Energy Density Laboratory Plasma Grant DE-SC0008693. The author thanks the organizers of Les Houches Winter School for the opportunity to contribute to the workshop. The author also thanks Prof. C.F. Driscoll, Prof. D.H.E. Dubin, and Prof. T.M. O'Neil for many years of enlightening guidance and theoretical support.

References

1. T. M. O'Neil, A confinement theorem for nonneutral plasmas, *Phys. Fluids* **23**, 2216–2218 (1980); D. H. E. Dubin and T. M. O'Neil, Trapped nonneutral plasmas, liquids, and crystals (the thermal equilibrium states), *Rev. Mod. Phys.* **71**, 87–172 (1999).
2. D. J. Heinzen *et al.*, Rotational equilibria and low-order modes of a non-neutral ion plasma, *Phys. Rev. Lett.* **66**, 2080–2083 (1991).
3. T. M. O'Neil and D. H. E. Dubin, Thermal equilibria and thermodynamics of trapped plasmas with a single sign of charge, *Phys. Plasmas* **5**, 2163–2193 (1998).
4. T. M. O'Neil, Cooling of a pure electron plasma by cyclotron radiation, *Phys. Fluids* **23**, 725 (1980).
5. B. R. Beck *et al.*, Temperature and anisotropic-temperature relaxation measurements in cold, pure-electron plasmas, *Phys. Plasmas* **3**, 1250 (1996).
6. J. R. Danielson *et al.*, Plasma and trap-based techniques for science with positrons, *Rev. Mod. Phys.* **87**, 247 (2015).
7. D. J. Larson *et al.*, Sympathetic cooling of trapped ions: A laser cooled two species non-neutral ion plasma, *Phys. Rev. Lett.* **57**, 70–73 (1986).
8. G. Gabrielse *et al.*, Cooling and slowing of trapped antiprotons below 100 meV, *Phys. Rev. Lett.* **63**, 1360–1363 (1989).
9. X. -P. Huang *et al.*, Steady-state confinement of non-neutral plasma by rotating electric fields, *Phys. Rev. Lett.* **78**, 875–878 (1997); F. Anderegg, E. M. Hollmann, and C. F. Driscoll, Rotating field confinement of pure electron plasmas using trivelpiece-gould modes, *Phys. Rev. Lett.* **78**, 4875 (1998).
10. J. R. Danielson *et al.*, High-density fixed point for radially compressed single-component plasmas, *Phys. Rev. Lett.* **99**, 135005 (2007).
11. X. -P. Huang *et al.*, Precise control of the global rotation of strongly coupled ion plasmas in a Penning trap, *Phys. Plasmas* **5**, 1656 (1998).
12. M. Affolter *et al.*, Cyclotron mode frequency shifts in multi-species ion plasmas, *Phys. Plasmas* **22**, 055701 (2015).
13. G. B. Andresen *et al.*, Centrifugal separation and equilibration dynamics in an electron–antiproton plasma, *Phys. Rev. Lett.* **106**, 145001 (2011).

CHAPTER TWELVE

CORRELATIONS IN TRAPPED PLASMA

François Anderegg
University of California San Diego, Physics Dept. 0319,
La Jolla CA 92093, USA
fanderegg@UCSD.edu

This chapter describes the effects of correlations on trapped plasma. When the potential energy between neighboring ions is larger than the thermal energy, the internal structure of trapped plasma changes, from plasma to liquid to Coulomb crystal. These Coulomb crystals are similar to solid state one but the inner particle spacing is of the order of 10 μm, significantly larger than solid state material. The structure of these Coulomb crystals is obtained not from X-ray scattering but from Bragg scattering of UV light ($\sim$ 300 nm). Correlations not only change equilibrium properties of a plasma but also dynamical properties, in particular, this chapter will describe the dramatic increase of the collision rate in the presence of correlations.

1. Introduction

The thermodynamic state of a one-component plasma is determined by its shape, size, and coupling parameter Γ:

$$\Gamma = \frac{1}{4\pi\epsilon_0}\frac{q^2}{a_{\rm ws}k_B T}, \tag{1}$$

where $a_{\rm ws}$ is the Wigner–Seitz radius:

$$a_{\rm ws} \equiv \left(\frac{3}{4\pi n}\right)^{\frac{1}{3}}, \tag{2}$$

$a_{\rm ws}$ is the radius of a sphere whose volume equals the volume occupied by one charged particle in a plasma of density n. The coupling parameter Γ represents the ratio of the potential energy between neighboring charged particles and the thermal energy. When $\Gamma > 1$, a one-component plasma is strongly coupled. A large value of the coupling parameter can be achieved with high density n, or large charge per particle q, or low temperature T.

Strongly coupled one-component plasmas are believed to exist in dense astrophysical objects such as giant planets interior ($T \sim 1\,\text{eV}$, $n \sim 10^{24}\,\text{cm}^{-3}, q = \text{e}$, resulting in $\Gamma \sim 10$), white dwarf stars ($T \sim 100\,\text{eV}$, $n \sim 10^{30}\,\text{cm}^{-3}, q = \text{e}$, resulting in $\Gamma \sim 10$) [1]. Strongly coupled plasmas also exist in less dense objects if the charge per particle is large, such as dust grain in a dusty plasma [2] ($T^{\text{dust}} \sim 1\,\text{eV}$, $n \sim 1\,\text{cm}^{-3}$, $q = 10^4$ e, resulting in $\Gamma \sim 10$), or if the temperature is low enough in laser cooled trapped ion plasma ($T \sim 10^{-5}\,\text{eV}$, $n \sim 10^7\,\text{cm}^{-3}$, and $q = e$, resulting in $\Gamma \sim 10$). One sees that these vastly different physical systems can all have a coupling parameter $\Gamma \sim 10$. Therefore, astrophysical effects depending on Γ can be studied with laser cooled trapped ions, as will be described in Section 3 of this chapter.

For coupling parameter $\Gamma \ll 1$ trapped ions are in a "plasma state", for $\Gamma > 1$ trapped ions are in a liquid state and for $\Gamma \gtrsim 172$ trapped ions are in a solid state called a Coulomb crystal.

2. Effect of Correlations on Equilibrium Properties

In a trapped ion plasma consisting of many particles ($N \gg 1$), even when the correlation parameter Γ is large, the mean electric potential is large compared to the potential energy between neighboring ions.

$$e\phi \gg \frac{e^2}{4\pi\epsilon_0 a_{\text{ws}}}. \tag{3}$$

The mean electric potential determines the equilibrium shape of the plasma in the trap. The plasma shape remains essentially unchanged by the presence of correlation, the correlations only change the internal structure of the plasma, not its shape.

In the absence of correlation, the "one" particle distribution function is a Boltzman distribution.

$$f(r, v) = C \exp\left(\frac{-1}{k_B T}[H + \omega P_\theta]\right), \tag{4}$$

where the Hamiltonian H is:

$$H = \frac{mv^2}{2} + e(\phi_T + \phi_p), \tag{5}$$

ϕ_T is the trap potential and ϕ_p is the plasma potential which is determined by Poisson's equation:

$$\nabla^2 \phi_p = \frac{-en}{\epsilon_0} \tag{6}$$

and the canonical angular momentum P_θ in a uniform magnetic field in the z-direction is:

$$P_\theta = mv_\theta r + \frac{eB}{2} r^2. \tag{7}$$

In contrast, when correlations are present, the N particle distribution is a Gibbs distribution:

$$f(r_1, v_1, r_2, v_2, \ldots, r_N, v_N) = C \exp\left(\frac{-1}{k_B T}\left[H^{(N)} + \omega P_\theta^{(N)}\right]\right), \tag{8}$$

where the N particle Hamiltonian is:

$$H^{(N)} = \sum_{i=1}^{N} \frac{mv_i^2}{2} + e\left(\phi_T(r_i) + \sum_{j>i} \phi_{ij}\right), \tag{9}$$

where ϕ_T is the trap potential and ϕ_{ij} the interaction potential:

$$\phi_{ij} = \frac{e^2}{4\pi\epsilon_0 |r_i - r_j|} + \text{“image charge”}, \tag{10}$$

ϕ_{ij} is a Green function when the image charges are included [3]. In this chapter, we assume that the image charge contribution is negligible, that is, the plasma is far from the wall of the trap.

The N particle canonical angular momentum is:

$$P_\theta^{(N)} = \sum_{i=1}^{N} \left(mv_{\theta i} r_i + \frac{eB}{2} r_i^2\right) \tag{11}$$

and the N particle distribution becomes:

$$\begin{aligned} f(r_1, v_1, r_2, v_2, \ldots, r_N, v_N) &= C \exp\left(\sum_{i=1}^{N} \frac{m}{2k_B T}\left[v_i + \omega r_i \hat{\theta}_i\right]\right) \\ &+ \tilde{C} \exp\left(-\sum_{i=1}^{N} \frac{1}{k_B T}\left[\frac{1}{2}\sum_{i\neq j} \frac{e^2}{4\pi\epsilon_0 |r_i - r_j|} + e\phi_T\right]\right). \end{aligned} \tag{12}$$

Useful quantities to be considered are the reduced distribution; for example, the spatial distributions are obtained by integrating over velocities, and the N particle spatial distribution is:

$$\rho^{(N)}(r_1, r_2, \ldots, r_M) = \int d^3 r_{M+1} \ldots d^3 r_N \, f(r_1, \ldots, r_N). \tag{13}$$

The density is simply the first reduced distribution:

$$n(r) = N \rho^{(1)}(r). \tag{14}$$

The two-particle distribution is:

$$\rho^{(2)}(r_1, r_2) = \rho^{(1)}(r_1)\, \rho^{(1)}(r_2) \left[1 + g(r_1, r_2)\right], \tag{15}$$

where $g(r_1, r_2)$ represents the two-body spatial correlations which measure the extra probability beyond what would be expected of a completely random distribution of finding particles at r_1 and r_2.

Since the Coulomb interaction is a binary interaction, only $n(r)$, T and $\rho^{(2)}(r_1, r_2)$ are necessary to describe thermodynamic functions. No higher order terms are necessary. Figure 1 shows the correlation function $g(r_1, r_2)$ for a one-component plasma for various values of the correlation parameter [4].

In the absence of correlation, the correlation function is equal to zero at large distance, and goes to -1 at short distance reflecting the effect of Debye shielding. As the correlation parameter Γ increases, $g(r_1, r_2)$ increases at a distance of about 1.7 Wigner–Seitz radius; for distance smaller than one Wigner–Seitz radius $g(r_1, r_2)$ decreases, indicating that short range order is appearing in the system. These oscillations are evidence of the beginning of a crystal lattice.

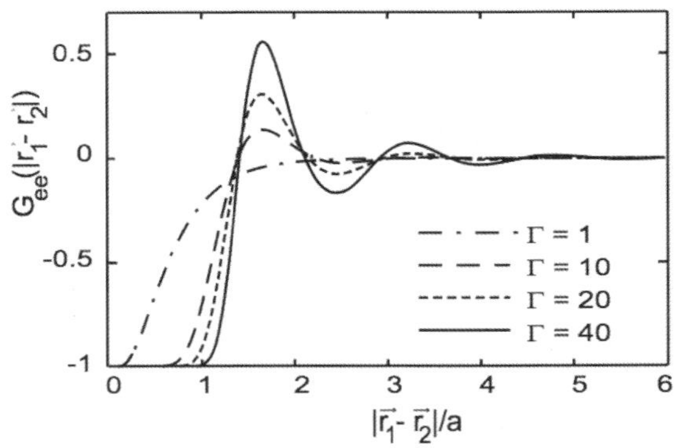

Fig. 1. Correlation function for one-component plasma.

2.1. *Correlation with small plasmas*

Early numerical simulations [5] solved the following equations for $N = 400$ ions:

$$\frac{dx_i}{dt} = \frac{E_i}{B} \times \hat{z} + U_i\hat{z},$$

$$\frac{dU_i}{dt} = \frac{mE_i}{e}\hat{z},$$

$$E_i = \frac{-\partial\Phi}{\partial x_i}, \tag{16}$$

$$e\Phi(x_i,\ldots,x_N) = \sum_{i>j} \frac{e^2}{4\pi\epsilon_0|x_i - x_j|} + \sum_i \frac{1}{2}m\omega_z^2\left(z_i^2 - \frac{\rho_i^2}{2}\right),$$

where one can see the potential Φ is the same as the first term of Equation (10) and that the trap potential is the standard quadratic potential of a Penning trap. These simulations show that for small plasmas, boundary effects dominate the geometry and inside the plasma ions are organized in a concentric shell structure.

The results of these simulations are shown in Figure 2(a), at low Γ the normalized spatial distribution is uniform, in contrast for large Γ sharp "onion-like shell" is predicted. Figure 2(b) is a measurement of such structure on a cloud of beryllium ions [6]. The number of shells observed depends on the number of ions N, with $N = 20$, one shell is observed and with $N = 15,000$, 16 shells are observed.

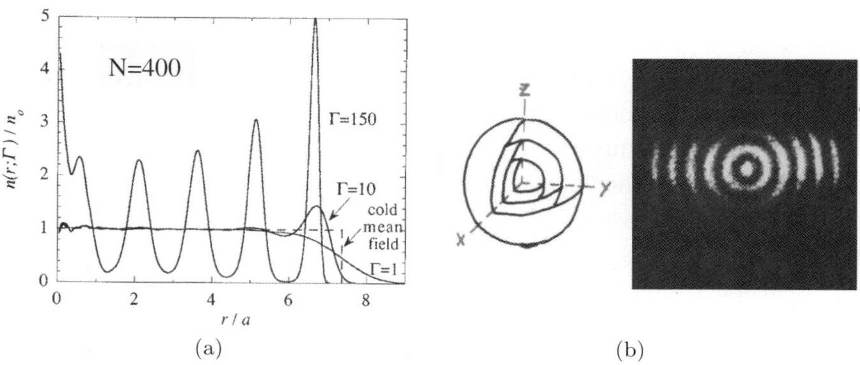

Fig. 2. (a) Density as a function of spherical radius; (b) observation of shell structure in Penning trap.

2.2. *Correlation with large plasmas*

The influence of the surface is limited for large plasma and its interior is comparable to an infinite size plasma. The lowest energy state for a Coulomb crystalline structure is a body center cubic (bcc) structure followed closely by a face centered cubic (fcc) and a hexagonal close packed (hcp). These different structures have very small fractional difference of Coulomb energies per ion, typically $< 10^{-4}$. Numerical simulations using a planar model [7] suggest that one needs at least 60 inter-particle spacings to observe bulk behavior; that is, $N > 10^5$ ions are necessary in a spherical plasma to exhibit bulk properties. More recently, numerical simulations of spherical plasma [8] have suggested that a bcc lattice may be present in small sections of a plasma with as little as 15,000 ions.

The inter particle spacing of Coulomb crystals is $\sim 10\,\mu$m, therefore Bragg scattering can be performed on them with ultraviolet light instead of X-ray as for solid state crystals. Since Coulomb crystals contain only a small number of ions compared to solid state crystals, the wavelength is chosen to be resonant with an atomic transition to increase the scattering cross-section.

Figure 3 shows the NIST trap designed to study large Coulomb crystals.

The inside diameter of the trap is 4.5 cm and the magnetic field $B = 4.5$ T. In this trap, Beryllium ions can be laser cooled down to $T <$ 1 mK. The Bragg scattering is done by an axial beam. The direct beam is deflected to avoid saturating the CCD camera, and crossed polarizers are used to further minimize unwanted scattering from the entrance window [9].

Scattering pictures are shown in Figure 4. The location of scattering rings indicates that the Coulomb crystal structure is bcc. Since the scattering picture is accumulated over several plasma rotations, it is not possible to distinguish a single crystal from several smaller crystals in the trap. Similarly, X-ray diffraction on powdered crystal results in diffraction rings. Locking the crystal rotation to the rotating wall and strobing the camera at the rotating wall frequency determines unambiguously that a single crystal is in the trap. Figure 7 in Chapter 11 describing the rotating wall technique shows a strobed diffraction pattern corresponding to a bcc crystal.

Real space images of the plasma also confirm a bcc crystal. Depending on the orientation of the probe laser beam, the (100) plane or the (111) plane can be illuminated as shown in Figure 5. The spacing of the ions in the (100) plane and the (111) plane is in agreement with a bcc crystal.

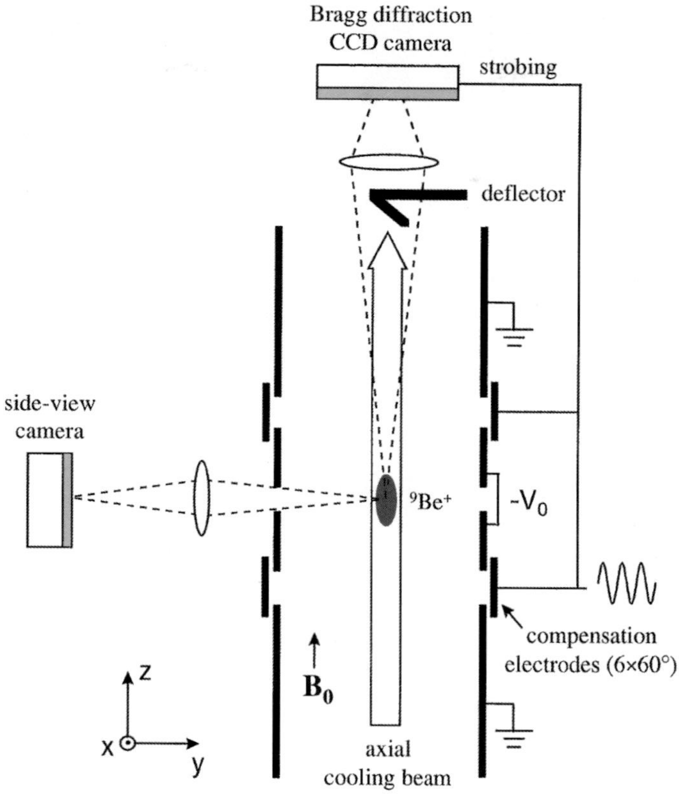

Fig. 3. NIST cylindrical Penning trap for large crystal.

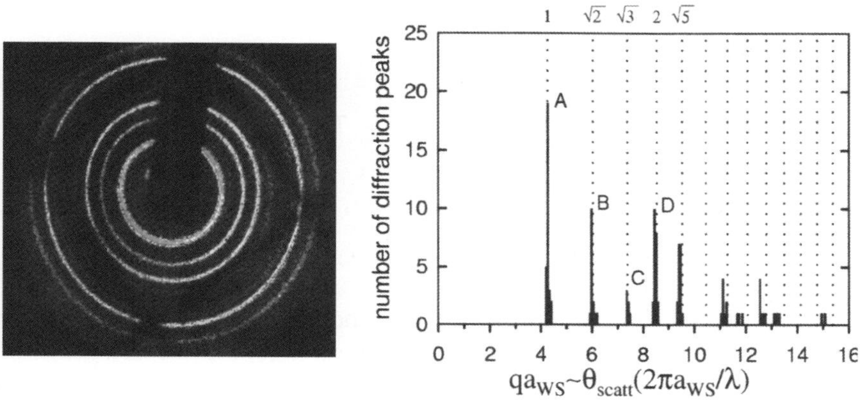

Fig. 4. Bragg scattering rings and frequency of ring location.

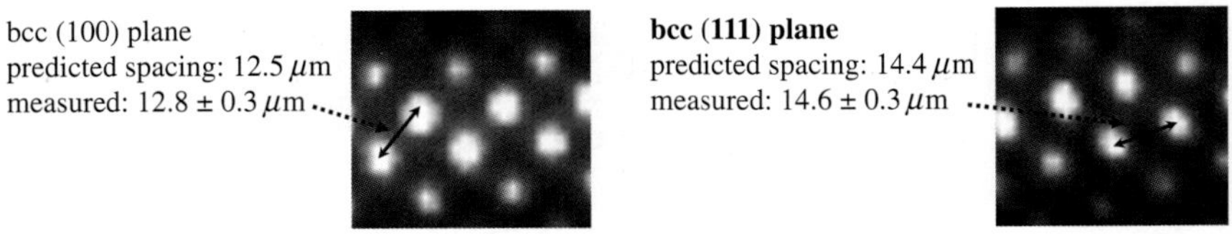

Fig. 5. Real space images of bcc Coulomb crystal.

2.2.1. *Summary of correlation on equilibrium properties*

For plasmas with $N < 10^4$ ions, boundary effects dominate and shell structure observed. For large plasmas, with $N > 10^5$ ions, bcc Coulomb crystals are observed in spheroidal plasma.

3. Effect of Correlations on a Dynamical Property

In this section, we will briefly describe theory results and measurements that use non-neutral plasmas to model aspects of the physics of nuclear fusion reactions in dense, correlated plasmas, such as in giant planets, degenerate stars, and laser fusion plasmas. Nuclear reaction rates in dense correlated plasmas are, according to theory, enhanced compared to rates predicted for reactions at lower density. In the astrophysics community, this theoretical effect is known as the Salpeter enhancement [10]. Here, we use an analogy between screened nuclear reactions in dense plasmas and perpendicular to parallel energy equipartition in strongly coupled and strongly magnetized non-neutral plasmas [11, 12].

In a magnetized plasma (i.e. $\Omega_c \gg \omega_p$) with a perpendicular temperature $T_\perp$ and a parallel temperature $T_\parallel$, we consider the perpendicular to parallel collision rate $\nu_{\perp\parallel}$ defined as:

$$\frac{d}{dt}T_\perp = \nu_{\perp\parallel}\,(T_\parallel - T_\perp) \tag{17}$$

with

$$\nu_{\perp\parallel} \equiv n\bar{v}b^2\,4\sqrt{2}I(\bar{\kappa})\,g(\Gamma). \tag{18}$$

Here, the "bare" collision rate $4\sqrt{2}\,n\bar{v}b^2$ is modified by a dynamical factor $I(\bar{\kappa})$ depending only on the magnetization parameter

$$\bar{\kappa} \equiv \sqrt{2}\,\frac{b}{r_c} \tag{19}$$

and modified by a correlation factor $g(\Gamma)$, depending only on the correlation parameter Γ, where b is the distance of closest approach

$$b \equiv \frac{e^2}{4\pi\epsilon_0 a_{ws} k_B T}. \tag{20}$$

$I(\bar{\kappa})$ suppress the perpendicular to parallel collision in the strongly magnetized regime of $\bar{\kappa} > 1$. In this regime, only rare energetic collisions mix the perpendicular energy $E_\perp$ and parallel energy $E_\parallel$.

The correlation factor $g(\Gamma)$ enhances these rare collisions due to particle correlations in the cryogenic liquid regime of $1 < \Gamma < 10$.

3.1. *Strong magnetization*

I will briefly review the strong magnetization regime results, a rigorous derivation can be found in Ref. [11]. For $r_c < b$, the perpendicular energy of two particles is an adiabatic invariant $E_\perp = E_{\perp 1} + E_{\perp 2}$, that is conserved by most collisions except by rare energetic (large $E_\parallel$) collision. The cross-section for sharing perpendicular and parallel energy is a function of $E_\parallel$:

$$\sigma(E_\parallel) \propto \exp\left[-\pi\left(\frac{b}{r_c}\right)\right] \approx \exp\left[-\pi\left(\frac{Cst}{E_\parallel}\right)^{\frac{3}{2}}\right]. \tag{21}$$

That is, the cross-section for $E_\parallel - E_\perp$ sharing increases exponentially for large $E_\parallel$. The collision rate is obtained by integrating the product of the maxwellian particle distribution and $\sigma(E_\parallel)$.

$$\nu_{\perp\parallel}^{\text{no corr}} = \int dE_\parallel \frac{1}{k_B T} \exp\left(-\frac{E_\parallel}{k_B T}\right) \sigma(E_\parallel) = n\bar{v}b^2 4\sqrt{2}\, I(\bar{\kappa}), \tag{22}$$

where $I(\bar{\kappa})$ is [13]:

$$I(\bar{\kappa}) \approx 1.5 \exp\left(-2.044\, \bar{\kappa}^{\frac{2}{5}}\right). \tag{23}$$

The Maxwellian has almost no particles at large $E_\parallel$ and the cross-section is large at large $E_\parallel$ as shown in Figure 6. Most of the collisions causing sharing of $E_\parallel$ and $E_\perp$ comes from the "Gamow" peak shown in Figure 6. For example, for $\bar{\kappa} = 20$, the Gamow peak is located at $4\bar{v}$ that is less than 2% of the particles participate in such "rare" collision. The cyclotron energy is released only by rare collisions, analog to fusion reactions where the energy stored in the nuclei is liberated only by rare energetic collisions.

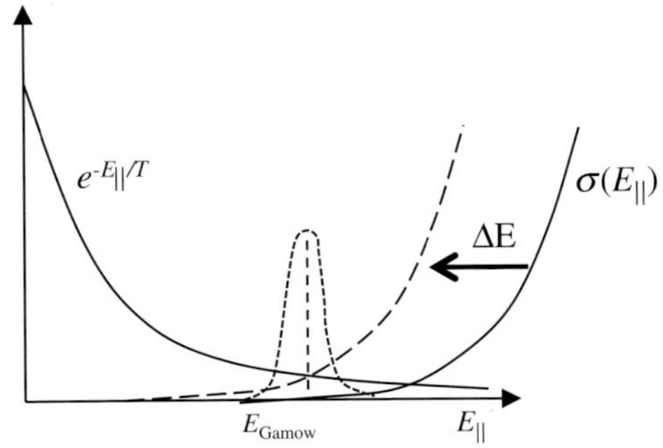

Fig. 6. Graphic description of the integrand of Equation (22) showing exponentially decaying Maxwellian particle energy distribution and the exponentially growing cross-section σ. The product of the particle distribution and the cross-section gives rise to the Gamow peak. Shifting σ by ΔE gives enhancement $\exp(\Delta E/k_B T)$.

3.2. *Correlations*

Correlations enhance the perpendicular to parallel collision rate through screening effects, by reducing the amount of parallel energy required by two ions to come within a distance ρ. In the absence of shielding, the energy required is:

$$E_{\|} = \frac{e^2}{4\pi\epsilon_0\rho}, \tag{24}$$

in contrast, with Debye screening the parallel energy required is smaller:

$$E_{\|} = \frac{e^2}{4\pi\epsilon_0\rho}\exp\left(\frac{-\rho}{\lambda_D}\right) \simeq \frac{1}{4\pi\epsilon_0}\left[\frac{e^2}{\rho} - \frac{e^2}{\lambda_D}\right]. \tag{25}$$

In other words, screening reduces the parallel energy required to come within a distance ρ. In the strong coupling regime of $\Gamma > 1$, the effective shielding distance is the inter-particle spacing, and the energy required for a collision at distance $\rho < a_{\text{ws}}$ is:

$$E_{\|} \simeq \frac{1}{4\pi\epsilon_0}\left[\frac{e^2}{\rho} - \frac{e^2}{a_{\text{ws}}}\right]. \tag{26}$$

This shifts the cross-section $\sigma(E_{\|})$ by $\Delta E_{\|} = e^2/(4\pi\epsilon_0 a_{\text{ws}})$ as shown in Figure 6. Equivalently, the Maxwellian in Equation (22) is shifted by $\Delta E_{\|}/(k_B T) = e^2/(4\pi\epsilon_0 a_{\text{ws}} k_B T) = \Gamma$, therefore Equation (22) becomes:

$$\nu_{\perp\|}^{\text{corr}} \simeq \int dE_{\|}\,\frac{1}{k_B T}\,\exp\left(-\frac{E_{\|}}{k_B T} - \frac{e^2}{4\pi\epsilon_0 a_{\text{ws}} k_B T}\right)\sigma(E_{\|}),$$

$$= \exp\left(\frac{e^2}{4\pi\epsilon_0 a_{\text{ws}} k_B T}\right) \int dE_{\parallel} \, \frac{1}{k_B T} \, \exp\left(-\frac{E_{\parallel}}{k_B T}\right) \sigma(E_{\parallel})$$

$$= \exp(\Gamma) \;\; \nu_{\perp\parallel}^{\text{no corr}}. \tag{27}$$

Correlation increases the perpendicular to parallel collision rate by a factor of roughly $g(\Gamma) = \exp(\Gamma)$. It is worth noting that the enhancement is independent of $\sigma(E)$, as in the fusion case, where this effect is known as the Salpeter enhancement.

3.3. *Experiments*

To test the theoretically predicted correlation enhancement of the collision rate, we use a magnesium ion plasma contained in a Penning–Malmberg trap. The plasma density for this experiment is controlled with a rotating wall ($0.12\times10^7 \leq n \leq 2\times10^7$ cm^{-3}), the temperature ($2.5\times10^{-6} \leq T \leq 1$ eV) is controlled by laser cooling, the uniform axial magnetic field was changed in the range of $1.2\text{T} \leq B \leq 3\text{T}$. The adiabaticity parameter $\bar{\kappa}$ is equal to one at a temperature $T = 5 \times 10^{-4}$eV and $B = 3\,$T. The coupling parameter is $\Gamma = 1$ for $n = 2 \times 10^7$cm^{-3} and $T = 6 \times 10^{-5}$ eV.

The measured perpendicular to parallel collision rate is plotted in Figure 7 for two densities $n = 2 \times 10^7$ and 0.12×10^7cm^{-3} labeled $n_7 = 2$ and $n_7 = 0.12$. In both cases, the collision rate is strongly suppressed when $\bar{\kappa}$ is larger than unity. The solid lines are theory curves obtained from Equation (22) using numerical values of $I(\bar{\kappa})$ from Ref. [13] with no adjustable parameters.

The dashed lines are from Equation (27). At lower density, the plasma is never strongly correlated, as shown by Γ which is also plotted for both densities. The $n = 2\times10^7$ cm^{-3} density labeled $n_7 = 2$ has $\Gamma > 1$ at low temperatures, and the measured collisionality is enhanced by several orders of magnitude over theory neglecting correlations. At low density, the collision rate is measured down to a rate of 1 sec^{-1}, setting an upper limit on extraneous collisional effects. Figure 8 shows the measured collision rate divided by the theoretical rate neglecting correlations, that is, the Salpeter enhancement $g(\Gamma)$. The enhancement depends on Γ but is independent of $\bar{\kappa}$, as predicted by theory. The measured correlation enhancement $g(\Gamma)$ is consistent with equilibrium shielding theories, and no support for alternative dynamic shielding effects is seen.

This work illustrates how laboratory non-neutral plasmas can be used to study high energy density plasmas where the same enhancement applies

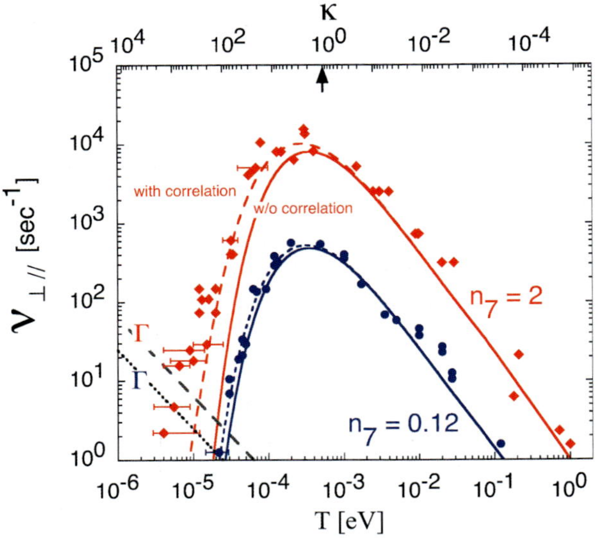

Fig. 7. Measured collision rates for two densities versus temperature (lower axis) and $\bar{\kappa}$ (upper axis) compared to theory with and without correlations. The correlation parameter Γ for high and low density is also shown.

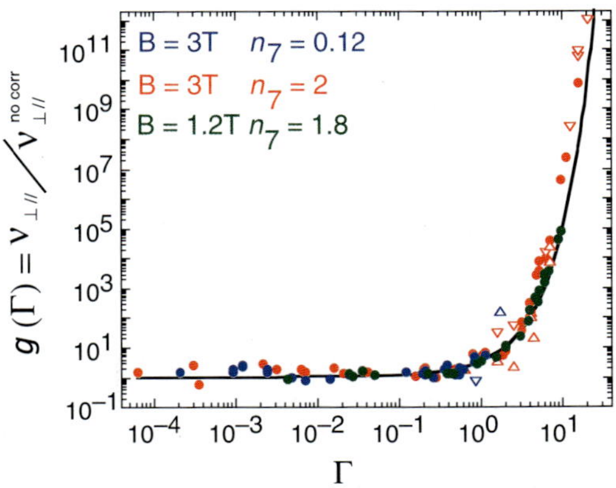

Fig. 8. Correlation enhancement $g(\Gamma)$ of the collision rate versus the correlation parameter Γ.

to rare energetic fusion collisions in hot, dense correlated plasmas such as stars.

3.3.1. *Summary of perpendicular to parallel collision rate*

The perpendicular to parallel collision rate is strongly suppressed in the "strong magnetization" regime of $\bar{\kappa} > 1$. Only rare energetic collisions cause $E_\perp$ to $E_\parallel$ energy exchange. These rare energetic collisions are strongly enhanced in the correlated liquid and crystal regimes. Enhancement of up to 10^9 over uncorrelated theory is observed. The same enhancement applies to rare energetic fusion collisions in hot, dense, correlated plasmas such as stars.

4. Tutorial Problem

Devise a technique to measure the perpendicular to parallel collision rate $\nu_{\perp\parallel}$ in a magnetized plasma. [*Hint*: look at Equation (17) to see which physical quantities have to be perturbed to measure the collision rate $\nu_{\perp\parallel}$].

A detailed description of two different techniques is given in Ref. [12]. The first technique directly observes $T_\perp$ and $T_\parallel$ as they relax to a common temperature. The parallel temperature is initially increased by small oscillating voltages applied at one end of the plasma. This direct measurement is practical only for slow rates ($\nu_{\perp\parallel} < 100\ \mathrm{s}^{-1}$) due to photon counting rate limitations, and is not accurate for low temperatures ($T < 10^{-4}$eV) since ion-neutral collisions give a heating rate which dominates the temperature evolution.

The second technique also uses small oscillating voltages applied at one end of the plasma. This acts as a piston and alternatively compresses and expands the plasma in the axial direction. If the oscillation frequency f_{osc} is large compared to the collision rate, the cycle is a reversible process since heat is not transferred to the perpendicular degrees of freedom (DoF). Similarly, if the oscillation frequency is low compared to the collision rate, the cycle is also reversible, since heat is fully shared with the perpendicular DoF. In contrast, if $f_{\mathrm{osc}} \sim \nu_{\perp\parallel}$, the process is not reversible: more work is done during the compression stroke and the excess appears as plasma heat. The maximum heat per cycle occurs when $2\pi f_{\mathrm{osc}} C \simeq \nu_{\perp\parallel}$, where C is the specific heat at constant density of a magnetized plasma. In the absence of correlations $C = 1/3$; and C increases slightly in the presence of correlations.

Acknowledgments

This work was supported by National Science Foundation Grant PHY-1414570, Department of Energy Grant DE-SC0002451 and Department of Energy High Energy Density Laboratory Plasma Grant DE-SC0008693. The author thanks the organizers of Les Houches Winter School for the opportunity to contribute to the workshop. The author also thanks Prof. C.F. Driscoll, Prof. D.H.E. Dubin, and Prof. T.M. O'Neil for many years of enlightening guidance and theoretical support.

References

1. R. C. Davidson *et al.*, *Frontiers in High Energy Density Physics*. NRC, Washington DC, The National Academies Press (2003).
2. V. E. Fortov *et al.*, Dusty plasmas, *Physics-Uspekhi* **47**, 447–492, (2004); H. Thomas *et al.*, Plasma crystal: Coulomb crystallization in a dusty plasma, *Phys. Rev. Lett.* **72**, 652–656, (1994).
3. D. H. E. Dubin and T. M. O'Neil, Trapped nonneutral plasmas, liquids, and crystals (the thermal equilibrium states), *Rev. Mod. Phys.* **71**, 87–172 (1999); T. M. O'Neil and D. H. E. Dubin, Thermal equilibria and thermodynamics of trapped plasmas with a single sign of charge, *Phys. Plasmas* **5**, 2163–2193, (1998).
4. S. G. Kuzmin and T. M. O'Neil, Numerical simulation of ultracold plasmas, *Phys. Plasmas* **9**, 3743 (2002).
5. D. H. E. Dubin and T. M. O'Neil, Computer simulation of ion clouds in a Penning trap, *Phys. Rev. Lett.* **60**, 511 (1988); D. H. E. Dubin, Effect of correlations on the thermal equilibrium and normal modes of a nonneutral plasma, *Phys. Rev. E* **53**, 5268 (1996).
6. S. L. Gilbert *et al.*, Shell-structure phase of magnetically confined strongly coupled plasmas, *Phys. Rev. Lett.* **60**, 2022–2025 (1988).
7. D. H. E. Dubin, Correlation energies of simple bounded Coulomb lattices, *Phys. Rev. A* **40**, 1140 (1989).
8. H. Totsuji *et al.*, Competition between two forms of ordering in finite Coulomb clusters, *Phys. Rev. Lett.* **88**, 125002 (2002).
9. W. M. Itano *et al.*, Bragg diffraction from crystallized ion plasmas, *Science* **279**, 686–689 (1998).
10. E. E. Salpeter, Electron screening and thermonuclear reactions, *Aust. J. Phys.* **7**, 373 (1954); E. E. Salpeter and H. Van Horn, Nuclear reaction rates at high densities, *Astrophys. J.* **155**, 916 (1969).
11. D. H. E. Dubin, Modeling nuclear fusion in dense plasmas using a cryogenic non-neutral plasma, *Phys. Plasmas* **15**, 055705 (2008).

12. F. Anderegg *et al.*, Measurement of correlation-enhanced collision rates, *Phys. Rev. Lett.* **102**, 185001 (2009).
13. M. E. Glinsky *et al.*, Collisional equipartition rate for a magnetized pure electron plasma, *Phys. Fluids B* **4**, 1156 (1992).

CHAPTER THIRTEEN

AUTORESONANCE*

J. Fajans

Department of Physics
University of California, Berkeley
Berkeley, 94720-7300, California, USA
joel@physics.berkeley.edu

L. Friedland

Racah Institute of Physics, Hebrew University of Jerusalem
91904, Jerusalem, Israel
lazar@mail.huji.ac.il

A weakly-driven pendulum cannot be strongly excited by a fixed frequency drive. The only way to strongly excite the pendulum is to use a drive whose frequency decreases with time. Feedback is often used to control the rate at which the frequency decreases. Feedback need not be employed, however, the drive frequency can simply be swept downwards. With this method, the drive strength must exceed a threshold proportional to the sweep rate raised to the 3/4 power. This threshold has been discovered only recently, and holds for a very broad class of driven nonlinear oscillators. The threshold may explain the abundance of 3:2 resonances and sparsity of 2:1 resonances observed between the orbital periods of Neptune and the Plutinos (Pluto and many of the Kuiper Belt objects), and has been extensively investigated in the Diocotron and other systems in single-species plasmas.

*This chapter was largely reproduced with permission from "Autoresonant (nonstationary) excitation of pendulums, Plutinos, plasmas, and other nonlinear oscillators", J. Fajans and L. Friedland, *Am. J. Phys.* **69**, 1096 (2001). Available at: http://dx.doi.org/10.1119/1.1389278. (Copyright 2001, American Association of Physics Teachers.)

1. Introduction

How can you excite a pendulum to high amplitude with a weak drive? The usual answer is to drive the pendulum at its linear resonant frequency, f_0. However, as the pendulum amplitude increases, its oscillation frequency decreases and the pendulum goes out of phase with its drive. As shown in Figure 1, the amplitude only attains a modest value before beating all the way back down to zero [1].

It is not surprising that driving at f_0 will not strongly excite the pendulum. As shown by the solutions of the pendulum equation,

$$\ddot{\theta} + (2\pi f_0)^2 \sin\theta = \bar{\epsilon}\cos(2\pi f t), \tag{1}$$

graphed in Figure 2 [2–4], the equilibrium response of the pendulum is large only when the drive frequency f is lower than the linear frequency f_0. Even this is not sufficient, however, because there exist two stable branches to the response, one with a much higher amplitude than the other. Suddenly

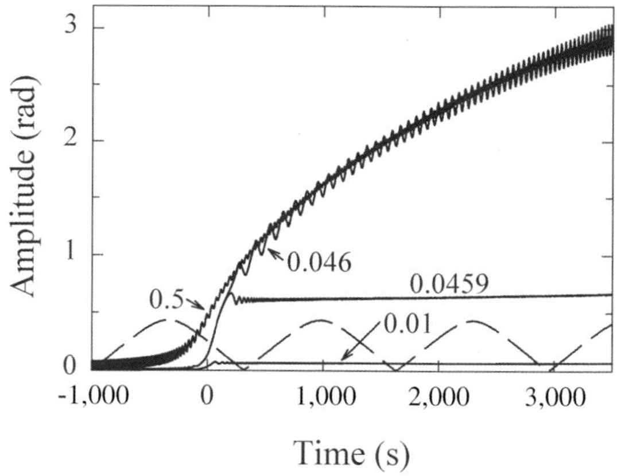

Fig. 1. The response of a pendulum to a drive sweeping at rate $\alpha = 0.001$ for four different values of the drive strength $\bar{\epsilon}$ (solid lines) and to a fixed frequency drive of strength $\bar{\epsilon} = 0.1$ (dashed line). The response to the $\bar{\epsilon} = 0.01$ drive is very small, and the response to the $\bar{\epsilon} = 0.0459$ drive is only somewhat greater. However, the response to the $\bar{\epsilon} = 0.0460$ drive, which is only 0.2% greater than the $\bar{\epsilon} = 0.0459$ drive, is large, and results in the pendulum swinging over its top. The response to the $\bar{\epsilon} = 0.5$ drive is qualitatively similar to the response to the $\bar{\epsilon} = 0.0460$ drive. Clearly there is a sharp threshold near $\bar{\epsilon} = 0.0460$. The oscillations in the $\bar{\epsilon} = 0.0460$ curve are the manifestations of the pseudoparticle oscillations in the pseudopotential wells. These curves come from numerically simulating Equation (2) with $\omega_0 = 2\pi$. For clarity, the timescale for the fixed frequency curve (the dashed line) has been expanded by a factor of 10.

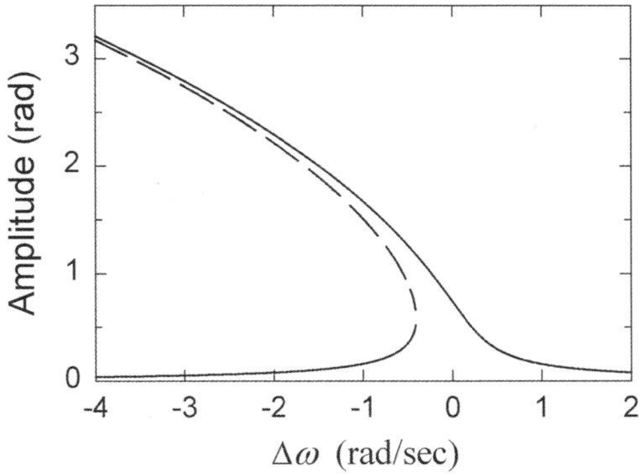

Fig. 2. Equilibrium pendulum amplitude as a function of the drive frequency detuning $\Delta\omega$, defined by $\omega = \omega_0 + \Delta\omega$, where ω is the drive frequency. (For the swept drive used in this paper, $\Delta\omega = -\alpha t$.) Only the first-order correction to the frequency is retained in this graph, so the equilibria come from solving for the steady amplitude solutions to the equation $\ddot{\theta} + \omega_0^2(\theta - \theta^3/6) = \bar{\epsilon}\cos[(\omega_0 + \Delta\omega)t]$. The two solid lines are stable equilibria, and the dashed line is an unstable equilibrium. Far from resonance, the low amplitude solutions reduce to the standard solutions of the linearized pendulum equation, $\ddot{\theta} + \omega_0^2\theta = \bar{\epsilon}\cos[(\omega_0 + \Delta\omega)t]$. The high amplitude solutions comes from balancing the nonlinearities in the next order equation. The θ^3 term introduces the possibility, realized for large negative $\Delta\omega$, of three equilibria at a given $\Delta\omega$. For this figure, the drive strength is $\bar{\epsilon} = 2$, and $\omega_0 = 2\pi$.

applying a low frequency drive to an initially quiescent pendulum results in oscillations around the low amplitude branch, not the high amplitude branch. Here, θ is the angle of the pendulum from vertical, and $\bar{\epsilon}$ is the drive strength.

The only way to strongly excite the pendulum from rest is to sweep the frequency downward and hope that the pendulum's response follows the response function's upper branch to high amplitude. Feedback can be used to appropriately sweep the frequency; this is how we excite a child's swing. But there are circumstances in which using feedback is impractical or undesirable. For instance, you might not be able to sense the phase of the pendulum well enough to apply feedback properly, or you might want to simultaneously excite several pendulums with the same drive. What can you do then? Simply starting the sweep at a frequency well above f_0, and sweeping downwards through the resonance at a sufficiently slow rate can strongly excite the pendulum [1]. We call this phenomenon autoresonance [5] because, at each instant in time, the pendulum automatically adjusts its amplitude so that its instantaneous nonlinear frequency matches the drive frequency. Autoresonant effects were first observed in particle accelerators [6], and have since been noted in atomic physics [5,7], fluid dynamics [8], plasmas [9,10], nonlinear waves [11,12], and planetary dynamics [13,14].

Autoresonance in pendulums and other systems has been used implicitly in many papers [15–23]. However, these papers do not address a very important question: how fast can the frequency be swept and still strongly excite the pendulum? Specifically, given a driven pendulum described by the equation,

$$\ddot{\theta} + \omega_0^2 \sin\theta = \bar{\epsilon}\cos(\omega_0 t - \alpha t^2/2), \tag{2}$$

how large can the sweep rate α be and still stay in resonance? Here, $\omega_0/2\pi = f_0$ is the pendulum's linear frequency, and the drive frequency is $\omega_0 - \alpha t$.

Recently, we have addressed this problem in a series of papers [9,10, 24–26] focused on a similar nonlinear oscillator, the Diocotron mode [27] in non-neutral plasmas. Here, we apply these results to the pendulum, and find that there is a very sharp threshold for autoresonance; if the drive amplitude $\bar{\epsilon}$ exceeds a threshold proportional to the sweep rate α raised to the three quarters power, the pendulum will follow the drive to high amplitude (see Figures 1 and 3). If the drive amplitude is below this threshold, the pendulum amplitude will stay very low. This $\alpha^{3/4}$ scaling applies to a very broad class of nonlinear oscillators, not just to the pendulum and to

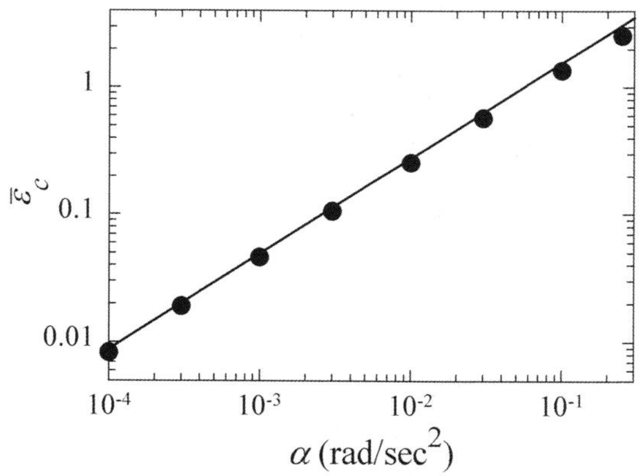

Fig. 3. The numerically determined critical drive strength as a function of the sweep rate α (dots) and the theoretical scaling from Equation (24) (line) for $\omega_0 = 2\pi$ The numeric data is in excellent agreement with the theory. Experiments [9,10] with the Diocotron mode in non-neutral plasmas have verified this scaling law over five orders of magnitude in α.

the Diocotron. Moreover, the scaling can be extended to drives at subharmonics of f_0 [24,28] and survives in the presence of damping [26].

We begin this chapter with the mathematical analysis of the threshold. Then we describe some of the Diocotron experiments in plasmas, and discuss how the threshold explains the Plutino resonances. We end with some concluding remarks.

2. Analysis

The complete threshold analysis is given in Refs. [8,10], so we will only give a precis here. The analysis divides into three regimes: the linear, phasetrapping regime where the pendulum amplitude is so low that its frequency does not significantly deviate from f_0, the weakly-nonlinear regime where we take only the lowest order amplitude correction to the frequency, and the strongly-nonlinear regime where we must use the complete expression for the pendulum frequency. We will consider each regime in turn.

2.1. *Linear, phase-trapping regime*

The pendulum will be in the linear regime from the time at which the drive is first applied, $t = t_s < 0$, to near the time at which the drive frequency crosses f_0, namely, $t \approx 0$. Since the system is effectively linear here, it reduces to a simple harmonic oscillator (SHO) subject to a swept frequency drive.

$$\ddot{\theta} + \omega_0^2\theta = \bar{\epsilon}\cos(\omega_0 t - \alpha t^2/2). \tag{3}$$

This system was solved exactly in terms of complicated Fresnel Sine and Cosine functions by Lewis [29]. However, the behavior of the solution can be understood quite readily. Like any SHO, the sudden application of the drive excites a driven mode at the drive frequency and an undriven, homogeneous mode at the linear frequency. Assuming that the pendulum is initially quiescent, the two modes have equal and opposite amplitude, are proportional to the drive, and inversely proportional to the deviation $\Delta\omega(t_s) = \omega(t_s) - \omega_0 = -\alpha t_s$ from the linear resonant frequency. Thereafter, just like in a steady-state SHO, the amplitude of the driven mode continues to be approximately inversely proportional to $\Delta\omega(t)$. Consequently, the driven mode grows proportional to $1/t$ as $t \to 0$. The homogeneous mode is not further excited by the sweeping frequency.

The net motion of the pendulum is the sum of the phase-locked driven mode and the free-running homogeneous mode. Initially, the net motion will not be phase-locked because the amplitudes of the two modes are comparable. But since the driven mode amplitude grows while the homogeneous mode amplitude is constant, the driven mode will soon dominate, and the net pendulum motion phase-locks to the drive.

2.2. *Weakly nonlinear regime*

In the weakly nonlinear regime, we need to retain the lowest order amplitude correction to the pendulum frequency. The set of weakly nonlinear equations describing our adiabatically driven pendulum can be derived as follows. We begin by replacing $\sin\theta$ by its truncated expansion in Equation (2):

$$\ddot{\theta} + \omega_0^2 \left(1 - \frac{\theta^2}{6}\right)\theta = \bar{\epsilon}\cos(\psi) = \bar{\epsilon}\mathrm{Re}(e^{i\psi}), \tag{4}$$

where $\psi = \omega_0 t - \alpha t^2/2$ is the driving phase. Then we seek solutions of Equation (4) of the form

$$\theta = a\cos\varphi = \mathrm{Re}(ae^{i\varphi}), \tag{5}$$

where $a(t)$ is the real amplitude, and $\varphi(t)$ is the phase of the pendulum, and we have neglected higher harmonics (i.e. the terms with $e^{2i\varphi}$, $e^{3i\varphi}$, etc.) By differentiating Equation (5), we find

$$\ddot{\theta} \approx \mathrm{Re}\left[(2i\dot{\varphi}\dot{a} + i\ddot{\varphi}a - \dot{\varphi}^2 a)e^{i\varphi}\right], \tag{6}$$

and by cubing Equation (5),

$$\theta^3 \approx \mathrm{Re}\left(\frac{3}{4}a^3 e^{i\varphi}\right), \tag{7}$$

where we have neglected the $\ddot{a}$ term in Equation (6) (slow amplitude assumption) and kept the first harmonic term only in Equation (7). With these approximations, Equation (4) becomes

$$2i\dot{\varphi}\dot{a} + i\ddot{\varphi}a - \dot{\varphi}^2 a + \omega_0^2\left(1 - \frac{1}{8}a^2\right)a = \bar{\epsilon}e^{i(\psi-\varphi)}. \tag{8}$$

On separating the real and imaginary parts in the last equation, we obtain:

$$\frac{d\left(a^2\dot{\varphi}\right)}{dt} = a(2\dot{\varphi}\dot{a} + \ddot{\varphi}a) = -\bar{\epsilon}a\sin\Phi, \tag{9}$$

and

$$\omega_0^2 - \dot{\varphi}^2 = \omega_0^2\frac{a^2}{8} + \frac{\bar{\epsilon}}{a}\cos\Phi, \tag{10}$$

where the phase mismatch is defined as $\Phi = \varphi - \psi$. Next, we assume that the system is nearly in resonance, i.e. that the pendulum frequency is close to the linear frequency, $\dot{\varphi} \approx \omega_0$. Then $\omega_0^2 - \dot{\varphi}^2 \approx 2\omega_0(\omega_0 - \dot{\varphi})$, and Equations (9) and (10) can be rewritten as:

$$\dot{a} = -\frac{\bar{\epsilon}}{2\omega_0} \sin \Phi, \tag{11}$$

$$\dot{\Phi} = \omega_0 - \frac{\omega_0}{16} a^2 - \dot{\psi} - \frac{\bar{\epsilon}}{2a\omega_0} \cos \Phi. \tag{12}$$

Finally, we define the action variable $I = a^2/2$, and the weakly nonlinear frequency of the pendulum $\Omega(I) = \omega_0 - \omega_0 a^2/16 = \omega_0(1 - \beta I)$, $(\beta = 1/8)$ and substitute the driving frequency $\dot{\psi} = \omega_0 - \alpha t$, arriving at [30]

$$\frac{dI}{dt} = -2\epsilon I^{1/2} \sin \Phi, \tag{13}$$

$$\frac{d\Phi}{dt} = \Omega(I) - \omega_0 + \alpha t - \epsilon I^{-1/2} \cos \Phi, \tag{14}$$

where $\epsilon = \bar{\epsilon}/(\sqrt{8}\omega_0)$ is the normalized drive strength.

It should be mentioned that the expression $I = a^2/2$ is just the small amplitude limit of the normalized action variable frequently used in describing nonlinear oscillators. More generally, the normalized action, in our case, is defined as

$$I = \frac{1}{2\pi\omega_0} \oint \dot{\theta}\, d\theta, \tag{15}$$

where the integration is over one period of oscillation of the unperturbed pendulum. The action I is a measure of the energy in the system, and, in combination with another variable called the "angle", Θ, is used to replace the phase space variables $(\theta, \dot{\theta})$ in studying nonlinear oscillators. The (I, Θ) representation is very convenient in studying weak perturbations of oscillators because the unperturbed motion in (I, Θ) variables is extremely simple, i.e. $I =$ const and $\Theta = \Omega(I)t$. Furthermore, the structure of Equations (13) and (14) is also preserved in a general nonlinear case, with Φ representing the phase mismatch $\Theta - \psi$, and $2I^{1/2}$ and $I^{-1/2}$ in the interaction terms in these equations replaced by some function $V(I)$ and dV/dI, respectively.

Equations (13) and (14) are easy to interpret. If the drive is turned off ($\epsilon = 0$), the action will be constant, and the phase mismatch Φ will advance appropriately. When the drive is on ($\epsilon \neq 0$), the action will increase or decrease depending on whether or not the pendulum is in phase or out of phase with the drive. The rate at which the action changes depends on the action itself, because the work done per cycle depends on the pendulum amplitude. Likewise the drive can "drag" the phase mismatch. When the pendulum amplitude is large, it is difficult for the drive to change the pendulum angle quickly, but when the pendulum amplitude is small, the drive can change the pendulum angle readily. Consequently, the rate of change of the phase mismatch is inversely proportional to (the square root of) the action.

The pendulum enters the weakly nonlinear regime from the linear regime at about $t = 0$. From the results of Section 2.1, we know that the system is phase-locked at this time, so Φ starts out near π. If the system is to stay in resonance, it must stay phase-locked and Φ must remain near π. Otherwise, the phase between the pendulum and its drive would stray and the drive would not be effectively coupled. If Φ is to stay near π, the right-hand side of Equation (14) must be close to zero. This requirement will be met if

$$0 = \alpha t - \beta\omega_0 I_0 + \frac{\epsilon}{I_0^{1/2}}, \tag{16}$$

where we have defined the action to be within a small deviation Δ of the equilibrium action I_0, $I = I_0 - \Delta$. Note that I_0 is a slow function of time: the action grows as time increases and the drive frequency gets further and further from the linear resonant frequency. If αt is considered to be the slowly varying detuning, this equation is identical (in action-angle variables) to the standard equation used to find the nonlinear response of a pendulum, and its solution is plotted in Figure 2.

Since I_0 is a slow function of time, we can expand the system [Equations (13) and (14)] around the instantaneous value of I_0, yielding two new equations:

$$\dot{\Delta} = 2\epsilon\sqrt{I_0}\sin\Phi + \frac{\alpha}{S}, \tag{17}$$

$$\dot{\Phi} = S\Delta, \tag{18}$$

where $S = \beta\omega_0 + \epsilon/2I_0^{3/2}$. Note that S is a function of time through I_0. Together, these two equations form a Hamiltonian system with

$$H(\Phi, \Delta) = S\Delta^2/2 + V_{\text{pseudo}}(\Phi), \tag{19}$$

where

$$V_{\text{pseudo}}(\Phi) = 2\epsilon I_0^{1/2}\cos\Phi - \frac{\alpha}{S}\Phi. \tag{20}$$

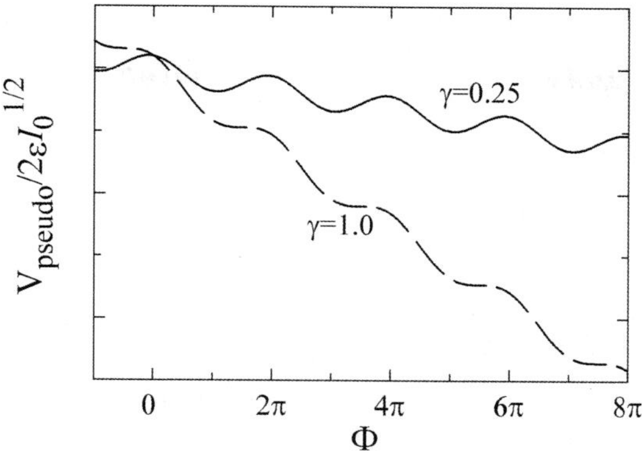

Fig. 4. Critical (dashed line) and typical above-threshold (solid line) normalized pseudopotentials $V_{\text{pseudo}}/2\epsilon I_0^{1/2} = \cos\Phi - \gamma\Phi$ as a function of the phaseslip Φ, where $\gamma = \alpha/2\epsilon I_0^{1/2}S$. The critical pseudopotential, defined by Equation (21), occurs when $\gamma = 1.0$.

Thus, the system reduces to a pseudoparticle of slowly-varying effective mass $1/S$ moving in a slowly-varying pseudopotential well.

The pseudopotential, V_{pseudo}, looks like a tilted series of potential wells (see Figure 4). Near $t = 0$, we know that the system is phase-locked and Φ is near π; for this to remain true, the pseudoparticle must be trapped at the bottom of one of the potential wells. If the pseudopotential and the effective mass change slowly, and the wells continue to exist, the pseudoparticle will stay trapped at the bottom of the well as time advances. The phase mismatch Φ will stay near zero, the equilibrium action will continue to satisfy Equation (16), and the system will stay in resonance. However, the pseudopotential wells will only exist if the pseudopotential tilt is less than the well depth, i.e. if

$$2\epsilon I_0^{1/2} > \alpha/S. \tag{21}$$

If this condition is not met, the wells will disappear, the pseudoparticle will escape, phase-locking will be lost, and the system will not stay in resonance [1]. By differentiating the quantity $SI_0^{1/2}$ (remember that S is itself a function of I_0), it is easy to show that there is a critical action at which condition (21) is most difficult to satisfy and the wells are most likely to disappear,

$$I_{0\text{crt}} = (\epsilon/\beta\omega_0)^{2/3}. \tag{22}$$

If the system makes it past this critical action, the wells will be retained effectively forever, and the system will grow to high amplitude. Thus, replacing I_0 with $I_{0\text{crit}}$ in Equation (21) yields the minimum drive amplitude for which the system stays in resonance:

$$\epsilon_c = \frac{1}{\sqrt{\beta\omega_0}}\left(\frac{\alpha}{3}\right)^{3/4}, \tag{23}$$

or

$$\bar{\epsilon}_c = 8\sqrt{\omega_0}\left(\frac{\alpha}{3}\right)^{3/4}. \tag{24}$$

This threshold has been verified numerically (see Figures 1 and 3) and, for the non-neutral plasma Diocotron mode, experimentally [9,10].

For most system parameters, $I_{0\text{crit}}$ is quite small. For ϵ near the critical value (Equation (23)), $I_{0\text{crit}}$ is approximately $(1/\beta)(3N)^{-1/2}$, where $N = \omega_0^2/\alpha$ measures the number of cycles in the sweep, so $I_{0\text{crit}}$ is indeed small for any reasonable sweep rate. Consequently, whether or not the system stays in resonance is determined at very low pendulum amplitude. Thus, the assumptions made at the beginning of this section, that we need only take the first order terms in the action-angle equations, and that only the first-order correction to the linear frequency is important, are valid. More importantly, we can generalize our results to *any* driven nonlinear oscillator whose nonlinear frequency dependence reduces to $\omega = \omega_0(1 + \beta I)$ for small I, i.e. when the equation of motion reduces to

$$\ddot{\theta} + \omega_0^2(\theta + a\theta^2 + b\theta^3) = \bar{\epsilon}\cos(\omega_0 t - \alpha t^2/2). \tag{25}$$

For the pendulum, $\beta = 3b/4 - 5a^2/6$ [3]. If $a = 0$, Equation (25) is called the Duffing equation, and is the low amplitude description of many physical systems. Systems that reduce to the Duffing Equation are very common because the "Duffing" term, $b\omega_0^2\theta^3$, is the first symmetric nonlinearity. Thus, any system whose potential goes like $U(\theta) = \bar{a}\theta^2 + \bar{b}\theta^4 + \cdots$, where $\bar{a}$ and $\bar{b}$ are constants, will reduce to a Duffing oscillator at low amplitude. The pendulum, the Diocotron (Section 3) [27], many mechanical systems [16–20], galvanometers [15], electronic oscillators [21], etc., all reduce appropriately. Some two-dimensional systems, like the Neptune–Plutinos systems (Section 5), also reduce appropriately.

2.3. *Strongly-nonlinear regime*

In the strongly-nonlinear regime, the action becomes large, and the small I assumption used to derive Equations (13) and (14) is not strictly valid.

Nonetheless, computer simulations of the original equation of motion [Equation (2)] and analysis of the corresponding action-angle evolution Equation (31) confirm that the phase-locking in the system continues, and the frequency of the oscillator decreases (i.e. its oscillation amplitude grows) to approximately match that of the drive, until the pendulum swings over the top. This usually happens before the drive frequency reaches zero, as the small oscillations around the equilibrium action will be sufficient to drive the pendulum over.

Intuition might lead one to believe that the drive amplitude would have to increase eventually to excite the pendulum to very high amplitude; perhaps, the most remarkable aspect of the strongly-nonlinear regime is that the drive amplitude can be *decreased* when the pendulum amplitude is large. This follows from the decreasing pseudopotential tilt once past the critical action, which makes the wells effectively deeper. Thus, the drive can be decreased while still maintaining the wells.

3. Autoresonance in the Diocotron Mode in Pure-electron Plasmas

Consider a column of electrons that is aligned along a strong magnetic field **B**, and confined within a conducting cylindrical wall. If the column is displaced from the cylindrical wall axis, it will orbit around the axis. This oscillation is called the Diocotron mode [27, see Chapter 10], and is found in electron beams in accelerators and in "pure-electron plasmas" confined in Malmberg–Penning traps (Figure 5). Understanding the Diocotron

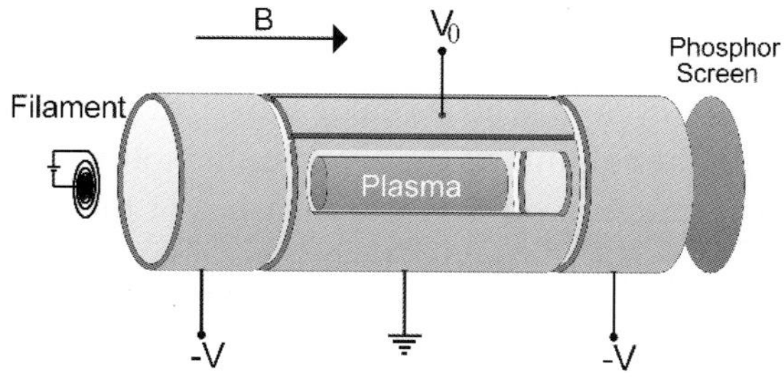

Fig. 5. Malmberg–Penning trap geometry. Electrons are confined axially by negatively biasing the end cylinders, and radially by a strong axial magnetic field. The electrons are emitted from the filament, and loaded into the trap by temporarily grounding the left cylinder. Portions of the wall are azimuthally segmented. Details of the trap operation can be found in [32].

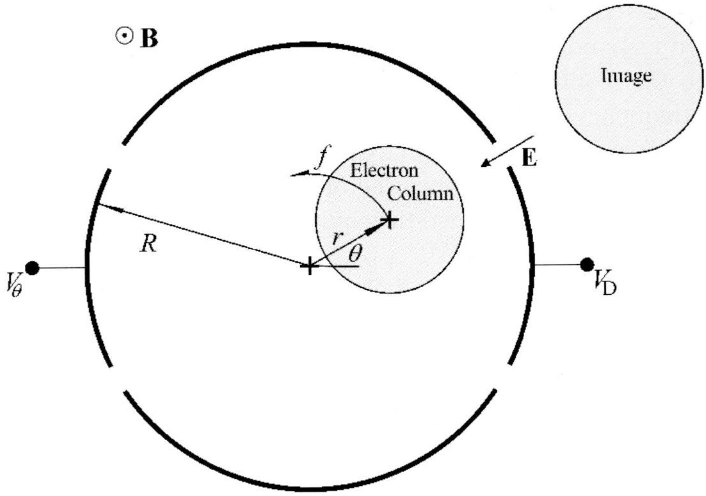

Fig. 6. Endview of the Malmberg–Penning trap showing the confining wall at R, the electron column a distance r from the trap center, the electron column image, the image electric field **E**, and the Diocotron drift at frequency f. The mode is detected by monitoring the image charge on the pickup sector V_θ and driven by applying a voltage to the drive sector V_D. Further details are given in [10].

has been crucial to understanding charged plasmas, and dozens of papers have been published on the subject. The Diocotron oscillation comes about because of an interaction between the electron column and its image. At any given instant, the electron column **E** × **B** drifts azimuthally in the electric field **E** of the image (See Figure 6). An electron subjected to crossed **E** and **B** fields will move perpendicular to both fields, hence the name **E** × **B** drift. The physics of the drift is simple: The electron is accelerated antiparallel to **E**, but the Lorentz force from **B** pushes the electron sideways. The net motion is a cycloid whose center moves at velocity (**E** × **B**.) The image moves with the column, so the net column motion is to orbit around the wall axis. The distance off-axis is a measure of the amplitude of the oscillation. The image electric field gets stronger nonlinearly as the column approaches the wall, so the oscillation frequency increases with amplitude, following the equation

$$\omega = \frac{\omega_0}{1 - r^2}, \tag{26}$$

where ω_0 is the linear frequency of the mode, and r is the suitably normalized oscillation amplitude. The oscillation is very robust, and very

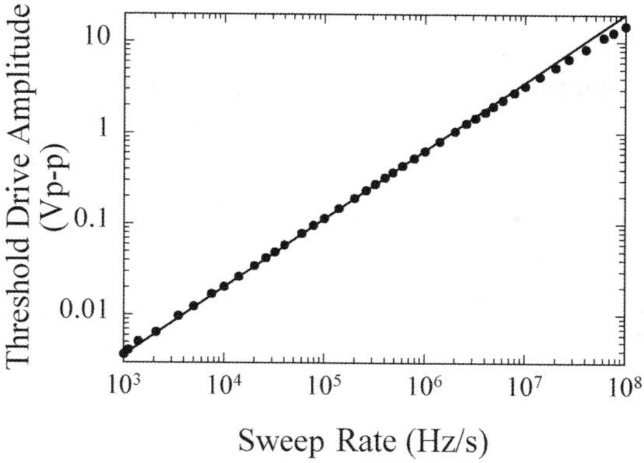

Fig. 7. Critical Diocotron drive amplitude versus sweep rate $\alpha/2\pi$. Measured results (•), and theoretical prediction from Equation (24) (solid line). For more information, see Ref. [10].

lightly damped; the column can orbit the trap hundreds of thousands of times.

At low amplitude (r small), the Diocotron reduces to a Duffing oscillator. It is easy to drive the Diocotron by impressing an oscillating voltage on an azimuthal section of the wall. By starting at a frequency below the linear frequency, and sweeping the frequency upwards, the Diocotron can be grown autoresonantly [9, 10, 24–26] to so large an amplitude that the electron column hits the wall. As show in Figure 7, the system obeys the sweep rate threshold scaling law Equation (24) over five orders of magnitude. Many other aspects of the autoresonant theory presented here have been tested with the Diocotron, including the behavior in the linear regime, the pseudopotential wells, and the possibility of lowering the drive strength once in the strongly-nonlinear regime.

4. Applications to Antimatter Plasmas

Autoresonant excitation of Diocotron waves has been employed to "park" positron plasmas off axis in multicell traps [33]. These traps contain large numbers of radially displaced Penning–Malmberg traps, and are designed to trap very large numbers of positrons. Autoresonant excitations of Diocotrons have also been studied as a means of transporting positrons off-axis into a particular positronium forming target in the AEgIS experiment [34]. Finally, autoresonant excitation of the axial motion of antiprotons is a key step in the synthesis of and trapping of antihydrogen by the ALPHA experiment [35–37] (see also Chapter 14).

5. The Problem of Plutinos

The autoresonance phenomenon and the threshold for capture into resonance described in Section 2.2 can be found in more complicated dynamical systems. One of the most remarkable examples is found in Nature in relation to early evolution of the trans-Neptunian region [38] of the solar system. In contrast to the nonlinear pendulum, the Keplerian two-body (Sun-planet) problem has two degrees of freedom (DoF) and yields elliptical orbits in a plane, given, in polar coordinates (r, φ), by equation $a/r = 1 + e\cos\varphi$, where e is the eccentricity of the orbit. It is well known that most planets in the solar system move roughly in one plane (the ecliptic) on nearly circular orbits with eccentricities $e < 0.09$. A notable exception is Pluto, the most distant planet in the solar system, which has a very eccentric orbit ($e = 0.25$). Furthermore, Pluto is observed to be in a 3:2 resonance with Neptune, i.e. Pluto completes two rotations around the sun during the time Neptune completes three rotations. According to present understanding, this peculiar synchronization has existed since the planetary formation several billions years ago.

Pluto is not the only trans-Neptunian body in the solar system. There exist a large number of smaller masses (estimated number of $\sim 100,000$) which comprise the Kuiper Belt, a disc shaped region at distances roughly between 35 AU to 100 AU from the sun (1 AU is the distance between the Earth and the Sun). Remarkably, about one-third of presently observed Kuiper Belt objects (KBO's) are also engaged in the 3:2 resonance with Neptune (these objects resemble Pluto and, thus, are called Plutinos) and also have very eccentric orbits $0.1 < e < 0.35$ [39]. How can one explain this anomaly? What is the origin of orbital eccentricity of the resonant trans-Neptunian objects?

It is now widely accepted that the resonances in the Plutino orbits are the result of Neptune's orbit migration during the last stage of planetary formation. Neptune's radius r_N experienced a slow increase (by roughly 30% during some time) due to some migration mechanism, and its orbital frequency decreased concomitantly. The force exerted by the orbiting Neptune acted as a quasi-periodic drive on the Plutinos, passing through, and capturing many of them in resonance [40], just like the pendulum phase-locks to its drive as described in Section 2.1. Beyond the trapping stage, as Neptune's radius continued to increase, the Plutinos entered autoresonance and their initially circular orbits developed growing radial oscillations, i.e. became increasingly eccentric (see the orbit equation above).

The theory of migrating planets explained a number of important features observed today, such as the distribution of eccentricities of Plutinos in the Kuiper belt, for example. Nevertheless, the early theory [41] could not explain the sparsity of KBO's in the similar, 2:1 resonance with Neptune. These early calculations yielded similar populations of 3:2 and 2:1 resonances. Astronomical observations, on the other hand, showed almost no 2:1 resonant KBO's. The sparsity of 2:1 resonant KBO's was one of the main remaining questions of the resonant KBO capture theory, with a possible explanation given only recently [14]. The explanation is related to the issue of thresholds for capture into resonance. We have shown that the governing equations describing orbital evolution of a KBO in the field of slowly migrating Neptune can be described by the reduced system of evolution equations identical to Equations (13) and 14, where I is replaced by e^2, while Φ represents the phase mismatch between the rotating Neptune and the KBO. In the $(j+1):j$ autoresonance, $(j+1)\Omega \approx j\omega_N(t)$, where Ω is the Keplerian frequency of the trapped KBO and $\omega_N(t)$ is the slowly varying frequency of migrating Neptune. Each resonance has a different coupling constant ϵ (see Equations (3) and (4)) and, thus, yields different Neptune migration timescale $t^{mig} = r_N(dr_N/dt)^{-1}$ thresholds for trapping into resonance. We have calculated these thresholds [14] and found that $t_{th}^{mig} = 2\times10^6$ and 2×10^7 years for capturing into 3:2 and 2:1 resonances, respectively. The order of magnitude difference between the thresholds is due to the Sun's rotation around the Sun–Neptune center of mass. Inclusion of this rotation required analysis of the associated three-body problem, but affected the timescale for capture into 2:1 resonance *only*, lowering the corresponding value of ϵ significantly, thus, increasing the threshold timescale by one order of magnitude. Therefore, if the actual migration timescale of Neptune is between 2×10^6 and 2×10^7 years, a large fraction of the KBOs would be captured into 3:2 resonance and none into 2:1 resonance, as observed in the present day solar system. Thus, these arguments allow us to find accurate bounds on the timescales involved in the early stage of the evolution of the solar system on the bases of present astronomical observations, and to discard slower Neptune migration models.

6. Conclusions

We have shown that a swept-frequency drive can strongly excite a pendulum. The initial drive frequency must be above the pendulum's linear frequency. The pendulum will phase-lock to the drive while the drive frequency is still above the linear frequency. If the pendulum remains locked to the drive past a critical drive frequency, the pendulum will be strongly excited as the drive continues to sweep downwards. In this circumstance, the pendulum's amplitude will automatically adjust itself so that the pendulum's nonlinear frequency will match the drive frequency: hence, the name autoresonance. The pendulum will remain locked to the drive only if the drive strength exceeds a threshold proportional to the sweep rate α raised to the 3/4 power (Equation (23)). The critical point occurs at a frequency which is only slightly lower than the linear frequency, where the pendulum amplitude is still quite low. Because the critical point occurs at such a low amplitude, only the lowest order corrections to the frequency are relevant, and the pendulum can be considered to be a Duffing oscillator (Equation (25)). Many if not most nonlinear oscillators reduce to the Duffing oscillator at low amplitude, so the analysis presented here is very general, and the same $\alpha^{3/4}$ drive strength scaling applies to all these systems.

In this chapter, we assumed that the oscillator is lightly damped, but recent calculations and experiments [26] show that the results still apply in the presence of appreciable damping. We demonstrated elsewhere [24,28] that a very similar scaling law holds if a system is driven near a subharmonic ω_0/n. In this case, the scaling law becomes $\alpha^{3/4n}$. Furthermore, autoresonance phenomena occur when *any* sufficiently slow change is made to the system [9]. Here, we have only discussed sweeping the drive frequency, but a pendulum can be autoresonantly excited by a fixed frequency drive if the pendulum bob length is continuously shortened such that the pendulum's linear resonant frequency passes through the drive frequency [1]. A similar scaling law will apply [10].

7. Problem

It is not easy to construct a system which is not linear to lowest order. Thus, most systems will obey the Duffing equation as the Duffing term is the first higher-order-in-amplitude correction to a linear system. Any Duffing system will exhibit autoresonance.

Consider the system shown in Figure 8, which consists of two identical springs of spring constant k held at their equilibrium length L. The springs are attached to a central mass m which can deviate sideways. Ignore gravity. What is the differential equation that describes small oscillations in this system? Does this system reduce to the Duffing equation?

Solution: One can solve this system by calculating the restoring force directly, or by using an energy method. We will do the latter. With a

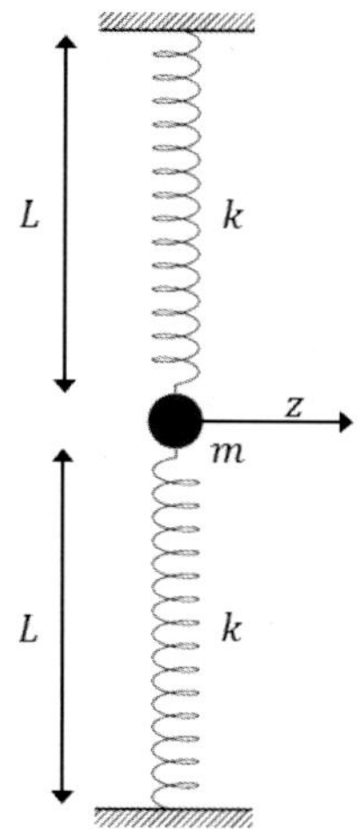

Fig. 8. An oscillating system with two identical springs attached to a sideways oscillating mass.

sideways deflection, the length of each spring is

$$\Delta L = \sqrt{L^2 + z^2} - L, \tag{27}$$

which reduces to

$$\Delta L = \frac{z^2}{2L} \tag{28}$$

for small z. Thus, the energy gained for a small deflection is

$$U(z) = 2\frac{1}{2}k\Delta L^2 = \frac{kz^4}{4L^2}, \tag{29}$$

where the extra factor of two comes from the existence of two springs. Then, the restoring force is

$$F(z) = -\frac{dU(z)}{dz} = -\frac{kz^3}{L^2}. \tag{30}$$

Finally, $F = ma$ yields the differential equation for small deflections in this system:

$$m\frac{d^2z}{dt^2} = -\frac{kz^3}{L^2}. \tag{31}$$

The system does not reduce to a linear system, and does not obey the Duffing equation. Nonetheless, it may still exhibit autoresonance, though the conditions for autoresonance will be different [42].

Acknowledgment

This research was funded by the Office of Naval Research and the Binational U.S.–Israel Science Foundation.

References

1. Four movies illustrating the phenomena described in this paper can be found at http://socrates.berkeley.edu/~fajans/Autoresonance/Autoresonance.htm. The movies show: (1) A pendulum driven at a its linear resonant frequency, (2) An autoresonantly pendulum driven by a swept frequency drive, (3) An autoresonantly driven pendulum with the corresponding pseudopotential wells, and (4) A pendulum with an ever shrinking length driven at a fixed frequency.
2. Y. A. Mitropolski, *Nonstationary Processes in Nonlinear Oscillatory Systems*. USSR, Izd-vo AN, Kiev (1955). (in Russian)
3. L. D. Landau and E. M. Lifshitz, *Mechanics*. New York, Pergamon Press (1960).
4. J. Marion and S. Thornton, *Classical Dynamics of Particles and Systems*. Fort Worth, Saunders (1995).
5. B. Meerson and L. Friedland, Strong autoresonance excitation of rydberg atoms: The rydberg accelerator, *Phys. Rev. A*. **41**, 5233 (1990).
6. M. S. Livingston, *High-energy Particle Accelerators*. New York, Interscience (1954).
7. W. K. Liu *et al.*, Nonlinear dynamics of chirped pulse excitation and dissociation of diatomic molecules, *Phys. Rev. Lett.* **75**, 1292 (1995).
8. L. Friedland, Control of kirchhoff vortices by a resonant strain, *Phys. Rev. E*. **59**, 4106 (1999).
9. J. Fajans *et al.*, Autoresonant (nonstationary) excitation of the diocotron mode in non-neutral plasmas, *Phys. Rev. Lett.* **82**, 4444 (1999). doi: 10.1103/PhysRevLett.82.4444.
10. J. Fajans *et al.*, Autoresonant (nonstationary) excitation of a collective nonlinear mode, *Phys. Plasmas* **6**, 4497 (1999).
11. I. Aranson *et al.*, Excitation of solitons by an external resonant wave with a slowly varying phase velocity, *Phys. Rev. A* **45**, 7501 (1992).
12. L. Friedland and A. G. Shagalov, Excitation of solitons by adiabatic multiresonant forcing, *Phys. Rev. Lett.* **81**, 4357 (1998).
13. R. Malhotra, Migrating planets, *Sci. Am.* **281**, 56 (1999).
14. L. Friedland, Migration timescale thresholds for resonant capture in the plutino problem, *Astrophys. J.* **547**(1) Part 2, L75 (2001).
15. E. Appelton, On the anomalous behavior of a vibrating galvanometer, *Philos. Mag.* **47**, 609–619 (1924).

16. C. A. Ludeke, An experimental investigation of forced vibrations in a mechanical system having a non-linear restoring force, *J. Appl. Phys.* **17**, 603 (1946).
17. D. P. Stockard *et al.*, Study of amplitude jumps, *Am. J. Phys.* **35**, 961 (1967).
18. J. N. Fox and J. J. Arlotto, Demonstration experiment using a dissectable anharmonic oscillator, *Am. J. Phys.* **36**, 326 (1968).
19. T. W. Arnold and W. Case, Nonlinear effects in a simple mechanical system, *Am. J. Phys.* **50**, 220 (1982).
20. H. J. Janssen *et al.*, Experimental demonstration of the resonance of an anharmonic oscillator, *Am. J. Phys.* **51**, 655 (1983).
21. H. J. Jannson *et al.*, An experimental look at the resonant behaviour of a nonlinear LC circuit, *Eur. J. Phys.* **5**, 94 (1984).
22. N. Alessi *et al.*, Measurements of amplitude jumps and hysteresis in a driven inverted pendulum, *Am. J. Phys.* **60**, 755 (1992).
23. R. D. Peters, Resonance response of a moderately driven rigid planar pendulum, *Am. J. Phys.* **64**, 170 (1996).
24. L. Friedland *et al.*, Subharmonic autoresonance of the diocotron mode, *Phys. Plasmas.* **7**, 1712 (2000).
25. J. Fajans *et al.*, Second harmonic autoresonant control of the l=1 diocotron mode in pure-electron plasmas, *Phys. Rev. E* **62**, 4131 (2000).
26. J. Fajans *et al.*, The effect of damping on autoresonant (nonstationary) excitation, *Phys. Plasmas.* **8**, 423 (2001).
27. R. C. Davidson, *Physics of Nonneutral Plasmas*. Redwood City, Addison-Wesley (1990).
28. L. Friedland, Subharmonic autoresonance, *Phys. Rev. E.* **61**, 3732 (2000).
29. F. M. Lewis, Vibration during acceleration through a critical speed, *Trans. ASME.* **54**, 253 (1932).
30. R. Z. Sagdeev *et al.*, *Nonlinear Physics: From the Pendulum to Turbulence and Chaos*. New York, Harwood Academic Publishers (1988).
31. L. Friedland, Autoresonant excitation and evolution of nonlinear waves: The variational approach, *Phys. Rev. E.* **55**, 1929 (1997).
32. J. H. Malmberg *et al.*, *Nonneutral Plasma Physics* (*Eds. C. Roberson and C. Driscoll*), chapter Experiments with Pure Electron Plasmas, vol. AIP 175, p. 28. American Institute of Physics (1988).
33. J. Danielson *et al.*, Plasma manipulation techniques for positron storage in a multicell trap, *Phys. Plasmas.* **13**, 123502 (2006).
34. C. Canali *et al.*, Off-axial plasma displacement suitable for antihydrogen production in aegis experiment, *The European Physical Journal D.* **65**(3), 499–504 (2011). ISSN 1434-6060. doi: 10.1140/epjd/e2011-20552-x. URL http://dx.doi.org/10.1140/epjd/e2011-20552-x.
35. G. B. Andresen *et al.*, Trapped antihydrogen, *Nature* **468**, 673–676 (2010). doi: 10.1038/nature09610.
36. W. A. Bertsche *et al.*, Antihydrogen formation by autoresonant excitation of antiproton plasmas, *Hyperfine Int.* **212**, 61 (2012).
37. I. Barth *et al.*, Autoresonant transition in the presence of noise and self-fields, *Phys. Rev. Lett.* **103**, 155001 (2009).
38. R. Gomes, On the edge of the solar system, *Science* **286**, 1487 (1999).

39. D. Jewitt and J. Luu, *Protostars and Planets IV (Eds. V. Mannings. et al.)*, pp. 1201–1229. Arizona U. Press (2000).
40. R. Malhotra, The origin of pluto's peculiar orbit, *Nature* **365**, 819 (1993).
41. R. Malhotra, The origin of pluto's orbit: implications for the solar system beyond neptune, *Astronom. J.* **110**, 420 (1995).
42. E. Nakar and L. Friedland, Passage through resonance and autoresonance in x^{2n}-type potentials, *Phys. Rev. E* **60**, 5479 (1999).

CHAPTER FOURTEEN

ANTIHYDROGEN PHYSICS

Niels Madsen

Department of Physics, College of Science, Swansea University, Singleton Park SA2 8PP Swansea, UK
n.madsen@swansea.ac.uk

Antihydrogen, the bound state of an antiproton and a positron, is now routinely made and trapped and the era of antihydrogen physics has started. This development owes much to physics of trapped charged particles. With a focus on this aspect, we discuss the various techniques used for making and trapping antihydrogen as well as some of the more peculiar issues that arise from the combined traps that must hold both charged and neutral species.

1. Antihydrogen From Trapped Charged Particles

As a neutral (anti)atom, antihydrogen, the bound state of an antiproton and a positron does not casually lend itself to a discussion on the physics of trapped charged particles. However, due to the puzzling absence of bulk antimatter in the Universe, those who wish to work with antihydrogen are obliged to make it themselves by first securing the constituents and then bringing these together such that the neutral antiatom can be formed. Efforts in this direction started at the LEAR machine at CERN in the 1980s and have since 2001 continued on its successor the Antiproton Decelerator (AD) also at CERN [1]. The AD remains the only source of the low energy antiprotons required by all current antihydrogen experiments. These efforts, as we shall see, require the use of almost all techniques described in this volume, and going through the process of synthesising, trapping, and studying antihydrogen is a fruitful way to demonstrate the application and implementation of many of the ideas discussed in this volume. We will endeavor to point out the particular variations on the techniques discussed elsewhere when applied to antihydrogen, as well as focusing on some of the more peculiar issues that arise due to the particular circumstances under and for which antihydrogen is produced.

2. Antiprotons

Antiprotons for these experiments are sourced from high energy collisions of protons with a target. The AD machine is supplied with 26 GeV/c protons from the CERN Proton Synchrotron (PS) and collisions with a sandwich target of carbon and iridium results in about 3×10^7 antiprotons at 3.5 GeV/c in the AD machine from an incident beam of 10^{13} protons [1]. The AD then, through a series of stages that take about 2 min, decelerates these antiprotons to a kinetic energy of 5.3 MeV at which energy they are ejected to the experiments in a ~100 ns long bunch. This is still too energetic to be trapped for further use and two overall strategies are used to moderate the antiprotons.

The most straightforward method lets the antiprotons pass through a thin foil (called a degrader) of ~0.2 mm of, e.g. aluminium. This not only degrades the antiprotons but also causes their energy spread to increase by several orders of magnitude (typically ~1 MeV). However, a sufficient fraction of the antiprotons emerge below a few keV, and they can then be trapped in a Penning–Malmberg trap located downstream of the degrader. A typical efficiency using traps with 5–10 kV fields is about 1%. A different method consists of building a linear decelerator which uses Radiofrequency (RF) fields to decelerate the bunched beam, and suitable structures to keep it focused over a couple of meters. This method has been demonstrated to be about 25% efficient [2], but is more expensive and space consuming to install and operate, and the emerging low energy antiprotons have a large divergence such that they do not lend themselves to be shared amongst several independent experiments. A superior strategy for increasing the number of low energy antiprotons is to use a deceleration ring. Such a device, called ELENA, is currently under construction as an addition to the AD and will, once operational in a couple of years, supply 100 keV antiprotons to the experiments, thereby allowing trapping efficiencies of ~50% using ultrathin foils for the final degrading [2].

Once the antiprotons are at a few keV, they are generally trapped following a scheme similar to the one shown in Figure 1. A tesla strength axial magnetic field confines the antiprotons radially and cylindrical electrodes

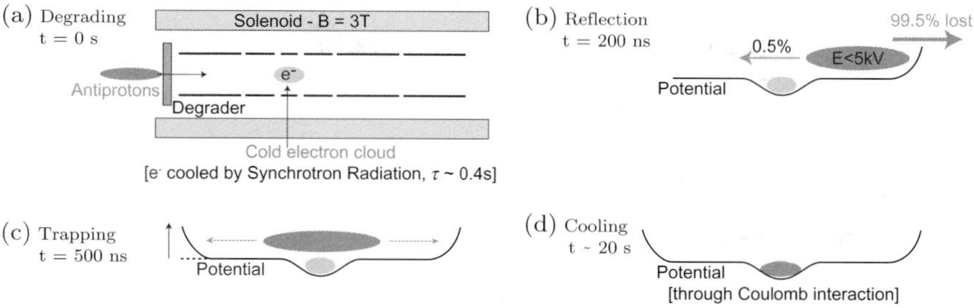

Fig. 1. Antiproton trapping and cooling. (a) Energic antiprotons are degraded in a thin foil and enter the trap region where an electron plasma has been preloaded. (b) A potential has been erected on the far side of the trap that will reflect some of the degraded antiprotons. (c) While the antiprotons are being reflected, a potential is erected on the incoming side that will trap the antiprotons. (d) The antiprotons cool through collisions with the cyclotron-cooled electrons.

assembled as a Penning–Malmberg trap can be excited to kVs and may secure confinement axially. Following the figure, the antiprotons arrive from the left through the degrader into the trap where those with a kinetic energy below 5 keV (in this example) reflect axially on electrode HVB. Before the antiprotons exit, the trap to the left HVA is quickly energized and the antiprotons are now trapped. Due to their mass (see Chapter 7.2), the antiprotons will lose very little energy through cyclotron radiation and the trap has therefore been pre-loaded with electrons, that cool efficiently through cyclotron radiation in the tesla strength magnetic field. The antiprotons are cooled through collisions with the continuously self-cooling electrons. When the antiprotons are cold enough, they will find themselves in a mixed-species non-neutral plasma with electrons. Typical experiments use tens of millions of electrons to cool hundreds of thousands of antiprotons in about a minute's time [2].

Once cooled, the antiprotons are in principle ready to use for making antihydrogen. However, a further few manipulations are usually conducted in order to increase the rate of antihydrogen formation, lower the antihydrogen temperatures or increase the efficiency of trapping [1].

2.1. *Ejection of electrons*

About an order or two of magnitude more electrons than antiprotons are usually used for the initial cooling of the antiprotons. The space charge effects of the electrons are significant and electrons may recombine with positrons to form Positronium (Ps). Both of these effects can be deleterious

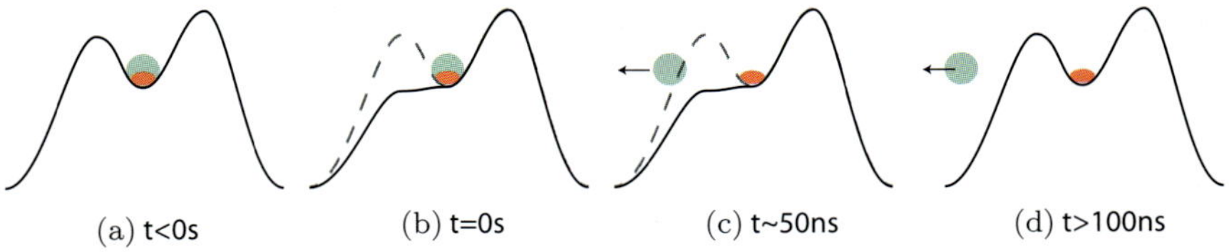

Fig. 2. Selective electron ejection from a mixed antiproton (red) electron (green) plasma. The particles are held in a positive potential well (a) such that when one side of the well is opened (b) by applying a short (∼100 ns) square pulse to the relevant electrode, it allows enough time for the fast electrons to escape (c) while the slower antiprotons remain (d).

to antihydrogen formation and most experiments eject all or most of the electrons from the mixed plasma before making antihydrogen. This can be accomplished by applying a fast (∼100 ns) pulse to one side of the well confining the mixed plasma, such that the fast electrons escape while the slower antiprotons remain. An example of this is given in Figure 2.

2.2. *Radial size of the antiprotons*

The radial size of the antiproton plasma can be important for several reasons. A typical concern is to ensure that all antiprotons are made to interact with the positrons when antihydrogen is made by merging plasmas of the two species (see Section 4.1). This is not the case if the radial size of the antiprotons is larger than that of the positrons. Other reasons for changing the plasma size are to control the plasma density as this influences, e.g. antihydrogen formation, and also to utilize the fact that small plasmas are less susceptible to the influence of transverse multipolar magnetic fields as discussed in more detail in Section 5. The radial size of the antiprotons can be changed by applying the rotating wall (RW) technique discussed in Chapter 11 or, if the density is low, by the axialization technique discussed in Chapter 1. The one caveat for using the RW on antiprotons is that the RW requires a cooling mechanism to function. This is often provided by laser, cyclotron, or buffer-gas cooling — for antiprotons, the typical "buffer gas" is cyclotron cooled electrons.

2.3. *Temperature of the antiprotons*

The kinetic energy of the antihydrogen atom is predominantly that of the antiproton. It is therefore important for forming cold antihydrogen that the antiproton has a low energy when it captures a positron. The temperature is also relevant for the formation rates, but is usually dominated by the positron temperature as we will discuss in Section 4. While electron cooling was sufficient for initial experiments on antihydrogen in the early 2000's [3], trapping as well as other proposed experiments have found it necessary, in order to achieve ~1 K temperatures, to apply additional cooling techniques after ejecting all or part of the electrons residing with the antiprotons [1]. Several of these are mentioned in this volume and we shall briefly discuss them in the context of antiprotons.

2.3.1. *Evaporative cooling*

Evaporative cooling is a standard technique for cooling atoms. Evaporative cooling works by letting particles hotter than the average temperature of the sample escape the sample and then let the remainder equilibrate to the new average. Obviously, this strategy implies losses, but if the loss-rate is controlled correctly relative to the re-equilibration rate, the phase-space density of cold particles will increase.

The process can be described by the following coupled rate equations:

$$\frac{dN}{dt} = -\frac{N}{\tau_{ev}}, \quad \frac{dT}{dt} = \alpha\frac{dN}{dt}, \tag{1}$$

where N is the number of atoms, τ_{ev} is the timescale of the evaporation, and α is the ratio of the average energy removed by an evaporating particle compared to that of a trapped particle. The evaporation timescale, τ_{ev}, is determined by the collision rate (also the equilibration rate), τ_{col}, and the truncation fraction of the well, parametrized by the ratio of the well depth to the temperature as $\eta = U_W/k_BT$. In a Penning trap where the losses are in one dimension only, the following relationship holds for $\eta > 4$:

$$\frac{\tau_{ev}}{\tau_{col}} = \frac{\sqrt{2}}{3}\eta e^{\eta}. \tag{2}$$

In practice, η tends to a constant value for a wide range of parameters, which leaves T to be a function of U_W only [4].

Evaporation in a Penning trap will occur only along the axis in one dimension as mentioned above. This leaves a hole in the particle cloud (plasma) which is refilled through collisions. However, since the total canonical angular momentum is conserved, this refilling will also lead to particles migrating outwards such that the ensemble radial extent increases following the expression:

$$\frac{N_0}{N} = \frac{\langle r^2 \rangle}{\langle r_0^2 \rangle}, \tag{3}$$

where N_0 and r_0 are the initial particle number and radius of the ensemble, and N and r the final values after evaporative cooling. The radial increase, together with the loss of particles, puts some limits to the applicability of the technique, it has however been a key factor and a workhorse for the success of the ALPHA experiment.

2.3.2. *Adiabatic cooling*

Adiabatic cooling relies on an adiabatic invariant. For trapped particles in a Penning trap, the axial bounce is such an invariant, and by adiabatically lengthening the well (e.g. increasing the volume), the particles will cool. The invariant quantity is given by

$$J = \int_a^b v_{||} dl, \tag{4}$$

where a and b are the turning points of the motion, and $v_{||}$ is the velocity component parallel to the magnetic field. For a one-dimensional harmonic potential $U_z = \frac{1}{2} m\omega_z^2 z^2$, this can be expressed as

$$J = \frac{E}{\omega_z}, \tag{5}$$

where E is the particle's energy. Thus, reducing ω_z in an adiabatic manner results in a corresponding reduction in E. Experimentally, this has been demonstrated by ATRAP to cool antiprotons to (3.5±0.7) K with a stretching of a factor 10 of the initial distribution [5]. The technique allows cooling without losses or radial size changes, but the lengthening of the plasma may make it more susceptible to magnetic field inhomogeneities, in particular, those intentionally introduced when trapping antihydrogen.

2.3.3. *Sympathetic cooling*

Electron cooling of antiprotons is a form of sympathetic or indirect cooling. However, one may in principle use any species that does not annihilate the antiprotons. Suggestions have been made to use laser-cooled negative ions and some research into a couple of ions has been done, but to date, no negative ions been laser-cooled. One of the limitations is the strongly limited number of negative ions that have any useful internal structure as they often only have a single bound state [21].

3. Positrons

Positrons are generally sourced from radioactive sources, for antihydrogen, predominantly from the radioactive isotope ^{22}Na. There are proposals to use pulsed beams of high energy electrons that may generate positrons through pair-production as well as reactor based sources, but since these are not (yet) in use for antihydrogen, we will not include these sources in our discussion here. For an exhaustive review of positron related trap and plasma techniques, see Ref. [6].

Positrons that emerge from ^{22}Na have too wide an energy spread to be practical (typically ranging from zero to $\sim$0.5 MeV). They are therefore moderated typically using a moderator, often of solid Neon. Passing through a moderator allows a fraction ($\sim$1%) of the positrons to emerge as a beam with an energy spread of typically a few eV [7]. Once moderated, a typical low energy beam intensity from such a source is 10^6 e^+/s [8].

Antihydrogen has been formed with anything between 10^6 and 10^8 positrons and to achieve these numbers, some accumulation from the slow beam is usually required. The standard approach uses a Surko-type accumulator where the positrons are slowed and cooled in a differentially pumped buffer gas arranged in such a fashion as to ensure that trapped positrons accumulate in the lowest pressure region of the system where their lifetime is the longest. Figure 3 shows an example of how such a device may look. The overall layout is a Penning–Malmberg trap with varying radius electrodes to secure the buffer gas gradient.

Once sufficient positrons are accumulated, they need to be brought to the place where antihydrogen can be formed. For reasons of longevity, antihydrogen is usually made in ultrahigh vacuum with typical pressures below 10^{-12} mBar. The antihydrogen formation region therefore needs to be well shielded from the positron accumulator with a vacuum in the 10^{-8} range. This can be accomplished either through differential pumping alone, or in combination with valves allowing short exposure times. Independent of how this is accomplished, positrons will need to be transferred from one region to another across some distance defined by the space available for the experiment. Typically, the transfer is done such that the positrons follow magnetic field lines from one trap to the next in a ballistic fashion, i.e. a quick change of potentials release the positrons in a bunch that is then

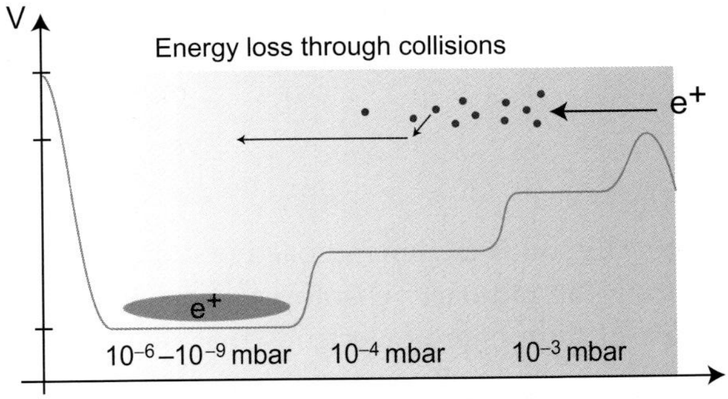

Fig. 3. Schematic of potentials (solid curve) and pressures (shading) in a Surko-type buffer gas positron accumulator. The beam of positrons arrives from the right and if a particle loses enough energy on the first return trip to be below the input barrier, the particle may continue to loose energy and be accumulated.

dynamically captured by a quick change of potentials in the receiving trap similar to how antiprotons are caught [8].

4. Antihydrogen Synthesis

There are a number of ways, both proposed and demonstrated, by which to make antihydrogen from the constituents at low energies. The basic physics idea is the same for all of them: Bring the antiproton and the positron close and remove the excess energy that keeps them from being bound. The processes can be summarized as follows:

$$\bar{p} + e^+ \rightarrow \bar{\mathrm{H}} + \gamma, \tag{6}$$

$$\bar{p} + e^+ + \gamma \rightarrow \bar{\mathrm{H}} + \gamma + \gamma, \tag{7}$$

$$\bar{p} + e^+ + e^+ \rightarrow \bar{\mathrm{H}}^* + e^+, \tag{8}$$

$$\bar{p} + Ps \rightarrow \bar{\mathrm{H}} + e^-, \tag{9}$$

$$\bar{p} + Ps^* \rightarrow \bar{\mathrm{H}}^* + e^-. \tag{10}$$

In the radiative recombination (RR) process, a spontaneously emitted photon carries away the excess energy and momentum (Equation (6)) in what is the inverse process of photo-ionization. The radiative process can be stimulated (SRR) by suitable light with a photon energy close to the ionization threshold of the state to be populated (Equation (7)). Rather than having a photon carry away the excess energy and momentum, a spectator positron can do the job in so-called three-body recombination (TBR) (Equation (8)).

In TBR, the energy exchange is typically given by the temperature of the positrons (as opposed to that of the antiprotons — see also Section 4.1) and the binding energy is therefore small, such that preferentially weakly bound states are populated. The two final strategies consist of first generating Ps, a bound state of a positron and an electron, either in its ground state (GSPS) (Equation (9)) or in an excited state (ESPS) (Equation (10)) in order for the electron to carry away the excess energy. The antihydrogen will in this case inherit the binding energy of the Ps. The cross-section for this process can be greatly enhanced with excited state Ps (Ps*), which also, due to the smaller overlap of positron and electron, has a longer lifetime. The lifetime of ground state Ps is dominated by annihilations of the electron and the positron, and the longest lived triplet state $^3S_1$ with parallel spins (ortho-positronium (o-Ps)) has a lifetime of 142 ns [7].

All of these processes have been attempted except the collision of $\bar{p}$ and ground state Ps [2]. The predominant process in terms of rates and applicability for further experimentation has so far been the TBR process which dominates in all experiments currently making antihydrogen on a regular basis. The RR process seems to have too low rates to be relevant for most experiments until now and attempts to stimulate have failed so far [9]. A demonstration experiment with excited state Ps has been carried out, but the rates were very low compared to TBR. There are potentially good physics reasons to continue trying to use Ps based methods as well as SRR as some proposed experiments are particularly sensitive to the initial state of the antihydrogen. We will discuss this in more detail later.

4.1. *Synthesis from merged plasmas*

The most successful method for antihydrogen synthesis to date is to merge a cold plasma of antiprotons with a cold plasma of positrons — the technique used for the first low energy antihydrogen in 2002 [3]. As mentioned earlier, these particles are typically manipulated in Penning–Malmberg traps (cylindrical Penning traps) that allow for easy access and transfer of the different species with minimal losses. The TBR process scales with the relative velocity of the two species as $\sim v_{\text{rel}}^{-9}$ (or, in temperature, as $T^{-9/2}$) and experimenters therefore chose to keep the positron plasma static for these experiments while manipulating the antiprotons such that they enter the positron plasma. As the positrons have the least mass, they will often be the limiting factor in the relative velocity of the two species. As the species are oppositely charged, they cannot be kept statically in the same volume, and in the standard Penning–Malmberg set-up used the positrons are therefore kept

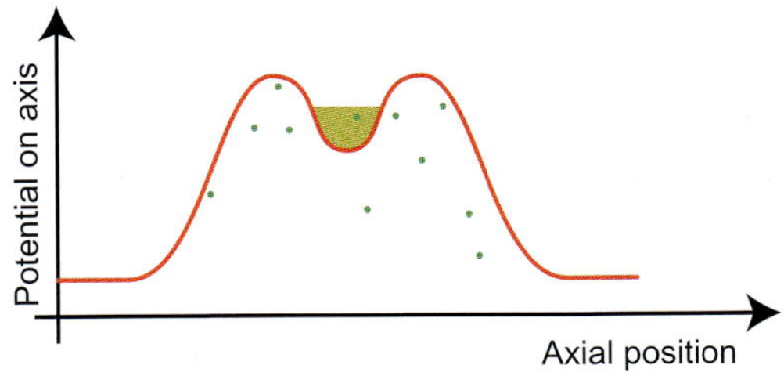

Fig. 4. Nested trap and $\bar{p}\,e^+$ mixing schemes. Example nested trap with positrons in yellow — sufficient to flatten the axial potential such that $\bar{p}$ may find themselves below the vacuum potential. The green dots show potential locations of trapped $\bar{p}$ in the well.

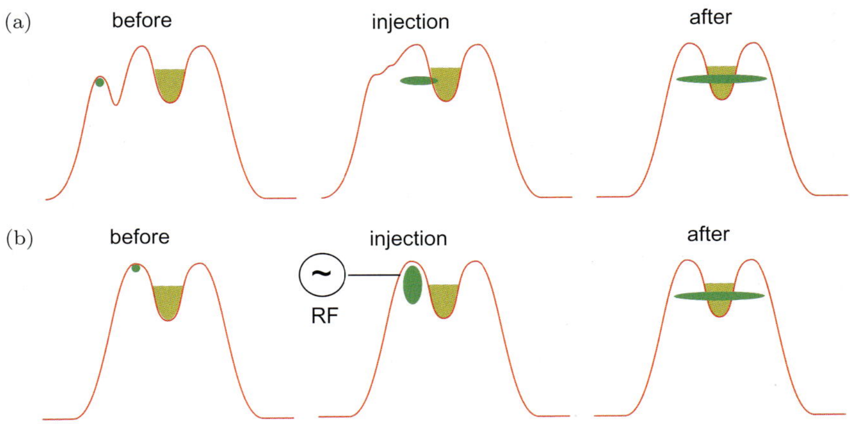

Fig. 5. Mixing scheme examples — see text for details. (a) Antiprotons (green) are brought into contact with positrons (yellow) by manipulating the confining electrostatic potentials. (b) Antiprotons are brought into contact by applying a specific type (see text) of RF signal to the confining potential.

in a negative potential centered in the middle of a positive potential that will contain the antiprotons — the so-called nested trap — as illustrated in Figure 4.

There are a number of ways in which to ensure that the antiprotons are brought into contact with the positrons. Figure 5 illustrates some of the various ways that have been demonstrated and/or are in use. The first experiment to successfully form antihydrogen at low energies was

ATHENA and they used the method depicted in Figure 5(a), which consists of using a fast potential manipulation to launch the antiprotons into their well at high enough energy that they will pass through the potential flattened by the positron space charge and thus through the positrons. This was the workhorse for a number of years, but ultimately, it was realized that this method produced antihydrogen that was too energetic to be trapped [13] and, at least for trapping experiments, different methods are now used. A second method, which is still in use, consists of initially containing the antiprotons in one side-well next to the positrons (so no contact initially) and then heat them using suitable electronic noise (Figure 5(b)). The third method is a variation of the first, in that it uses potential manipulations, but in this case, it starts out with the antiprotons trapped in a side well and slowly moves the potentials such that the antiprotons and the positrons are brought together. The fourth and final method mentioned here consists of again starting with the antiprotons in a side-well and then exciting them with a chirped RF drive matched to the bounce frequencies in the side well. This technique uses autoresonance as discussed in Chapter 13, and allows the antiprotons to collectively be injected at low relative energy into the positron plasma. This technique was successfully used in the first demonstration of antihydrogen trapping in 2010 [10].

Many details have been measured and published regarding the details of the synthesis process and we will not discuss all of these here. However, it is worth noting that the key to trapping $\bar{\mathrm{H}}$, to be discussed in the next section, is the kinetic energy of the nascent antihydrogen atoms. Typically, kinetic energies of less than about 1 K k_B are required and many of the effects we have mentioned in this and previous sections conspire against this. Merging plasmas using any scheme will likely always have the additional hurdle of the space charge of the plasma as an issue to overcome. However, results from the ALPHA collaboration using the autoresonant mixing scheme seem to indicate that at least in that experiment, the antiprotons thermally equilibrate with the positrons faster than they form antihydrogen, thus changing the problem of cold antiprotons to one of cold positrons. In the original work in 2002 where the antiprotons were launched into the positron, the opposite was true and relatively hot antihydrogen was produced [13]. The current technique's strong dependence on positron temperature was one of the motivations behind the use of the evaporative cooling technique also on positrons and has motivated efforts towards making even colder positrons through sympathetic cooling by positive ions [14].

4.2. *Synthesis using Ps*

As several experiments have demonstrated the ability to cool antiprotons to the kelvin level, an alternative route to cold antihydrogen that is being pursued is that using the intermediary of Ps. By using Ps, there is no need to worry about the often significant space charge of the positron plasma in the plasma mixing techniques discussed above, nor the equilibrating collisions inside the positron plasma, and the problem of final kinetic energy of the antihydrogen is reduced to a problem of the temperature of the antiprotons. While these features are highly motivating, this formation scheme is yet to be in regular use. Demonstration experiments have produced comparatively little antihydrogen, and so far, no attempts have been made to trap and measure the energy distribution of the thus produced antihydrogen.

5. Antihydrogen Trapping

Atoms, while neutral, may be trapped if they have a magnetic moment ($\boldsymbol{\mu}$). The potential energy associated with a dipole in a magnetic field is given by

$$U = -\boldsymbol{\mu} \cdot \mathbf{B}. \tag{11}$$

It is thus possible to confine a diamagnetic atom (with moment antiparallel to the magnetic field) in a three-dimensional (3D) minimum in magnetic field strength. These so-called low–field seekers thus have minimum energy at low-field. For the ground state of (anti)hydrogen, this can be depicted as a Breit–Rabi diagram showing the splitting of the two zero B-field states into four non-zero B-field states as shown in Figure 6. The magnetic moment of a ground state (anti)hydrogen atom is about 1 Bohr magneton, which gives an effective trap depth of 0.67 K per tesla of well depth, where kelvin is used as an energy unit.

A 3D magnetic minimum can be made using a Ioffe–Pritchard geometry, where four parallel bars generate a transverse magnetic quadrupole with zero field at zero radius and two end coils result in an axial-minimum in the center [2]. In practice, for antihydrogen to be trapped, tesla strength fields are needed as the antihydrogen is at best tens of kelvin discussed previously, and therefore, super-conducting magnets with many coils are used. When these ideas were first floated, it was realized that the neutral atom trap must be energized before antihydrogen is formed, and that these strong transverse fields would strongly perturb the otherwise homogeneous magnetic field needed for the Penning–Malmberg traps used. It was already well known that magnetic imperfections reduce the lifetime of

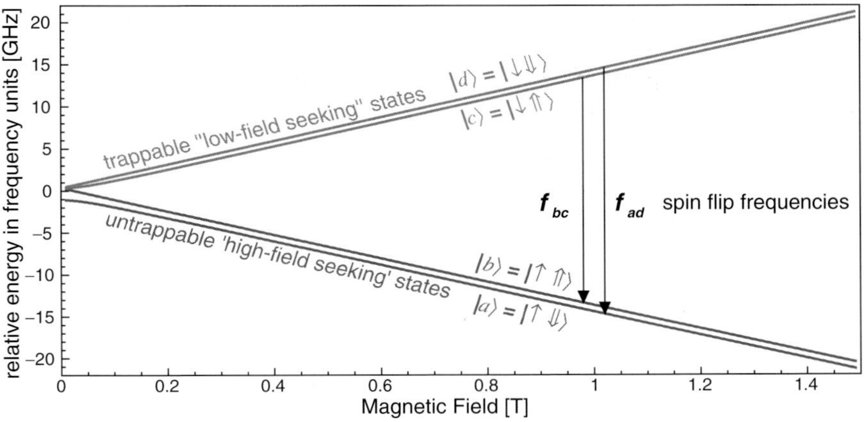

Fig. 6. Breit–Rabi diagram showing the energy levels of ground state (anti)hydrogen as a function of magnetic field strength. The two hyperfine states are split into four as both the positron and the antiproton magnetic moments interact with the magnetic field. The four states are traditionally labeled $|a\rangle$, $|b\rangle$, $|c\rangle$, and $|d\rangle$ as shown. Atoms in the states $|c\rangle$ and $|d\rangle$ may be trapped in a magnetic minimum.

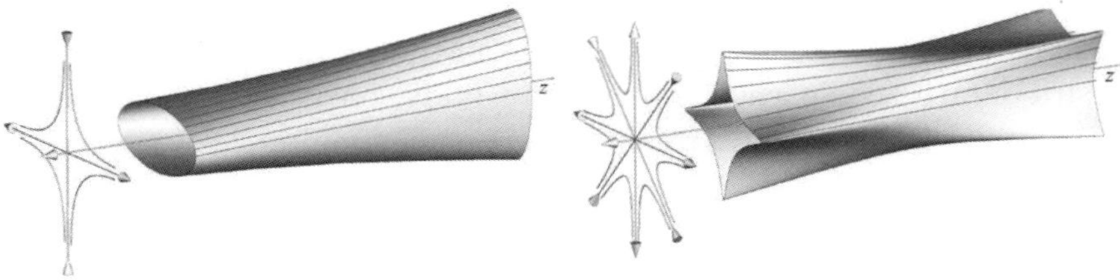

Fig. 7. Magnetic field lines for a transverse quadrupole (left) and octupole (right), superimposed on a uniform axial field. The vectors on the left represent directions of the axially invariant multipole and axial field components. The surfaces are created by following the field lines from a centered circular locus, and the lines shown within the surfaces are field lines [18].

non-neutral plasmas in Penning traps (see e.g. Chapter 11), and it was soon established that introducing strong transverse magnetic fields had a detrimental effect on the Penning trap. Without going into great detail, we can illustrate the basic problem with a simple field line figure (Figure 7) which shows how the field lines are distorted by the introduction of a multipole on top of a homogeneous solenoidal field.

As we can see in Figure 7, the multipole makes the field-lines diverge radially in one axial direction and converge in the other. The low energy particles used for antihydrogen formation all, essentially, follow the field-lines, and thus, if this distortion is strong enough, their paths can be made to intersect the walls of the apparatus and cause the particles to be lost. This can be expressed as a dynamic aperture, a radius beyond which particles stored in a well of a certain axial length l will not survive [18]. The critical radius, expressed in terms of the wall radius R_w, the axial path length L, the axial magnetic field B_z, and the multipole field at the wall B_w is given by

$$r_{crit} = R_w \exp\left(-\frac{1}{2}\frac{B_w}{B_z}\frac{L}{R_w}\right) \tag{12}$$

for a quadrupole and

$$r_{crit} = \frac{R_w}{\sqrt{1 + \frac{B_w}{B_z}\frac{L}{R_w}}} \tag{13}$$

for an octupole. For a typical 2 cm long well in a 1 T solenoidal field with a quadrupole of 2 T and a wall radius of 2 cm, the critical radius is 7.4 mm, already comparable to typical radii of plasmas in these experiments. This result is increased to 1.2 cm for an octupole. It is interesting to note that this aperture can be used as an *in situ* diagnostic of the radial particle distribution if good particle loss detection is available, like it is for antiprotons. ALPHA demonstrated this by sweeping their multipole magnet while recording particle losses [20].

For higher-order multipoles, the field varies stronger with radius as illustrated in Figure 8. This results in larger critical radii (compare e.g.

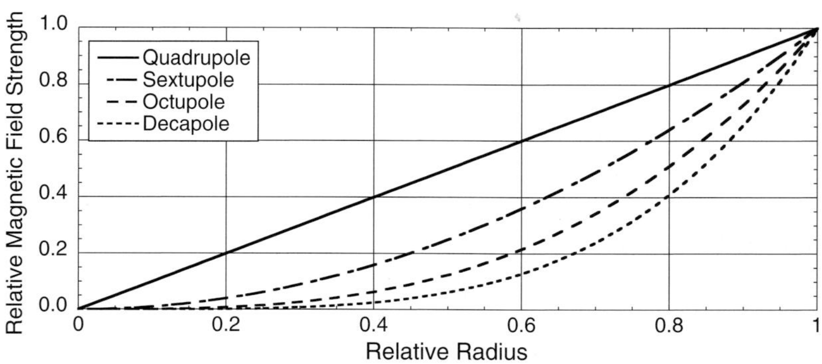

Fig. 8. Comparison of relative transverse magnetfic field strength from different poled transverse multipoles. The plot is normalized such that they all have strength one at the wall which is at radius one.

Equations (12) and (13)) and motivated the ALPHA collaboration to build a magnetic trap using an octupole for transverse confinement. While the critical radius imposes a strict upper limit to the radius of a plasma, detrimental effects have also been observed at smaller radii, where the main influence is increased radial expansion rates and associated temperature increases of the plasma. While these effects have not been studied in great detail, they are in qualitative agreement with expectations that field inhomogeneities are a cause of plasma expansion and heating in Penning traps (see Chapter 11).

The first trapped antihydrogen, using these techniques, was reported by the ALPHA collaboration in 2010 [10]. The initial experiment observed on average one trapped antihydrogen per nine experiments, but improvements in plasma temperatures and densities later increased this to about one trapped atom per experiment [19]. The experiments reportedly had a cycle of about 15 min. While a single experiment, which includes several stages of cooling of both antiprotons and positrons, as well as radial compression, took about 7 min, the second half of the period was dominated by letting the Penning–Malmberg trap electrodes cool after they had been heated by the rapid shutdown of the neutral trap used to detect the antihydrogen.

Without going into great detail, antihydrogen may be detected by detecting the annihilation of the antiproton, and using spatial filtering to determine the neutrality of the detected annihilation. If the antiproton annihilation can be determined to stem from a neutral system, it originates from antihydrogen. As the annihilation of an antiproton results in a number of energetic pions, it is comparatively easy to detect (typically more than 90% efficiency in the detector used by ALPHA). The full reconstruction of the origin of the pions and thereby the annihilation vertex reduces the efficiency to about 50%. By imposing an axial electric field across the trap, ALPHA ensured that any bare antiprotons that remained in the system (they were in principle cleared out by the application of a range of electrical pulses) would annihilate in regions where neutral antihydrogen would not. The dynamics of a trapped antiproton is very different from that of a neutral antihydrogen atom, also because the few remaining $\bar{H}$ atoms that may be around will necessarily have an energy below the 0.5 K trap depth, whereas any antiproton with energy below 20 eV would have been cleared out. This elaborate procedure was deemed necessary as bare antiprotons could be trapped on their motional magnetic moment. The motional magnetic moment is an adiabatic invariant and trapping depends on the ratio of their axial ($E_{\text{kin},||}$) and transverse ($E_{\text{kin},\perp}$) kinetic energies following the magnetic mirror equation,

$$B_{\text{max}} = B_0 \left(1 + \frac{E_{\text{kin},||}}{E_{\text{kin},\perp}}\right), \tag{14}$$

which defines the largest total magnetic field B_{max} to which an antiproton that starts at a field B_0 can propagate. The problem can at least partially be overcome by increasing the parallel energy by applying strong axial fields along the trap before searching for trapped antihydrogen. Such a procedure is standard in the trapping experiments ALPHA and ATRAP, but the effectiveness is limited by the available electric field. To ensure complete unambiguity, the ALPHA experiment utilize their ability to detect the antiproton annihilation vertex (position) by applying a bias field along the trap while de-energising the magnetic minimum trap. The bias field would deflect any trapped antiprotons such that they would preferentially exit the trap at a location determined by the applied bias.

Figure 9 shows a collection of results from these experiments and clearly demonstrates the lack of bias in the detected annihilations, and therefore that the annihilations stem from antihydrogen that was trapped. Even without the bias, it is possible to detect the difference between a trapped antihydrogen atom and a mirror-trapped antiproton as their trajectories in the magnetic fields are very distinct, not least because the

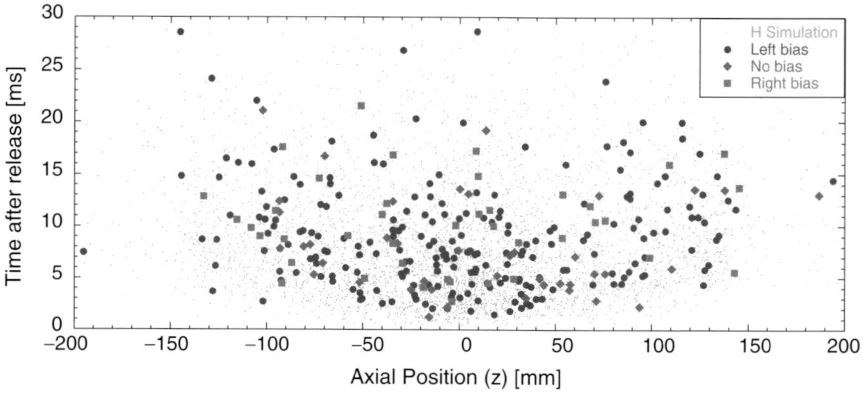

Fig. 9. Time and axial z distribution of annihilations on release of $\bar{\text{H}}$ from the neutral trap for different bias fields (see legend) and comparison with simulation (grey dots).

antihydrogen necessarily has a very low energy and effectively only undergoes one or two bounces in the 30 ms it takes to de-energize the magnetic minimum trap.

ALPHA's first trapping demonstration in 2010 was followed up by the observation that the trapped atoms survived up to 1,000 s in the trap, thus guaranteeing that they were in their ground state (requiring about 1 s to be reached by the initially weakly bound trapped antiatoms) and amenable to study. The competing ATRAP collaboration reported the observation of trapped antihydrogen in 2012 [2].

6. Antihydrogen Physics

The first spectroscopic investigation of antihydrogen was announced by the ALPHA collaboration in 2012 [15]. The ALPHA team reported observing resonantly excited positron spin-flips in trapped antihydrogen. The experiment consisted of illuminating trapped antihydrogen with microwaves, and noting that when the microwave frequency matched that of either of the two transitions $|d\rangle \rightarrow |a\rangle$ or $|c\rangle \rightarrow |b\rangle$, corresponding to positron spin-flip, loss of antihydrogen from the trap occurred (e.g. Figure 10). Recall from Figure 6 that the $|a\rangle$ and $|b\rangle$ states are high-field seekers and

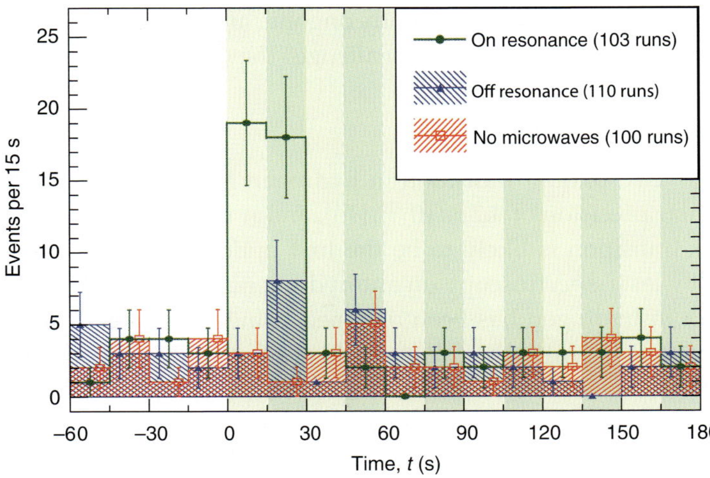

Fig. 10. Antihydrogen spin-flip signal from the ALPHA experiment. The microwaves are turned on at time zero (beginning of background shading). The microwaves are applied for six segments of two blocks of 15s each. The two 15s blocks address first the $|d\rangle \rightarrow |a\rangle$ transition and then the $|c\rangle \rightarrow |b\rangle$ [15].

will thus not be confined in the ALPHA magnetic minimum trap. Mainly due to uncertainties in the determination of the magnetic field the resolution of this first measurement was limited to four parts in 10^{-3}, but the observed spin-flip frequencies were consistent with those of hydrogen. The magnetic field was measured *in situ* using microwaves resonant with the cyclotron frequency to heat a plasma of cold electrons. By monitoring the temperature response of the plasma through the quadrupole mode ($m = 2$ — see Chapter 10), it was possible to determine the absolute magnetic field in a homogenous field region to a precision of 3.4×10^{-4} at 1 T. Issues with induced localized currents in the super-conducting magnets and ambiguity of the cyclotron technique in non-homogeneous fields (e.g. the minimum-B trap) put some practical constraints on the technique and set the final absolute precision of the measurement to the above.

For these microwave measurements, ALPHA conducted ~300 experiments (see Figure 10). Each experiment took about 20 min, and the typical trapping rate was about one atom per experiment. Assuming no mishaps this is 100 h of successful experimental time to acquire essentially three data points (on resonance, off resonance, and no microwaves). This aptly demonstrates the difficulties faced by antihydrogen experiments; the flux is low and new ways have to be invented to do these experiments. We will briefly discuss experiments currently ongoing and in preparation and look at some aspects of the particular challenges they may face.

6.1. *Laser spectroscopy*

The 1s–2s two photon transition in hydrogen has been measured to the spectacular precision of 4.2×10^{-15} [16], and it is therefore not surprising that this transition is likely to be the first optical transition that will be probed by laser-spectroscopy on antihydrogen. However, the spectacular precision in hydrogen has been obtained using a cold beam with a flux of 10^{17} atoms/s [16], something not likely for antihydrogen. Instead, it seems far more likely that antihydrogen will be probed in a trap, where the increased interaction time makes it possible to probe a single atom, though we shall not underestimate the difficulties faced. Hydrogen has also been probed in a trapped state, and doing so raises particular issues due to the magnetic fields used for the trapping. The best measurement so far on trapped hydrogen was done with a precision of 10^{-12} [17].

While not trying to exhaust the issues surrounding these measurements, some basic calculations give us an insight into the challenges to be faced. The first challenge is to excite the antiatom to the 2s state. The 1s–2s transition is forbidden, and requires two counter-propagating 243 nm photons, which does hold the advantage that the first-order Doppler shift will cancel out. There will likely be only very few atoms moving in a large volume relative to the size of the laser beam (in ALPHA, the trap is 274 mm long with a radius of 22 mm and a laser with enough intensity to be relevant will be 100's of μm in diameter at most), therefore significant time (10–100 of second) may be needed for a transition to occur. Trap lifetime measurements in ALPHA indicated lifetimes of order 1,000 s [19]. In addition, once a transition has happened, it must be detected. In ALPHA's microwave measurement, the detection method was ejection caused by positron spin-flip. However, there is no spin-flip when the atom decays from 2s to 1s. In hydrogen experiments, the 2s state is quenched with an electric field to 2p and the 121.5 nm photon from the spontaneously decay is detected. With a single atom, and the geometric constraints of antihydrogen experiments detection of this photon will be very difficult at best. A promising alternative is to consider photo-ionising the 2s antihydrogen and either, like in the microwave experiment detect the laser induced reduced number in antiatoms released when the trap is shut down, or in addition to that, capture and detect the antiproton left over after the ionization.

An alternative is to induce a transition from 1s to 2p using a pulsed 121.5 nm laser. This transition has been used for laser-cooling of hydrogen, an additional cooling that could prove useful for studies of trapped antihydrogen [2]. However, the 1s–2p transition with the short lifetime of the 2p state is not a good candidate for precision measurements. Other optical transitions have been proposed [11], but currently no known plans exist to address these.

6.2. *Microwave spectroscopy*

The hyperfine splitting of the ground state hydrogen atom has long ago been measured to an amazing precision of 10^{-12} [12]. There exist theoretical model arguments that indicate that the sensitivity to some specific potential symmetry violations is enhanced in this transition such that it would be a good test bed for symmetry breaking in antimatter [11]. As previously mentioned, the ALPHA collaboration has made a first measurement on this transition, albeit in the strong magnetic field of a trap, which together with other factors colluded to reduce the precision of the measurement to 4×10^{-3}.

There are therefore good reasons to attempt to make this measurement in zero magnetic field and work is on the way by the ASACUSA collaboration towards this [2]. The difficulty with such an experiment is that it requires removing the antihydrogen from its formation region, and the interesting state is the ground state. As we discussed earlier, antihydrogen is typically formed in weakly bound states that must first decay.

6.3. *Antimatter gravity*

A number of experiments aim to measure the gravitational acceleration of antihydrogen. Without going into great detail of the proposed experiments, we note that this can in principle be done in a trap, based experiment, but proposals also exist to use beams. The crucial point here is that, in general, very low temperatures are needed. The gravitational acceleration of a 1 m height difference at the Earth's surface corresponds to a kinetic energy of 10^{-3} K k_B. In a trap environment, one may envisage achieving low temperatures with laser-cooling of the antihydrogen itself as discussed above. Alternatively, one may trap antihydrogen ions (with two positrons) and cool them through collisions with a laser-cooled positive ion species. This idea is pursued by the GBAR collaboration and was originally proposed by Waltz and Hänsch [2]. Finally, as is pursued by the Aegis collaboration [2], one may try to start with ultracold antihydrogen by using the Ps path to antihydrogen using ultracold antiprotons. Ultracold antiprotons can in principle be obtained with evaporative or adiabatic cooling mentioned previously, or as alternatively discussed by sympathetic cooling with a laser-cooled anion.

7. Summary

The making and trapping of antihydrogen is motivated by fundamental questions about the Universe. The road to the recent successes with both trapping antihydrogen and starting the first measurements has required many developments in the area of trapped charged particles using techniques described throughout this volume. We have discussed the background and the various developments that have led to these successes with emphasis on the techniques particularly related to the physics with trapped charged particles. This includes some reference to techniques discussed in detail elsewhere in this volume, motivating many of these as well as discussion of some aspects that are unique in the physics of antihydrogen formation and trapping. We close the chapter by a brief discussion of the first physics results and results to come in the future.

8. Tutorial problems

(1) Calculate the cyclotron radius for a 5 keV antiproton in a 3 T magnetic field. Discuss the implications for the design of a trap to catch antiprotons from the AD antiproton beam.

Solution

The cyclotron radius (r_{cyc}) is given by equating the Lorentz force on the particle (charge q and mass m) and the centripetal force and we find

$$qvB = m\frac{v^2}{r} \Rightarrow r_{cyc} = \frac{mv}{qB}, \tag{15}$$

and as 5 keV is much smaller than the rest-mass of the antiproton, we can use the non-relativistic kinetic energy to determine the velocity as in $E_{kin} = \frac{1}{2}mv^2$ and find that

$$r_{cyc} = \frac{\sqrt{2E_{kin}m}}{qB}, \tag{16}$$

which for an antiproton at 5 keV and $B = 3$ T equals 3.4 mm.

The relatively large cyclotron radius found above means that it is often beneficial to create relatively large radius traps, and ensure that there are no radial constraints after the degrader foil (which there could be as the last part of the degrading material often forms part of a Faraday cup). In addition, it explains why it is beneficial to run at relatively strong fields (above 1 T) for successful antiproton trapping, as lower fields would require larger traps, and hence larger electron plasmas for the electron cooling — all things that would complicate the effort. Finally, it also gives a good size scale of how much the incoming antiproton beam needs to be focused onto the final degrader. If the bulk of the degrading material is located right before the trap, in the strong field, the "size" of the degraded antiprotons will reflect the beam size, which therefore does not need to be focused much better than the cyclotron radius. It is worth pointing out that this is far from true if even a small part of the degrading material is located at a significant distance from the trap as this will cause increase in the divergence of the incoming beam, and therefore a large beam size.

(2) Calculate the rotation frequency of a plasma of 5×10^6 positrons with a radius r_p of 1 mm and a half-length l_p of 1 cm in a 1 T field. Compare the velocity of the outermost positrons to the velocity of an antihydrogen atom with a kinetic energy of $0.5\,\mathrm{K}\cdot k_B$. Discuss why this is of interest.

Solution

The plasma is much smaller than it is long ($r_p \ll l_p$), so for simplicity, we will consider it a cylinder. The equilibrium rotation velocity in the plasma is given by an equilibrium between the outward electrostatic force from the space charge and the inward centripetal force from the rotation in the B-field. Since in equilibrium, we know that the plasma is a rigid rotator, we can use the electric field at the radial plasma edge. Assuming that the length $l_p \gg r_p$, we use Gauss' law on an infinite cylinder of constant density,

$$\int_S E_\perp dA = \frac{Q_{\text{enclosed}}}{\epsilon_0} \Leftrightarrow E_\perp = \frac{Ne}{4\pi r_p l_p \epsilon_0}, \tag{17}$$

where e is the elementary charge.

The rotation frequency can now be calculated by finding the equilibrium between the force due to $E_\perp$ and B as follows:

$$qE_\perp = qvB \Rightarrow \nu = \frac{v_{\text{surface}}}{2\pi r_p} = \frac{eN}{8\pi^2 l_p r_p^2 \epsilon_0 B}, \tag{18}$$

which for our given numbers gives 115 kHz, or a surface velocity of $720\,\mathrm{m\cdot s^{-1}}$. An antihydrogen atom with a kinetic energy of $0.5\,\mathrm{K}\cdot k_B$ has a velocity of $90\,\mathrm{m\cdot s^{-1}}$.

The particle number and size of the positron plasma given in the question is not far from typical parameters in, e.g. the ALPHA experiment for the positron plasmas used for antihydrogen synthesis for trapping. Typical trap depths of the ALPHA and ATRAP magnetic minimum traps for neutral atoms are of the order of 0.5 K, with kelvin as an energy unit ($\sim 50\,\mu\mathrm{V}$). The fact that the rotation velocity of the positron plasma is significant compared to the velocity of an atom with a kinetic energy equivalent to the trap depth is relevant as antiprotons injected into a positron plasma will equilibrate with the positrons, who are the dominant space charge contributor, and thus end up rotating at the same velocity and thereby potentially increasing their initial kinetic energy with a significant amount compared to the trap depth. This means that making trappable antihydrogen from merging plasmas requires careful optimization of parameters, as e.g. an increased positron density will increase the formation rate, but now also, potentially drastically increase the kinetic energy of the nascent antihydrogen.

References

1. N. Madsen, Cold antihydrogen: A new frontier in fundamental physics, *Phil. Trans. Roy. Soc. A* **368**, 3671–3682 (2010).
2. W. A. Bertsche *et al.*, Physics with antihydrogen, *Jour. Phys. B* **48**, 23 (2015).
3. M. Amoretti *et al.* (ATHENA), Production and detection of cold antihydrogen atoms, *Nature* **419**, 456–459 (2002).
4. G. B. Andresen *et al.* (ALPHA), Evaporative cooling of antiprotons to cryogenic temperatures, *Phys. Rev. Lett.* **105**, 013003 (2010).
5. G. Gabrielse *et al.* (ATRAP), Adiabatic cooling of antiprotons, *Phys. Rev. Lett.* **106**, 073002 (2011).
6. J. R. Danielson *et al.*, Plasma and trap-based techniques for science with positrons, *Rev. Mod. Phys*, **87**, 247–296 (2015).
7. M. Charlton and J. W. Humberston, *Positron Physics*, pp. 454. Cambridge, Cambridge University Press (2000).
8. L. V. Jørgensen *et al.* (ATHENA), New Source of Dense, Cryogenic Positron Plasmas, *Phys. Rev. Lett.* **95**, 025002 (2005).
9. M. Amoretti *et al.* (ATHENA), Search for laser-induced formation of Antihydrogen atoms, *Phys. Rev. Lett.* **97**, 213401 (2006).
10. G. B. Andresen *et al.* (ALPHA), Trapped antihydrogen, *Nature* **468**, 673–676 (2010).
11. V. A. Kostelecký and A. J. Vargas, Lorentz and CPT tests with hydrogen, antihydrogen, and related systems, arXiv:1506.01706v1 (2015).
12. H. Hellwig *et al.*, Measurement of the unperturbed hydrogen hyperfine transition frequency, *IEEE Trans. Inst. Meas.* **IM-19**, 200 (1970); L. Essen *et al.*, Frequency of the hydrogen maser, *Nature* **229**, 110 (1971).
13. N. Madsen *et al.*, Spatial distribution of cold antihydrogen formation, *Phys. Rev. Lett.* **94**, 033403 (2005).
14. N. Madsen *et al.*, Antihydrogen trapping assisted by sympathetically cooled positrons, *New Jour. Phys.* **16**, 063046 (2014).
15. C. Amole *et al.* (ALPHA), Resonant quantum transitions in trapped antihydrogen atoms, *Nature* **483**, 439–443 (2012).
16. C. G. Parthey *et al.*, Improved Measurement of the Hydrogen $1S-2S$ Transition Frequency, *Phys. Rev. Lett* **107**, 203001 (2011).
17. C. L. Cesar *et al.*, Two-photon spectroscopy of trapped atomic hydrogen, *Phys. Rev. Lett.* **77**, 255–258 (1996).
18. J. Fajans *et al.*, Critical loss radius in a Penning trap subject to multipole fields, *Phys. Plas.* **15**, 032108 (2008).

19. G. B. Andresen *et al.* (ALPHA), Confinement of antihydrogen for 1,000 seconds, *Nat. Phys.* **7**, 558–564 (2011).
20. G. B. Andresen *et al.* (ALPHA), A novel antiproton radial diagnostic based on octupole induced ballistic loss, *Phys. Plas.* **15**, 032107 (2008).
21. C. W. Walter *et al.*, Candidate for laser cooling of a negative ion: Observations of bound-bound transitions in La^-, *Phys. Rev. Lett.* **113**, 063001 (2014).

CHAPTER FIFTEEN

ION COULOMB CRYSTALS AND THEIR APPLICATIONS

Michael Drewsen
Department of Physics and Astronomy, Aarhus University, Ny Munkegade 120, DK-8000 Aarhus C, Denmark
drewsen@phys.au.dk

The following text will give a brief introduction to the physics of the spatially ordered structures, so-called Coulomb crystals, that appear when confined ions are cooled to sufficiently low temperatures. It will as well briefly comment on the very diverse scientific applications of such crystals, which have emerged in the past two decades. While this document lacks figures and many specific references, it is the hope, not the text will stimulate the reader to dig deeper into one or more of the discussed subjects, and inspire her/him to think about new potential applications. A fully referenced journal article of essentially the same text can be found in *Physica B* **460**, 105 (2015) [1].

1. Introduction

Coulomb crystals constitute a special class of spatial ordered structures of matter. While usual solid matter ranging from simple molecules through clusters to solids with long range ordered structures form through the quantum delocalized nature of electrons and hence are governed by the laws of quantum mechanics, Coulomb crystals are exclusively based on classical electromagnetic interactions between confined charged particles of the same sign of charge, and hence relying only on the classical laws of physics.

The first elaborated consideration of Coulomb crystals was made by E. Wigner in the 1930s [2], where he was interested in understanding the change in the electronic structure and properties of matter when the density of electrons becomes so low that despite the rather large DeBroglie wavelength of electrons, their individual wavefunctions do not overlap. Under such conditions, Wigner suggested the formation of regular structures with each electron taking up a particular position in space.

Wigner never managed to realize such crystals of electrons, but Coulomb crystallization of two-dimensional (2D) electron gases was demonstrated both on the surface of super fluid helium in the late 1970s [3] and within GaAs/GaAlAs quantum well structures around 1990 [4]. Three-dimensional (3D) Coulomb crystals of electrons have though still not been realized. When considering Coulomb crystals made up of electrons, such structures are also often referred to as Wigner-crystals.

Coulomb crystals can as well be composed of positively charged particles such as atomic ions at various charge stages. For decades, people within the astrophysical community have been considerably interested in such objects. This is due to the fact that when a star dies, it will eventually turn into one of the two very exotic stellar objects named White Dwarfs and Neutron Stars, which to various extents are assumed to incorporate Coulomb crystallized matter [5].

In case the mass of the original star is below a certain critical value after the nuclear burning processes has terminated, the remaining parts of the star will contract under the influence of gravity until the point where all the electrons form a degenerate gas which will be able to produce an equalizing quantum pressure. Such a remnant star with a radius of typically a few hundreds of kilometers will mainly consist of fully stripped oxygen and carbon atoms embedded in the degenerated electron gas. When eventually the so-called White Dwarf cools down by thermal radiation to a temperature, which becomes lower than the very high Fermi-energy of such a dense electron gas (typically equivalent to millions of Kelvin), quantum mechanics prohibits collisional energy exchanges between the ions and electrons. The ions can though still exchange energy through their Coulomb interactions within the confining potential created by the degenerated electron gas, and eventually at sufficiently low temperatures, Coulomb crystals of the fully stripped ions will be formed.

In the case of initially more massive stars, the quantum pressure of the degenerated electron gas cannot counteract the gravitational contracting forces, and eventually most of the materials of the star will be turned into a degenerated gas of neutrons which then provide a quantum pressure that can counteract a gravitational collapse. This situation leads to a so-called neutron star of the size of only a few tens of kilometers in diameter. While nuclear burning in White Dwarfs typically stops with the formation of mainly oxygen and carbon, in Neutron Stars, fusion processes continue until the formation of iron after which no further energy can be released through fusion. While the main part of Neutron Stars is made up of neutrons, it is believed that their crusts will still have fully stripped iron ions Fe^{26+} present, which even under the extreme high density conditions still is believed to form ion Coulomb crystals!

Due to the required conditions for formation of Coulomb crystals of ions, as will be revisited in the next section, it was first with the development of laser cooling techniques in the late 1970s and early 1980s that it became possible to form ion Coulomb crystals in laboratories. However, since these first demonstrations by the groups of Dr. Wineland, NIST, Boulder, USA [6] and Walther, Max-Planck-Institute for Quantum Optics, Garching, Germany [7], the number of groups and the breath of scientific investigations based on ion Coulomb crystals created in the laboratory have gone through an amazing development.

The rest of this contribution is organized as follows: in Section 2, a discussion of the condition for Coulomb crystallization will be provided, and in Section 3, how these requirements can be met in the case of positively charged ions will be presented. Structural properties of Coulomb crystals of various dimensionalities will be the focus of Section 4 with examples in the form of crystals of atomic ion species. In Section 5, some of the dynamical properties of Coulomb crystals will be discussed briefly. The many applications of ion Coulomb crystals in a large variety of scientific investigations will be the theme of Section 6. Section 7 will finally conclude the presentation.

2. Conditions for Coulomb Crystallization

The condition for Coulomb crystallization is often formulated in terms of the so-called plasma coupling parameter, Γ, which is defined in the following way:

$$\Gamma \equiv \frac{Q^2}{4\pi\epsilon_0 a k_B T}. \tag{1}$$

where Q is the charge of the particle involved, a is the Wigner–Seitz radius, determined by the particle density, and T is the temperature of the particles. Essentially, Γ is just a measure of the ratio of the inter-particle Coulomb energy to their kinetic energy,

$$\Gamma \sim \frac{E_{\mathrm{Coul}}}{E_{\mathrm{kin}}}. \tag{2}$$

For infinitely large 3D identical charged particle systems, often also referred to as one-component plasmas (OCPs), it can be shown that many of the thermodynamical properties scale with the value of Γ [8].

With respect to Coulomb crystallization, it has been proven by several groups [9] that the criterion is given by

$$\Gamma \geq 175, \tag{3}$$

or, as can be shown by introducing the local single ion oscillation frequency, or similarly, the plasma frequency ω_{plas},

$$\omega_{\text{plas}} = \sqrt{\frac{nQ^2}{\epsilon_0 M}}, \tag{4}$$

by the condition,

$$\Delta r_{\text{exc}}/a < 0.1, \tag{5}$$

where Δr_{exc} is the root-mean-square single particle excursion around its equilibrium position due to its kinetic energy. This inequality is very similar to the Lindemann criterion for usual solids with respect to the motion of the atomic nuclei.

For valence electrons in usual solids, even at the absolute zero temperature, the quantum mechanical excursion of the individual electrons makes it impossible to fulfill inequality (5), and delocalizing electrons leading to specific energy band structures emerge as a consequence. More generally, one can derive a rather simple approximate condition for this "quantum melting" to happen at absolute zero temperature (unpublished):

$$a \geq 10^4 \times \frac{h^2 \epsilon_0}{Q^2 M}, \tag{6}$$

where M is the mass of the charged particles.

For exotic stellar objects like White Dwarfs with interior ions being mainly C^{6+} and O^{8+}, and neutron star crusts with Fe^{26+} ions, the critical Wigner–Seitz radii for quantum melting become $a \sim 10^{-12}$ m and $a \sim 10^{-14}$ m, respectively. Surprisingly, despite the high density of such objects, quantum melting is not a problem, and classical Coulomb crystallization happens already at temperature in the million-kelvin range (see problem) [5]!

In contrast to short-range interacting particles leading to closed packed crystal lattices, the ground state of a infinite Coulomb crystal is a body-centered cubic (*bcc*) structure [9]. Hexagonal closed packed (*hcp*) and face centered cubic (*fcc*) structures correspond, however, only to slightly excited states.

In the case of effective harmonic confinement potentials, it is straightforward through the application of Poisson's equation to prove that finite size one-component systems will also have constant particle density at low temperatures.

For such finite systems, one finds that the condition for reaching Coulomb crystallization, defined as the temperature at which there is a maximum in the specific heat, is first reached at larger values of Γ, or equivalently at lower temperatures. For instance, for isotropic confined systems ranging from $\sim$100 to $\sim$10,000 particles, the corresponding critical values of Γ varies from $\sim$500 to $\sim$200. So far, criteria for crystallization under various anisotropic confinement conditions have not been studied in detail, but a variation in the values of Γ can be expected even for the same number of ions due to changes in the surface effects.

3. Ion Coulomb Crystals in Laboratories

By standard ion trapping techniques, either in the form of Penning traps (see Chapter 1) or radiofrequency (RF) traps also named Paul traps (see Chapter 2), the highest practical reachable particle density of singly charged ions is $\sim 10^{15}\,\mathrm{m}^{-3}$, corresponding to $a \sim 10\,\mu\mathrm{m}$. With this value of a, inequality (3) and the definition of Γ in Equation (1) lead to the following requirement in terms of temperature to obtain Coulomb crystallization (see Problem Set):

$$T \leq T_{\mathrm{CC}} \sim 10\,\mathrm{mK}. \tag{7}$$

Consequently, before the advent of laser cooling techniques, it was impossible to reach the condition for ion Coulomb crystallization since until then, all other cooling techniques were limited by the temperature of liquid helium, and hence typically to temperatures in the range of a few kelvins. On the other hand, for standard laser Doppler cooling, the minimum temperature is effectively given by

$$T_{\mathrm{Dopp}} \sim \frac{\hbar\Gamma_{\mathrm{cool}}}{k_B} \sim 0.1 - 1\,\mathrm{mK}, \tag{8}$$

where Γ_{cool} is the spectral width of the cooling transition. This temperature is clearly below T_{CC}, and even low enough to create crystals of the smallest finite systems.

The production of ion Coulomb crystals through laser cooling of ions (see Chapter 6) was pioneered by the groups of David Wineland (NIST,

Boulder, Colorado, USA) and Prof. H. Walther (MPQ, Garching, Germany) in the 1980s, and the past decades an ever increasing number of groups worldwide have taken part in the further development, exploration and application of these exotic crystalline structures.

An interesting issue concerning Coulomb crystallization in both Penning and RF traps is the fact that in both cases, the crystallized ions in addition to their random thermal motion perform synchronized driven motion, either in the form of rotation (Penning traps) or quadrupolar oscillations (RF traps). Interestingly, the corresponding averaged kinetic energy can easily exceed the thermal energy by a factor of 10^4-10^6!

4. Structural Properties (One-dimensional, Two-dimensional, and Three-dimensional Structures)

While the lowest energy state of infinite constant density Coulomb crystals is a *bcc* structure [9,10], the structures of finite size crystals depend strongly on the number of ions as well as the shape of the trapping potential. Even in the case of trapping conditions leading to constant density (i.e. 3D harmonic trapping potentials), 3D crystals can have many different features.

For the isotropic confinement case, where the confining force can be written in terms of a single force constant κ,

$$F_{\text{trap}}(r) = -\kappa r, \tag{9}$$

the overall structure of the Coulomb crystals must be spherical due to spherical symmetry. However, what is not obvious is the fact that for crystals (or more correctly clusters) containing up to a few thousand ions, the total potential energy is minimized by having the ions organized in concentric shells with a specific "magic" numbers of ions [11] as the temperature goes to zero. Within each shell, the ions furthermore form closed 2D structures, which to a high degree is like a hexagonal lattice, the minimum energy state for an infinite 2D planar crystal.

Already with more than a few ions present, it is essentially impossible to predict the ground state configuration, and Monte Carlo or Molecular Dynamics (MD) simulations have to be introduced to find those [11]. However, since it is well known from cluster physics that the number of metastable configurations increases roughly exponentially with the number of particles forming the cluster, it soon becomes extremely difficult to ensure that a particular simulation has reached the minimum energetic state.

The uncertainty in the predicted magic numbers of ions from MD simulations within each shell is though so small that for a given spherical shell structure, the number of ions can be determined with an uncertainty much smaller than the square-root of the total number of ions [11]. Hence, comparing MD simulations with projection images of crystals recorded in the laboratories constitutes a reliable method to obtain information on the number of ions as well as the ion density in experiments.

Since the ions will always have a finite thermal energy in the laboratories, it is indeed possible also to observe the formation of energetically excited metastable configurations which may even have extended long range ordered structures with *bcc* or *fcc* character at ion numbers much smaller than $\sim$10,000, expected from theoretical investigations to be the minimum number in order to have such structures as the ground states. Sometimes, crystals composed of domains of both *fcc* and *bcc* structures can even appear.

In another special trapping situation, where the ions are confined by an isotropic harmonic potential in two dimensions while being free to move along the third direction, concentric cylindrically shell structures represent the minimum energy states. In this situation, the number of shells depends rather on the linear density of particles along the unconfined axis than on the total number of ions. In the laboratories, this specific situation can effectively be realized by choosing a ring shaped 2D RF quadrupole trap as has been pioneered by Prof. H. Walther, MPQ [12], or by letting the ion species of interest (the low mass species) be part of a two-species crystal in a standard linear RF quadrupole trap [13]. In the first case, the ring shaped confinement will lead to an effective periodic boundary condition for the ions along the ring, which will not deviate substantially from the infinitely long 2D confinement situation, when the circumference is much larger than the typical ion–ion distance and diameter of the crystal. In the two-species case, the heavier ion species will feel an effective confining force which is weaker than for the lighter mass one in the plane with RF field confinement, and hence, the lighter mass ions will segregate within a cylindrical volume along the RF field free axis. Empirically, it has been shown that the shell structure of this inner component of the two-species crystal to a very high degree mimics the infinite case due to the effective electrical shielding by the surrounding heavier species [13]. In an extreme case, a string of 43 equidistantly spaced $^{24}Mg^{+}$ ions was situated within a crystal of $\sim$3,000 $^{40}Ca^{+}$ ions [13].

In the more general case of harmonic confinement with an isotropic potential in two dimensions, but a different force constant in the third one ($\kappa_z \neq \kappa_x = \kappa_y$), the equipotential surfaces are described by concentric spheroids. While a weakly interacting gas of ions in thermal equilibrium would have a spatial distribution with contour surfaces of the density corresponding to the equipotential surfaces of the confining potential, this is not true for Coulomb crystallized ion ensembles [13,14]. In cases where the number of ions in a Coulomb crystal is so large that the extension in all three dimensions exceeds significantly the spacing of the individual ions, it can be expected that the shape of the crystal should be very similar to the case of a confined cold charged fluid with a constant charge density. For this latter situation, it is indeed possible to find an analytic expression for the outer spheroidal shape of such a fluid in a potential with spheroidal equipotential surfaces. However, due to the Coulomb repulsion, the shapes deviate from the equipotential surfaces of the trapping potential. In a series of experiments, it has been verified that the outer contour of Coulomb crystals indeed follow the same shape as the cold charged liquid model, except at extreme confinement cases leading to the formation of real 2D (pancake) or 1D (string) structures [13]. For the number of ions reaching up to a few thousand, the ions will as in the isotropic confining case furthermore be organized in concentric spheroidal shells.

The 2D planar structures [15] and 1D string structures [16,17] constitute special cases, where the liquid model does not suffice to describe the shape. Here, different approaches including MD simulations have to be used to obtain more detailed structural information.

Both in theory and by experiments, it has been shown that under specific trapping conditions, Coulomb crystals can have negative Poisson coefficients, meaning that when the crystal is stretched along one direction, it will lead to a lateral expansion.

Another interesting situation is the one where two ion species with the same charge-to-mass ratio are simultaneously crystallized in, e.g. a linear RF trap. In this situation, both ion species feel the same effective potential and *a priori* could be expected to mix. On a gross scale, this is also true according to MD simulations, and for large systems, one indeed finds a simple cubic lattice (as in CsCl salt) as the minimum energy state [18]. For smaller finite systems of a few thousand ions, common shell structures like for a single-species are formed, however, with the common shells consisting of slightly displaced sub-shells of the two species [18]. It was also found by MD simulations that the degree of mixing is very sensitive to the exact values of the charge-to-mass ratios of the two ion species. A difference of only one per mille is essentially enough to observe at least partial segregation of the two species [18]. As we will discuss briefly in Section 6, such segregation effects may be studied in detail by experimenting with Highly Charged Ions (HCI), and may turn out to have relevance for the composition of Coulomb crystals within White Dwarfs, where $^{16}O^{8+}$ and $^{12}C^{6+}$ ions, which have nearly the same charge-to-mass ratio, are present.

Coulomb crystals with non-constant particle densities can as well be created and studied through the application of higher-order pole RF traps, like hexapole and octopole traps. Recently, Coulomb crystallization of ions in particular octupole traps have been considered both theoretically [19] and experimentally [20]. In such higher-order traps, the ground state configuration of the ions will never be a single string, but rather ring/tube-like structures or multi-string-like structures depending on the trapping conditions. For few ions where near hexagonal lattice-like pancake structures appear for 2D systems under RF quadrupole confinement, in higher-order traps, rings of ions are instead formed. These new types of structure may, for instance, find applications within the field of quantum simulations (see Section 6).

5. Dynamical Properties

Like usual solids, Coulomb crystals have a series of vibrational modes (phonon modes). In general, if a Coulomb crystal consists of N ions then such a crystal will have $3N$ normal modes with corresponding distinct eigenmode frequencies [21].

For smaller crystals, the individual modes can be found either through direct computations [17] or through the analysis of the motions of ions in MD simulations after the introduction of a motional excitation [21].

For larger spheroidal crystals which may in real experiments actually be found to be a series of isomeric configurations each with their particular mode pattern and spectrum, a simpler way to gain information on mode structures and frequencies is once again to approximate the real granular Coulomb crystals by a cold charged liquids with the same shape and size, and find such object's eigenfrequencies and eigenmodes. As has been shown by Prof. Dan Dubin, UCSD, USA, the modes of such cylindrical symmetric objects can be characterized by two quantum numbers (l, m), where m describes the azimuthal part of the eigenmode and l the longitudinal part with $l - 1$ indicating the number of nodal planes along the symmetry axis [22].

As long as the characteristic length scale for the (l, m)-modes exceeds significantly the ion–ion spacing within the Coulomb crystals, these modes may provide a good description of the real crystal modes. Experiments conducted both in Penning [15] and linear RF traps [23] have in fact proved that the modes like the (l, m)-modes can be excited in ion Coulomb crystals.

For highly anisotropic trapping conditions leading to either 1D string structures or 2D pancake-like structures a sub-set of 1D [17] and 2D [24] modes can be found more easily. As we shall discuss in the next section, various modes of such dimensionally restricted crystals have found applications within quantum information processing as well as quantum simulation.

6. Applications

As should be clear from this section, the applications of Coulomb crystals in carrying out research beyond the studies of the basic properties of such crystals are extremely broad.

6.1. *Nonlinear dynamics*

The fact that the interaction between confined ions by the nature of the Coulomb interaction is nonlinear, made already around 1990s the smallest non-trivial ion systems consisting of two ions an interesting platform for the study of chaotic behavior in RF traps [25]. The appearance of bifurcation in the motional state of the ions as well as the existence of instability of two-ion crystals within the usual parameter range for single ion stable motion was studied. Later, experiments with larger ($\sim$1,000 ions) systems furthermore showed that when the plasma frequency of such crystals reached half the RF drive frequency, parametric excitation would lead to crystal melting [26]. In some cases, the parametric resonance could be switched off by induced crystal rotation [26], which led to lower particle densities and consequently lower plasma frequencies.

6.2. *Statistical physics and thermodynamics*

Coulomb crystals in the form of ion-strings and so-called zig-zag configurations have recently also found applications within statistical physics [27]. For instance, several groups have recently investigated the formation of defects (often referred to as kinks) in zig-zag configurations when formed through fast changes in the trapping parameters leading to a change in the equilibrium configurations from string to zig-zag structures. Through these experiments, universal scaling laws for the number of defects have been shown to follow predictions of the Kibble–Zurek model in the special inhomogeneous case [28,29].

From a thermodynamics perspective, ion Coulomb crystals constitute as well an interesting "playground". Recently, e.g. the thermal diffusion of a single impurity ion in a chain of ions has been investigated experimentally, and models to study heat transport in such systems have been proposed [30]. Also recently, it has been proposed to use strings of trapped ions in combination with periodic corrugated potentials in the form of induced dipole forces to study fundamental issues related to friction [31] as well as quantum phase transitions [32] in connection with a Coulomb-version of the Frenkel–Kontorova model [31].

6.3. *Solid-state physics*

As mentioned already, Coulomb crystals constitute a special class of solids, which make them natural objects for studies of various structural formations and dynamics. In the future, the combination of trapping of ions in harmonic traps with periodic corrugated potentials in the form of standing wave dipole potentials should make it possible not only to pin specific metastable structures by addressing selected lattice planes but also well make it feasible to make controlled changes in the lattice structure, e.g. from a *bcc* to a *fcc* structure and vice versa, through only changes in the overall trap potential [33]. While such experiments have not yet been carried out, first experiments of optical trapping and pinning of few ions within the nodal/antinodal planes of an optical standing wave field has recently been demonstrated.

6.4. *Plasma physics*

By nature, Coulomb crystals are the solid-state representation of OCP [8], and hence are in this respect an interesting special state of such plasma. By performing experiments in Penning as well as RF traps, it becomes indeed possible to study OCPs under both magnetized and non-magnetized conditions. By introducing different ion species in the same trap, it becomes furthermore possible to study multi-species OCPs in or in the vicinity of Coulomb crystallization (see Chapters 9–13).

6.5. *Nuclear fusion*

When laser-cooled ions collide with hotter impurity ions within a magnetized plasma in a Penning trap, the correlated collision dynamics resembles to a high degree the processes governing thermal nuclear fusion in dense stellar interiors [34]. Hence, in the future, Penning trap experiments may actually be used to model nuclear fusion in hot dense plasmas.

6.6. *Geoscience*

Another not immediate connection of Coulomb crystals to other branches of science is the observed stick-slip motion of the orientation of ion Coulomb crystals in Penning traps with respect to the phase of a rotating dipolar or quadrupolar perturbation. However, it turns out that the probability distributions of the amplitude of the slips are well described by power law relations, similar to those found in experiments on avalanches and slips in granular systems, as well as in models of earthquakes [35].

6.7. *Exotic stellar objects*

Besides being of fundamental plasma physics interest, OCPs in the form of fully ionized atoms are expected to play an important role for the cooling mechanisms of White Dwarfs [5]. Since such stellar objects are supposed to consist mostly of $^{16}O^{8+}$ and $^{12}C^{6+}$ ions, which have nearly identical charge-to-mass ratios, it would be interesting to carry out experiments with two species with nearly the same charge-to-mass ratio. By performing experiments with HCIs (e.g. $^{27}Al^{3+}$, $^{36}Ar^{4+}$, $^{45}Sc^{5+}$, $^{54}Fe^{6+}, \ldots, {}^{180}Hf^{20+}$, $^{189}Os^{21+}, \ldots$) cooled sympathetically through Coulomb interactions with simultaneously trapped and laser-cooled $^{9}Be^{+}$ ions, one can explore the effect of tiny differences in the charge-to-mass ratio on the segregation of the species. In such experiments, the fact that different species will crystallize at different temperatures (see Equation (1)) may play an important role. In previous two-species MD simulations of ions in a linear RF trap, it was found that the degree of mixing is very sensitive to the exact values of the charge-to-mass ratios [18]. However, much more detailed work has to be carried out in order to provide results of high enough quality to be relevant for the investigations of the cooling of White Dwarfs.

6.8. *Test of quantum mechanics*

Ion Coulomb crystals in the form of few ion systems are quite unique objects for studying fundamental consequences of quantum mechanics. One of the first things to be studied was the concept of quantum jumps, i.e. the observation of the abrupt jumps in the quantum state of a single quantum system upon measurements during induced dynamics. In a series of experiments with single atomic ions, this concept was verified by driving narrow transitions between the ground and a metastable excited electronic state [36]. The fact that spontaneous decay is in fact also a very fundamental quantum phenomenon has beautifully been demonstrated by altering the boundary conditions for the light emission of a single ion, either by introducing a single mirror [37] or an optical cavity [38] to establish single photon self-interference. The interference of single photons in scattering processes involving two ions has furthermore led to the observation of super-/sub-radiant states [39] as well as Young's double slit like results [40]. Experiments focused on the investigation of the so-called quantum Zeno effect has additionally been carried out with ion Coulomb crystals [41].

6.9. *Cavity QED related experiments*

Ion Coulomb crystals are as well extremely interesting objects for the study of cavity QED effects. For a single atomic ion, laser-cooled to its quantum mechanical motional ground state of a harmonic trap potential with oscillation frequencies of 0.1–1 MHz, the resulting ground state wavefunction will have a spatial extension of only a few nanometers, and hence much smaller than the wavelength of light in the optical or near optical range (NIR–UV range). Consequently, it is possible to position a single ion very precisely with respect to the nodes and antinodes of a standing wave cavity field [38,42], and hence control the effective coupling between the ion and the cavity field [38]. In the recent past, there has been a series of experiments demonstrating and exploiting the strong spatial localization even with ions cooled only to the Doppler limit [38,42,43].

Larger Coulomb crystals are as well interesting objects when the goal is the investigation and exploitation of the collective effect in the coupling of atoms to cavity fields. Recently, collective strong coupling, where the rate of exchange of a collective electronic excitation of ions in a Coulomb crystal with a photon in the cavity field exceeds both the excited state decay rate as well as the decay rate of photons out of the cavity was demonstrated [44]. This is an interesting regime since it enables the study of the fundamental quantum dynamics of the combined photon-ensemble system without decoherence, as well as open for, e.g. the realization of a quantum memory for light and novel photon counters.

6.10. *Quantum information processing*

Due to the existence of common normal modes of vibration for the particles constituting a Coulomb crystal, quantum correlated states can be created between the internal states of ions in such crystals through the application of spatially localized laser beams addressing narrow line transitions in the individual ions. By detuning an excitation laser frequency up (blue) or down (red) by a common mode frequency with respect to the transition frequency, deterministic entanglement can be created between the internal states of an ion and the common motional state. Let's for simplicity consider a string of ions where one of the normal modes are cooled to the ground state $|0\rangle$ mode, and all N ions is in a particular state $|g\rangle$:

$$\Psi_{\text{in}} = |0\rangle_{\text{mode}} \prod_{i=1}^{N} |g\rangle_i. \tag{10}$$

Then, we apply a laser beam to the qth ion, which is blue detuned. This means that if the ion gets internally excited, it also leads to an excitation of the common mode. If the laser irradiation lasts for a period such that the internal state of the qth ion is brought into an equal superposition state of being in $|g\rangle$ and an excited state $|e\rangle$, the new state of the ion system will then be

$$\Psi_{\text{new}} = \frac{1}{\sqrt{2}} \left(|0\rangle_{\text{mode}} |g\rangle_q \prod_{i \neq q}^{N} |g\rangle_i + |1\rangle_{\text{mode}} |e\rangle_q \prod_{i \neq q}^{N} |g\rangle_i \right). \tag{11}$$

Clearly, this is a maximal entangled state between the internal state of the qth ion and the common motional state. Now, if finally, we apply a red detuned laser beam to the pth ion for a time leading to the transition $|g\rangle_p |1\rangle_{\text{mode}} \rightarrow |e\rangle_p |0\rangle_{\text{mode}}$ (due to being off-resonant, it will not excite $|g\rangle_p |0\rangle_{\text{mode}}$), we then get the state,

$$\begin{aligned} \Psi_{\text{final}} &= \frac{1}{\sqrt{2}} \left(|0\rangle_{\text{mode}} |g\rangle_p |g\rangle_q \prod_{i \neq p,q}^{N} |g\rangle_i + |0\rangle_{\text{mode}} |e\rangle_p |e\rangle_q \prod_{i \neq p,q}^{N} |g\rangle_i \right), \\ &= \frac{1}{\sqrt{2}} |0\rangle_{\text{mode}} \left(|g\rangle_p |g\rangle_g + |e\rangle_p |e\rangle_q \right) \prod_{i \neq p,q}^{N} |g\rangle_i. \end{aligned} \tag{12}$$

This final state represents a maximum entanglement between the internal states of the pth and qth ion, but without entanglement with the common motional mode! The common mode has merely been used as a quantum communication channel.

By carefully addressing individual ions with appropriate laser pulses, it was shown by Cirac and Zoller in 1995 [45] that universal quantum gate operations can be performed between any two qubits represented by the internal states $|g\rangle \equiv |0\rangle$ and $|e\rangle \equiv |1\rangle$ of the ions. Hence, an ion Coulomb crystal in the form of a string of N ions can be used as a quantum register of N qubits in a general purpose quantum computer. Since this first proposal for quantum computing with cold ions, several other schemes have been proposed, and an impressive series of important results have been obtained experimentally regarding multi-particle entanglement [46] and quantum gate operations [47].

6.11. *Quantum simulations*

The possibility of performing universal gates between any pairs of ion qubit states in a N qubit system as briefly discussed above makes it in principle also possible to emulate the quantum dynamics of any Hamilton operator acting on a quantum system in a Hilbert space of dimension 2^N [48]. While such emulations can in principle be carried out on classical computers, the dimension of the Hilbert space increases exponentially with the number of qubits involved, and eventually becomes intractable. On the other hand, using quantum gates to represent the dynamics, this problem can be solved [48] though the concatenation of many gate operations can become rather inefficient. In some cases, like e.g. the study of magnetism and more generally spin–spin interactions at the quantum level, much more effective simulations can be carried out through emulating the two states of a magnetic dipole or spin by the two internal states of the ions, and applying appropriate light fields, which illuminate all the ions, to mimic magnetic fields [24, 49]. By such quantum simulators, one can simplify the number of operations needed considerably compared to "digital" quantum computing. Whereas digital quantum processing procedures always will need some kind of individual addressing of all the ions, "analogue" quantum simulators have a larger potential to eventually be extended to 2 and 3D Coulomb crystals.

6.12. *High precision spectroscopy*

The fact that ions within Coulomb crystals are both spatially very localized and motionally cold makes such crystals ideal for high-resolution spectroscopy. In particular, at such low temperatures where the quantized excitation of the normal modes is negligible, extremely narrow electronic transitions in the ions can be probed with ultrahigh precision [50]. Today, one of the most precise measurements of an optical transition in an atom has been performed in a $^{27}Al^+$ ion being sympathetically cooled by a single laser-cooled $^{24}Mg^+$ ion to form a two-ion Coulomb crystal. Since a large range of ion species, including ions of exotic isotopes, super-heavy element ions [51], HCI [52] as well as molecular ions can be effectively sympathetically crystallized through Coulomb interactions with laser-cooled ions, such refined spectroscopy techniques may in the near future lead to a vast amount of new and improved spectroscopic data of importance for a variety of fundamental physics investigations ranging from nuclear to astrophysics (see also Chapter 18).

6.13. *Cold molecular ion research*

Sympathetic cooling of molecular ions through the Coulomb interaction with simultaneously trapped laser-cooled atomic ions has the past years opened for a broad range of molecular investigations of both physical and chemical interest [53,54]. By bringing the molecular ions into a crystalline state, it is indeed possible to exploit the specific properties of two-species Coulomb crystals to learn about the number of molecular ions present without being able to observe them directly since the fluorescence from the atomic ions will reveal the total size of the crystal [53]. By monitoring the growth in the number of dark ions in a reaction experiment, one can, e.g. infer reaction rates [53], and by recording the reduction in the size of the crystal through photodissociation of the molecular ions, one can, e.g. determine the internal state distribution of the molecular ions. This latter method has been implemented to directly prove that though the translational motion of the molecular ions can be brought into the millikelvin range, the internal rovibrational temperature of the molecular ions is hardly changed due to the very distant ($\sim$10 μm) Coulomb interactions. Indeed, the cooling of the internal degrees of freedom (DoF) of the molecules is so weak that they typically get in equilibrium with the radiation field in the trapping region, which for a room temperature trap means $\sim$300 K. In the past years, several methods have though been devised to produce cold rovibrational molecular ions by the direct production of homonuclear molecular ions in specific internal states through Resonance Enhanced Multi-Photon Ionization, laser-induced rotational cooling and buffer gas cooling either by laser-cooled atoms or a cryogenic helium gas. While the lowest internal temperatures have so far been obtained with a helium buffer gas ($\sim$8 K) [54], buffer gas cooling by an ensemble of laser-cooled atoms has the prospect to bring the internal temperature into the microkelvin range (see also Chapter 7). Combined with sympathetic sideband cooling to translational temperatures in the microkelvin regime, this will enable investigations of ion chemistry in a whole new ultracold regime.

7. Conclusion

By this brief introduction to ion Coulomb crystals and their applications, I hope, I have managed to show how extremely versatile these objects are. Clearly, there is material enough for a whole book, however, the aim of this work has primarily been to provide the reader with a text and references from which more detailed knowledge can be acquired elsewhere.

Remark

It should be noted that the present text has been published in slightly different formats in the proceedings for the International School of Physics (Enrico Fermi), Course CLXXXIX, 2013 and for ECRYS — International School — Workshop on Electronic Crystals [1].

8. Problem Set

In the following, we will consider Coulomb crystallization of an ensemble of identically charged particles.

A *necessary condition* for a classical description of motion of the charged particles, and hence for Coulomb crystallization, is that the Wigner–Seitz radius significantly exceeds the spatial spread of the quantum mechanical wavefunction of the particles.

It is often a reasonable approximation to assume that the particles locally feel a harmonic potential characterized by an oscillation (plasma) frequency ω_p given by

$$\omega_p^2 = Q^2 n/(\epsilon_0 m),$$

where n is the particle number density related to the Wigner–Seitz radius a in the following manner:

$$a = (3/(4\pi n))^{1/3}.$$

The spatial extension of the quantum mechanical wavefunction in such a potential is roughly given by the size of the ground state wavefunction, i.e.

$$\Delta r = (h/(8\pi\omega_p m))^{1/2},$$

where m is the mass of the particles and h is Planck's constant.

We will in the following assume that crystallization takes place when the equality sign in Equation (3) in the text is met.

Questions

Question 1

Let the density of an ensemble of $^{40}Ca^+$ ions in an ion trap be 5×10^8 cm^{-3}.

(1) Show that the above necessary condition for a classical description is met.
(2) What is the critical temperature for Coulomb crystallization?

Question 2

Consider now a lump of copper with a density of conducting electrons given by 10^{23} cm^{-3}.

(1) Can the motion of the electrons be considered classical, and be Coulomb crystallized?

Question 3

Finally, consider the crust of a Neutron Star. Here, fully stripped Fe-nuclei ($^{56}Fe^{26+}$) are supposed to be found in densities of 10^{10} g/cm^3.

(1) Assuming an atomic mass of 56 a.m.u. for the iron nuclei, show that the necessary condition for a classical description of the plasma is fulfilled.
(2) What is the corresponding Coulomb crystallization temperature?
(3) Do you believe the crust of the Neutron Star can become a Coulomb crystal?

Solutions

Question 1

(1) From the information given, one finds $\Delta r = 9.2$ nm and $a = 7.8\,\mu$m. Since a is nearly 1,000 times larger than Δr, the classical condition is clearly met.
(2) Using Equations (1) and 3 with the equality sign, one finds a critical temperature of 12.2 mK.

Question 2

(1) From the information given, one finds $\Delta r = 40$ pm and $a = 134$ pm. Since Δr is nearly as large as a, the classical condition is not met, and Coulomb crystallization is not possible.

Question 3

(1) From the information given, one finds $\Delta r = 2.5\,\text{fm}$ and $a = 130\,\text{fm}$. Since a is nearly 100 times larger than Δr (as well as more than an order of magnitude larger than the radius of the ^{56}Fe nucleus, which equals 5 fm), the classical condition is clearly met.
(2) Using Equations (1) and (3) with the equality sign, one finds a critical temperature of 500 MK — very high!
(3) Since a Neutron Star will eventually cool to a temperature below 500 MK, the crust of this object should by time Coulomb crystallize.

References

1. M. Drewsen, Ion Coulomb crystals, *Physica B: Condens. Matter* **460**(0), 105–113 (2015).
2. E. Wigner, On the interaction of electrons in metals, *Phys. Rev.* **46**, 1002–1011 (1934).
3. C. C. Grimes and G. Adams, Evidence for a liquid-to-crystal phase transition in a classical, two-dimensional sheet of electrons, *Phys. Rev. Lett.* **42**, 795–798 (1979).
4. V. J. Goldman *et al.*, Evidence for two-dimensional quantum Wigner crystal, *Phys. Rev. Lett.* **65**, 2189–2192 (1990).
5. H. M. Van Horn, Dense astrophysical plasmas, *Science* **252**(5004), 384–389 (1991).
6. D. J. Wineland *et al.*, Atomic-ion Coulomb clusters in an ion trap, *Phys. Rev. Lett.* **59**, 2935–2938 (1987).
7. F. Diedrich *et al.*, Observation of a phase transition of stored laser-cooled ions, *Phys. Rev. Lett.* **59**, 2931–2934 (1987).
8. S. Ichimaru, Strongly coupled plasmas: High-density classical plasmas and degenerate electron liquids, *Rev. Mod. Phys.* **54**, 1017–1059 (1982).
9. E. L. Pollock and J. P. Hansen, Statistical mechanics of dense ionized matter. II. Equilibrium properties and melting transition of the crystallized one-component plasma, *Phys. Rev. A* **8**, 3110–3122 (1973).
10. W. M. Itano *et al.*, Bragg diffraction from crystallized ion plasmas, *Science* **279** (5351), 686–689 (1998).
11. R. W. Hasse and V. V. Avilov, Structure and Madelung energy of spherical Coulomb crystals, *Phys. Rev. A* **44**, 4506–4515 (1991).
12. G. Birkl *et al.*, Multiple-shell structures of laser-cooled $^{24}Mg^{+}$ ions in a quadrupole storage ring, *Nature* **357**(6376), 310–313 (1992).
13. L. Hornekær *et al.*, Structural properties of two-component Coulomb crystals in linear Paul traps, *Phys. Rev. Lett.* **86**, 1994–1997 (2001).
14. S. Mavadia *et al.*, Control of the conformations of ion Coulomb crystals in a Penning trap, *Nat. Commun.* **4**, 2571 (2013).

15. T. B. Mitchell *et al.*, Direct observations of structural phase transitions in planar crystallized ion plasmas, *Science* **282**(5392), 1290–1293 (1998).
16. J. P. Schiffer, Phase transitions in anisotropically confined ionic crystals, *Phys. Rev. Lett.* **70**, 818–821 (1993).
17. D. F. V. James, Quantum dynamics of cold trapped ions with application to quantum computation, *Applied Physics B* **66**(2), 181–190 (1998).
18. T. Matthey *et al.*, Coulomb bicrystals of species with identical charge-to-mass ratios, *Phys. Rev. Lett.* **91**, 165001 (2003).
19. F. Calvo *et al.*, Crystallization of ion clouds in octupole traps: Structural transitions, core melting, and scaling laws, *Phys. Rev. A* **80**, 063401 (2009).
20. K. Okada *et al.*, Crystallization of Ca^+ ions in a linear rf octupole ion trap, *Phys. Rev. A* **75**, 033409 (2007).
21. D. H. E. Dubin and J. P. Schiffer, Normal modes of cold confined one-component plasmas, *Phys. Rev. E* **53**, 5249–5267 (1996).
22. D. H. E. Dubin, Theory of electrostatic fluid modes in a cold spheroidal non-neutral plasma, *Phys. Rev. Lett.* **66**, 2076–2079 (1991).
23. A. Dantan *et al.*, Noninvasive vibrational mode spectroscopy of ion Coulomb crystals through resonant collective coupling to an optical cavity field, *Phys. Rev. Lett.* **105**, 103001 (2010).
24. J. W. Britton *et al.*, Engineered two-dimensional ising interactions in a trapped-ion quantum simulator with hundreds of spins, *Nature* **484**(7395), 489–492 (2012).
25. J. Hoffnagle *et al.*, Order-chaos transition of two trapped ions, *Phys. Rev. Lett.* **61**, 255–258 (1988).
26. N. Kjærgaard *et al.*, Stability of Coulomb crystals in a linear Paul trap with storage-ring-like confinement, *Phys. Rev. E* **66**, 015401 (2002).
27. S. Fishman *et al.*, Structural phase transitions in low-dimensional ion crystals, *Phys. Rev. B* **77**, 064111 (2008).
28. S. Ulm *et al.*, Observation of the Kibble–Zurek scaling law for defect formation in ion crystals, *Nat. Commun.* **4**, 1–7 (2013), DOI: 10.1038/ncomms3291.
29. K. Pyka *et al.*, Topological defect formation and spontaneous symmetry breaking in ion Coulomb crystals, *Nat. Commun.* **4**, 1–6 (2013), DOI: 10.1038/ncomms3291.
30. A. Bermudez *et al.*, Controlling and measuring quantum transport of heat in trapped-ion crystals, *Phys. Rev. Lett.* **111**, 040601 (2013).
31. A. Benassi *et al.*, Nanofriction in cold ion traps., *Nat. Commun.* **2**, 236 (2011).
32. E. Shimshoni *et al.*, Quantum zigzag transition in ion chains, *Phys. Rev. Lett.* **106**, 010401 (2011).
33. P. Horak *et al.*, Optically induced structural phase transitions in ion Coulomb crystals, *Phys. Rev. A* **86**, 043435 (2012).
34. D. H. E. Dubin, Measurement of screening enhancement to nuclear reaction rates using a strongly magnetized and strongly correlated non-neutral plasma, *Phys. Rev. Lett.* **94**, 025002 (2005).
35. T. B. Mitchell *et al.*, Stick-slip dynamics of a stressed ion crystal, *Phys. Rev. Lett.* **87**, 183001 (2001).

36. W. Nagourney *et al.*, Shelved optical electron amplifier: Observation of quantum jumps, *Phys. Rev. Lett.* **56**, 2797–2799 (1986).
37. J. Eschner *et al.*, Light interference from single atoms and their mirror images, *Nature* **413**(6855), 495–498 (2001).
38. A. Kreuter *et al.*, Spontaneous emission lifetime of a single trapped Ca^+ ion in a high finesse cavity, *Phys. Rev. Lett.* **92**, 203002 (2004).
39. R. G. DeVoe and R. G. Brewer, Observation of superradiant and subradiant spontaneous emission of two trapped ions, *Phys. Rev. Lett.* **76**, 2049–2052 (1996).
40. U. Eichmann *et al.*, Young's interference experiment with light scattered from two atoms, *Phys. Rev. Lett.* **70**, 2359–2362 (1993).
41. W. M. Itano *et al.*, Quantum zeno effect, *Phys. Rev. A* **41**, 2295–2300 (1990).
42. G. R. Guthohrlein *et al.*, A single ion as a nanoscopic probe of an optical field, *Nature* **414**(6859), 49–51 (2001).
43. A. Stute *et al.*, Quantum-state transfer from an ion to a photon, *Nat. Photon.* **7** (3), 219–222 (2013).
44. P. F. Herskind *et al.*, Realization of collective strong coupling with ion Coulomb crystals in an optical cavity, *Nat Phys.* **5**(7), 494–498 (2009).
45. J. I. Cirac and P. Zoller, Quantum computations with cold trapped ions, *Phys. Rev. Lett.* **74**, 4091–4094 (1995).
46. H. Haffner *et al.*, Scalable multiparticle entanglement of trapped ions, *Nature* **438**(7068), 643–646 (2005).
47. F. Schmidt-Kaler *et al.*, Realization of the Cirac–Zoller controlled-NOT quantum gate, *Nature* **422**(6930), 408–411 (2003).
48. B. P. Lanyon *et al.*, Universal digital quantum simulation with trapped ions, *Science* **334**(6052), 57–61 (2011).
49. D. Porras and J. I. Cirac, Effective quantum spin systems with trapped ions, *Phys. Rev. Lett.* **92**, 207901 (2004).
50. P. O. Schmidt *et al.*, Spectroscopy using quantum logic, *Science* **309**(5735), 749–752 (2005).
51. M. Drewsen, Cooling, identification and spectroscopy of super-heavy element ions, *Eur. Phys. J. D.* **45**(1), 125–127 (2007).
52. L. Gruber, Evidence for highly charged ion Coulomb crystallization in multicomponent strongly coupled plasmas, *Phys. Rev. Lett.* **86**, 636–639 (2001).
53. M. Drewsen *et al.*, Ion Coulomb crystals: A tool for studying ion processes, *Int. J. Mass Spectrom.* **229**(1–2), 83–91 (2003).
54. A. K. Hansen *et al.*, Efficient rotational cooling of Coulomb-crystallized molecular ions by a helium buffer gas, *Nature* **508**(7494), 76–79 (2014).

CHAPTER SIXTEEN

COLD MOLECULAR IONS IN TRAPS

Roland Wester

Institute for Ion Physics and Applied Physics,
Universität Innsbruck,
Technikerstraße 25, 6020 Innsbruck, Austria
roland.wester@uibk.ac.at

This chapter discusses the trapping of molecular ions and provides an introduction to the cooling of their translational and internal degrees of freedom (DoF). We will describe two main approaches that are employed in current research, quadrupole and multipole radiofrequency ion traps. Different cooling techniques are employed in these traps that have been established to prepare the trapped molecular ions at low translational and internal temperature.

1. Introduction: Why Put Molecular Ions in Traps?

In our natural environment, most atoms are bound to molecules because the formation of chemical bonds releases substantial amounts of energy compared to available thermal energies. The only exception to the rule is the rare gas atoms because they feature a closed-shell electronic configuration. The study of the structure, the optical properties and the collision dynamics of molecules are therefore old topics in physics research. It overlaps closely with chemical research on the rules and mechanisms of molecular bond formation. Still today, many fundamental questions are open because detailed experiments require a high degree of control and most theoretical calculations still rely on substantial approximations.

Ion traps have come to be ideal tools to localize the position of charged atomic-scale particles. These ions are spatially confined for very long times and thereby available for precise experiments. A lot of research has been carried out with atomic ions. Optical spectroscopy, laser cooling, and coherent manipulation techniques have been developed to interrogate and manipulate these ions. This has brought important advances over the years to laser spectroscopy, ion cooling quantum computation and simulation, precision measurements of fundamental constants and optical clock development. In principle, molecular ions can be trapped by the same techniques as atomic ions, but their different structure requires additional approaches. During the last two decades, a lot of development has happened to make use of the long interrogation times in ion traps for molecular ions and perform studies of their structure and dynamics.

Molecules differ qualitatively from atoms, in their spectrum of quantum mechanical eigenstates. In atoms, different energy eigenstates correspond to different electronic wavefunctions, including spin–orbit interactions, which typically need several electronvolts to excite. In molecules in addition to electronic excitation, the vibrational and rotational motion leads to additional series of quantum mechanical eigenstates. For diatomic molecules, the energy spacing for these different excitations scales roughly as $1 : \sqrt{m_e/\mu} : m_e/\mu$, where m_e is the electron mass and μ the reduced mass of the molecule. In small molecules, this amounts to few hundred millielectronvolt for vibrational motion and a few millielectronvolt for rotational motion. In ion traps, all these different degrees of freedom (DoF) of molecular ions may be studied. Rovibrational spectroscopy provides accurate energy values from which molecular structures can be extracted and compared with calculation. Ion–atom or ion–molecule collisions deliver insight into the interaction potential, the rate for energy transfer between excited molecular ions, or the probability for chemical reactions to occur. However, for precision experiments, the different DoF of molecular ions also require additional techniques to probe and control them.

The following section of this chapter will discuss how radiofrequency (RF) ion traps are employed to prepare and study molecular ions. The focus will be on RF ion traps, which have become a workhorse for many applications. This will be illustrated with reference to selected original research publications. More details are found in recent review articles, e.g. Refs. [1,2]. For a description of other ion storage devices that are used to study molecular ions, in particular electrostatic resonator ion traps [3] or ion storage rings [4], the reader is referred to the respective literature. In the subsequent section, different approaches to cool and state-prepare molecular ions are explained.

2. Radiofrequency Traps for Molecular Ions

Trapping in RF ion traps only depends on the charge-to-mass ratio of a particle. Thus, RF ion traps operate in the same way for molecular ions as for atomic ions of the same mass and charge. However, for molecular ions, other ion trap configurations are employed than for atomic ions. Essentially, two general types of trap designs have evolved, quadrupole ion traps, where molecular ions are co-trapped with atomic ions, and multipole ion traps, which trap molecular ions and surround them by a neutral buffer gas.

2.1. *Molecular ions in quadrupole traps*

The operation principle of quadrupole ion traps is described in Chapter 2. Today, the most common design is the linear quadrupole trap. It consists of two pairs of symmetrically arranged electrodes to which the opposite phases of an RF generator are connected. This creates the ion confinement in the radial direction with typical trap depths of several electronvolt. Small repulsive static potentials provide the ion confinement along the axis of the trap. Typical depths of the effective trapping potential of an RF trap lie in the range of few electronvolts. Ions with less kinetic energy than the depth are confined in the trap. Provided the stability condition for quadrupole traps is fulfilled, the ions remain trapped until collisions with residual background gas accelerate them and ultimately drive them out of the trap.

In quadrupole traps, the key to study molecular ions is to co-trap them with atomic ions that can be laser-cooled. The latter are usually alkaline earth atoms, for example, Be^+, Mg^+ or Ca^+. Due to the strong reduction in translational temperature, these atomic ions form Coulomb crystals (see Chapter 15). The crystals are observable with a sensitive imaging camera because the atomic ions fluoresce during the laser cooling cycle. Co-trapped molecular ions collide elastically with the atomic ions and are thereby translationally cooled as well. In this way, they become part of the Coulomb crystal. However, molecular ions do not fluoresce because of the lack of closed optical cycling transitions. Therefore, their locations remain dark on the camera image. This is shown in the left part of Figure 1. The effective trapping potential in an RF trap is inversely proportional to the ion mass (see next section). The positions of the molecular ions in the Coulomb crystal therefore depend on the ratio of the molecular mass to the co-trapped atomic ion mass. If the molecular mass is smaller than the atomic mass, the molecular ions are found in the center of the crystal (which is the case

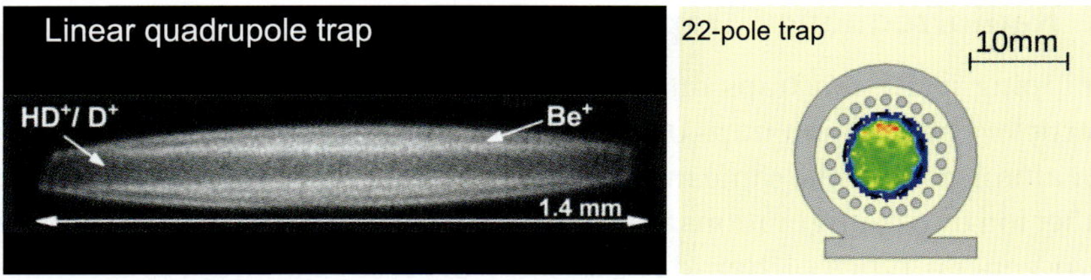

Fig. 1. Left panel: Image of a Coulomb crystal of laser-cooled Be^+ ions that are co-trapped with HD^+ molecular ions. The molecular ions do not fluoresce and therefore only show up on the camera image as the darker region in the center of the crystal. Some HD^+ ions are converted into D^+ ions after vibrational excitation and subsequent photofragmentation (see Ref. [12] for details). Right panel: Cut through a 22-pole ion trap perpendicular to the RF electrodes. Inside the trap, a measured density distribution of OH^- ions at room temperature is superimposed (see Ref. [13] for details).

depicted in Figure 1), if the molecular mass is larger than the molecular ions gathered outside the atomic ions at large radii.

By taking high resolution fluorescence images of a Coulomb crystal and comparing them to numerical simulations, one can obtain the number of trapped atomic and molecular ions, respectively, even though the molecular ions remain dark [5]. If different "dark" molecular ions are trapped together in the same crystal, additional techniques are needed to differentiate them. This can either be done by driving resonant oscillations of the ions in the trap [6], the frequency of which depends on the mass of both ions, or by extracting the ions from the trap and passing them into a time-of-flight mass spectrometer [7,8].

Different techniques exist to bring molecular ions into the ion trap. In the first experiments with molecular ions in Coulomb crystals, the ions were produced by a chemical reaction of a laser-cooled atomic ion with a neutral molecule in the residual gas of the vacuum chamber. In this way, MgH^+ or CaO^+ form in reactions of Mg^+ or Ca^+ with hydrogen or oxygen molecules, respectively [9]. Other molecular ions are being passed as neutral molecules into the trapping region and are then ionized by electron impact ionization, for example HD^+ to be co-trapped with Be^+ [5], or are ionized by a multi-photon process in a strong laser field, for example, aniline cations $C_6H_5NH_2^+$ to be co-trapped with Ca^+ [10]. Even larger molecular ions or ions that cannot be directly formed from a stable neutral precursor have to be produced in an external ion source. Electrospray ionization has been successfully employed to load the protonated Alexa Fluor 350 ion ($C_{16}H_{14}N_2O_9SH^+$) into a Coulomb crystal co-trapped with Ba^+ [11].

2.2. *Molecular ions in multipole traps*

Instead of co-trapping molecular ions with laser-cooled atomic ions, they can also be kept in an ion trap that is filled with a neutral gas. In this case, collisions with the neutral gas are used to cool the molecular ions. Multipole RF ion traps are most useful for cooling with neutral buffer gas, which is a consequence of the shape of the effective trapping potential. This will be explained at the end of the section. As introduced in Chapter 2, multipole traps typically employ linear RF electrode geometries as used for linear quadrupole traps, but instead of two pairs of electrodes, one uses n pairs of electrodes and with a π phase shift of the RF drive between neighboring electrodes (see Figure 1). For $n = 2$, this comes back to the linear quadrupole trap.

An analytical expression for the time-varying electric potential of an ideal linear multipole trap with infinite extension along the trap axis is given by

$$V(r, \phi, t) = V_0 \cos(n\phi) \left(\frac{r}{R_0}\right)^n \sin(\omega t), \tag{1}$$

where V_0 is the RF amplitude, R_0 the inscribed radius of the RF electrodes and ω denotes the angular frequency. In practice, this potential is created by $2n$ cylindrical electrodes of radius ρ arranged on a cylinder of inscribed radius R_0. To achieve a potential that optimally approximates the curvature of the ideal multipole potential of Equation (1) to first and second order, the diameter of the rods has to fulfil the relation [14] $\rho = R_0/(n-1)$. For a trap diameter of $2R_0 = 10$ mm and a rod diameter of $2\rho = 1$ mm, this leads to $n = 11$ and represents the widely-used 22-pole ion trap [15].

The dynamics of ions in the time-dependent field of a multipole ion trap cannot be solved analytically. This is different from the dynamics in a quadrupole or Paul trap because for multipole traps, the equation of motion becomes nonlinear in the position coordinate. Instead, the best way to describe the dynamics is with the aid of the effective potential approximation, introduced by Dehmelt [16]. It assumes that the position coordinate of a trapped ion is composed of a rapid oscillation $\vec{\xi}(t)$ that follows the RF, which is referred to as micromotion, and a slowly varying drift motion $\vec{R}(t)$, also referred to as the secular motion, $\vec{r}(t) = \vec{R}(t) + \vec{\xi}(t)$. For the drift motion, one obtains an equation of motion that includes a time-independent effective potential. For the ideal linear multipole trap described by Equation (1), the effective potential is given by

$$V_{\text{eff}}(\vec{R}) = \frac{n^2 q^2 V_0^2}{4m\omega^2 R_0^2} \left(\frac{R}{R_0} \right)^{2n-2} . \tag{2}$$

For large n, this potential increases rapidly with increasing radius R. This approximates an effective potential with a large almost field-free central region and steep walls. The effective potential actually corresponds to the time-averaged kinetic energy of the micromotion. During trapping, the kinetic energy of the drift motion in the center of the trap is converted into kinetic energy of the micromotion near the turning points of the ions' trajectories and re-converted to drift motion kinetic energy on the way back to the trap center. In this way, stable confinement of the ions is reached.

The driven micromotion is a potential source of heating for the translational motion of the ions in the trap. The perfectly reversible conversion of energy only holds in the absence of collisions. If a collision with a neutral buffer gas atom occurs, micromotion kinetic energy can be converted to translational energy of the secular motion. This effect is referred to as RF heating [1, 17]. As described above, the effective potential is very small up to large radii in multipole ion traps and only reaches substantial values near the turning points of the ions. Thus, the higher the multipole order n the lower the RF heating. The heating rate also depends on the mass ratio of the buffer gas atoms to the trapped ions. For large mass differences, the heating rate is suppressed. Overall, one expects a typical temperature increase of a few percent in 22-pole ion traps ($n = 11$) [1, 17], see also the next section.

To load molecular ions into multipole ion traps, an external ion source is the most commonly used approach. Depending on the choice of molecular ions, different ion sources are selected. Electron impact ionization is used to create various cations from neutral precursors or subsequent ion–molecule reactions in the source, for example H_2^+, N_2^+, H_3^+, HCO^+, and CH_5 [15]. Negative ions, such as OH^-, NH_2^-, CN^-, C_2^-, C_2H^-, C_4H^-, and C_6H^- are efficiently created in a pulsed-discharge supersonic expansion ion source [18, 19]. For large molecular ions, such as the protonated amino acids tryptophane-H^+ or tyrosine-H^+, an electrospray ionization source is employed [20]. About 10^2–10^4 trapped ions are typically used in experiments. Given the trap volume of more than a cm^3, Coulomb interaction between the trapped ions is usually not significant in multipole ion traps.

3. Cooling Trapped Molecular Ions

For applications in high resolution spectroscopy or in quantum-state-resolved chemical dynamics experiments, cold translational temperatures as well as controlled internal quantum states are required. Thus, in the cooling of molecular species, one has to consider the translational motion and the internal DoF due of the molecules. Different methods have to be explored to cool them, which are discussed in the following subsections.

3.1. *Collisional cooling in quadrupole traps*

Translational cooling of ions in quadrupole and multipole traps has already been introduced in the previous section since it is essential for trapping the molecular ions. In both quadrupole and multipole ion traps, elastic collisions provide the translational thermalization (see also Chapter 7 by Hilico). The Coulomb interaction between laser-cooled atomic ions and the co-trapped molecular ions determines the cross-section for the elastic collisions. In a Coulomb crystal, the laser-cooled atomic ions are localized in a small volume in the center of the trap. Elastic collisions can therefore only happen when the molecular ions are also localized in the vicinity of the atomic ions. The timescales for translational cooling vary substantially depending on the conditions under which the molecular ions are produced and passed into the ion trap. MgH^+ produced from laser-cooled Mg^+ is formed at almost the same position and with very similar translational energy as the precursor ion. Thus, it reaches its stationary state within milliseconds. In contrast, HD^+ ions that are formed by ionizing room temperature neutral gas require several seconds to cool and localize in a Coulomb crystal.

It would be convenient to describe the stationary state of the trapped ions in the Crystal by a temperature. Such an assignment of a temperature to the trapped ions is difficult because the time-dependent RF field drives the rapidly oscillating micromotion of the ions in the trap. Nevertheless, it has been found that an effective or secular temperature can be defined for the ions in a quadrupole potential, which is based on the pure secular motion of the ions in the effective trapping potential [21]. Experimentally, values near 10 mK can be reached if the mass ratio of atomic and molecular ion are similar. But even for large mass ratios of about 10, an effective temperature of below 1 K has been reached [2].

The long-range Coulomb interaction between trapped cations prohibits encounters at short distance. Therefore, anisotropic contributions to the ion–ion interaction that depend on the orientation or the internal excitation of the molecular ion can be fully neglected. As a consequence, the Coulomb interaction does not affect the population of the internal quantum states. This has been shown for MgH^+ where the translational effective temperature was cooled below a Kelvin, but the rotational quantum states were populated according to the Boltzmann statistics for a room temperature ion ensemble. In this case, the thermalization of the rotational states is caused by the ambient blackbody radiation [22].

3.2. *Collisional cooling in multipole traps*

In multipole traps, the molecular ions are usually cooled in collisions with neutral buffer gas. Most commonly, one uses helium because it is the only gas that remains gaseous down to few kelvin trap temperature. The elastic collision cross-section that describes the translational cooling process is given by the long-range ion-induced dipole interaction. A semiclassical formulation of it has been derived by Cote and Dalgarno [23]. They obtained the cross-section as a function of the relative collision energy,

$$\sigma(E_{\rm rel}) = \pi \left(\frac{\mu C_4^2}{\hbar^2}\right)^{1/3} \left(1 + \frac{\pi^2}{16}\right) E_{\rm rel}^{-1/3}, \tag{3}$$

where C_4 is the coefficient of the long-range ion-induced dipole interaction and μ is the reduced mass of the collision system. At room temperature and for a typical buffer gas density of $n = 10^{13}/\text{cm}^3$ helium atoms, this leads to collision rates $\Gamma = n\sigma v_{\rm rel}$ ($v_{\rm rel}$ is the relative velocity) of about $2 \cdot 10^4$ /s, which is rather independent of the ion mass for masses significantly larger than that of helium. Numerical simulations show that approximately 3–10 collisions with the buffer gas are sufficient to thermalize the translational motion [1]. Thus, a typical timescale for translational cooling is a few milliseconds. At low temperature, the weak dependence of Γ on $E_{\rm rel}$ leads to slightly longer cooling timescales.

In multipole traps, such as the 22-pole ion trap, the ions' velocity distribution is generally well described by a Maxwell–Boltzmann distribution. Only for very large velocities, enhanced probabilities are found compared to the Boltzmann distribution caused by the effect of the micromotion [14]. This enhancement becomes smaller the higher the order n of the multipole trap. The translational temperature may be obtained by measuring the Doppler profile of absorption lines in high resolution. This has been done for N_2^+ and good agreement with the buffer gas temperature has been obtained down to 50 K [24]. Due to RF heating (see Section 2.2), the translational temperature, which has been obtained by fitting numerical simulations of the ion velocity distribution to a Maxwell–Boltzmann distribution, is larger by several percent than the buffer gas temperature [1,17]. At very low temperatures (below 20 K), the buffer gas and ion temperature may deviate even more [25]. This is attributed to distortions of the trapping potential due to the potential that confines the ions axially or due to surface patch potentials, but it is not fully understood quantitatively yet.

3.3. *Cooling internal molecular quantum states*

To control the internal quantum states of trapped molecular ions, different approaches may be taken, depending on the properties of the quantum state. High-lying excitations, in particular, bound excited electronic states and high-frequency vibrational levels, decay by spontaneous radiative emission. For example, the lifetime of the electronic A-state in N_2^+ is about 10 μs [24] and the lifetime of the $v = 1$ vibrational level in OH^- is about 3 ms. In both cases, the numbers depend slightly on the respective rotational quantum state. For low-lying excitations, the radiative decay rates drop substantially, the $J = 1$ state of HD^+ already has a radiative lifetime of 140 s [26] and for molecules composed of heavy atoms these become years. Furthermore, many rovibrationally excited states do not decay by dipole radiation due to the molecular symmetry and are thus extremely long-lived. This applies in particular to all homonuclear diatomic molecular ions, such as H_2^+ and N_2^+.

Molecular ions are typically formed in a range of different quantum states since during ionization and in some cases of subsequent ion–molecule reactions, a lot of energy is distributed among the final products. To prepare these molecular ions in selected rotational and vibrational quantum states, the most straightforward approach is to use cold neutral buffer gas to cool the ions. This is the standard approach in multipole RF ion traps [1,15]. The ion trap is typically mounted on a cryostat so that the buffer gas, usually helium, inside the ion trap is cooled to a temperature around 4–10 K.

To estimate the rates for inelastic collisions of ions with buffer gas atoms, the Langevin or capture model [27] is usually employed. The assumption of this model is that a collision occurs with 100% probability when the two collision partners come closer to each other than a critical distance. The latter is defined by the requirement that the relative kinetic energy is sufficient to surmount the centrifugal barrier at this impact parameter. This yields a velocity- and temperature-independent rate coefficient

$$k = \frac{|q|}{2\epsilon_0}\sqrt{\frac{\alpha}{\mu}}, \tag{4}$$

where α is the neutral polarizability, μ is the reduced mass of the two-body system, q is the ion charge and ϵ_0 the electric constant. Note that this Langevin rate coefficient is not dependent on temperature.

For collisions with helium atoms, one obtains Langevin rate coefficients of about $5 \cdot 10^{-10}$ cm^3/s, again with only a weak dependence on the ion mass. For the typical buffer gas density introduced in the previous section, this would lead to an inelastic collision rate of about $5{\cdot}10^3$/s. However, during the close encounter of the two collision partners that is described by the Langevin rate, an efficient conversion of internal excitation to translational energy is not guaranteed. For neutral molecules measurements, suggest that rotational cooling occurs with rate coefficients that are around 10–100% of the capture rate, and that vibrational cooling rate coefficients may even be suppressed by several orders of magnitude [27]. For molecular ions, direct experimental information on inelastic rate coefficients exists for N_2^+ and OH^-. The obtained rate coefficients are a few percent of the Langevin rate [24,28]. To cool a range of rotational quantum states in collisions with cold helium gas, one therefore has to estimate a timescale of 10–100 ms. The cooled molecular ions can then be studied further, e.g. by performing spectroscopy, or following bimolecular or cluster-forming reactions.

In quadrupole ion traps, the Coulomb interaction between atomic and molecular ions does not cool the internal DoF, as discussed in Section 3.1. To overcome this, either optical techniques can be employed (see Section 3.4) or neutral buffer gas collision can be invoked. The latter approach has recently been utilized to cool the internal quantum states of MgH^+ molecular ions in a Coulomb crystal [29]. The ion-neutral collision rate was carefully adjusted to be small enough not to affect the translational cooling by ion–ion interaction, but fast enough to win over blackbody-induced radiative transitions. In this way, a rotational temperature of 7.5 K was achieved.

3.4. *Optical state preparation*

Electromagnetic radiation offers an alternative and very well controllable means to change the internal quantum state of a molecular ion.

Experimentally, however, it has proven to be challenging to implement. In atoms, optical pumping is routinely employed to change the population of internal quantum states, for example, different hyperfine ground states. For molecular ions, there are usually no suitable electronic transitions because excited states either dissociate rapidly or their transition frequencies lie in the ultraviolet spectral range. Thus, optical state preparation has to involve vibrational transitions. Alternatively, quantum state control may be achieved by state-selective ionization or by selective removal of quantum states.

Rotational state preparation by pumping on a vibrational transition has been achieved for MgH^+ and HD^+ [30,31]. In MgH^+, the cooling laser drove the transition from $(v, J) = (0, 2)$ to $(1, 1)$, which either decays back to the same state or to the optically dark rovibrational ground state $(0, 0)$. The other rotational states couple to the $J = 2$ state by blackbody radiation-induced transitions and are thereby cooled as well. Within 120 s, about 37% of the ions were pumped into the ground state [30]. In HD^+, a very similar scheme was employed, only that two cooling laser were used that drove transitions to the $v = 1$ and 2 states, respectively [31]. In both cases, the rotational population of the ground state corresponded to an effective rotational temperature between 20 and 30 K.

An alternative method for preparing molecular ions in the rovibrational ground state has been demonstrated for N_2^+ [32]. Here, the ions were produced by state-selective photo-ionization at threshold by resonantly-enhanced multiphoton ionization (REMPI) using 2+1 photons of a short, intense laser pulse. Rotational state selection can also be achieved by removal of unwanted quantum states [28]. Recently, direct laser cooling of molecular ions has been proposed [33], which if successful will provide interesting new opportunities for translational as well as internal state control.

4. Summary

In this chapter, the trapping of molecular ions in RF traps has been discussed. The focus of the chapter has been on explaining the key concepts that have been developed by many research groups over the last years in order to handle and control molecular ions, in particular, at low temperature. The different cooling techniques have been described, which are needed to address the translational and the internal DoF of trapped molecular ions.

5. Problems

5.1. *Population of excited states*

Estimate the relative population of excited rotational and vibrational levels in HD^+ and CN^- for 4 K and 300 K. Assume the molecules to be rigid rotors with rotational constants $B = 22.5$ and $1.89\,\text{cm}^{-1}$. The vibrational frequencies are 1,913 and 2,035 cm^{-1}, respectively.

Solution

The relative population of a rovibrational level (v, J) is given by

$$(2J + 1)\exp(-E_{(v,J)}/k_B T),$$

where T is the absolute temperature, k_B is Boltzmann's constant, and $E_{(v,J)} = (v + 1/2)\hbar\omega + J(J + 1)B$. For selected low-lying levels, one obtains:

	(0,0)	(0,1)	(0,2)	(0,3)	(1,0)
HD^+ — 4 K	1.00000	0.00000	0.00000	0.00000	0.00000
HD^+ — 300 K	1.00000	2.41752	2.61648	1.91687	0.00010
CN^- — 4 K	1.00000	0.77000	0.08454	0.00200	0.00000
CN^- — 300 K	1.00000	2.94609	4.73527	6.27838	0.00006

5.2. *Cooling with different buffer gas*

How is the buffer gas cooling of the translational DoF of N_2^+ ions affected when the buffer gas is changed from helium to argon in a multipole ion trap?

Solution

The cooling of N_2^+ in helium leads to an ion translational temperature that is slightly higher than the neutral gas temperature. Changing to argon buffer gas inverts the mass ratio from 7:1 to 7:10. This leads to much stronger RF heating and thereby a significantly higher ion temperature.

References

1. R. Wester, Radiofrequency multipole traps: Tools for spectroscopy and dynamics of cold molecular ions, *J. Phys. B* **42**, 154001 (2009).
2. S. Willitsch, Coulomb-crystallised molecular ions in traps: methods, applications, prospects, *Int. Rev. Phys. Chem.* **31**(2), 175–199 (2012).

3. D. Zajfman *et al.*, Electrostatic bottle for long-time storage of fast ion beams, *Phys. Rev. A* **55**, 1577 (1997).
4. S. P. Møller, ELISA, an electrostatic storage ring for atomic physics, *Nucl. Instrum. Methods A* **394**, 281 (1997).
5. P. Blythe *et al.*, Production of ultracold trapped molecular hydrogen ions, *Phys. Rev. Lett.* **95**, 183002 (2005).
6. M. Drewsen *et al.*, Nondestructive identification of cold and extremely localized single molecular ions, *Phys. Rev. Lett.* **93**, 243201 (2004).
7. S. J. Schowalter *et al.*, An integrated ion trap and time-of-flight mass spectrometer for chemical and photo-reaction dynamics studies, *Rev. Sci. Instr.* **83**(4), 043103 (2012).
8. N. Deb *et al.*, Coulomb crystal mass spectrometry in a digital ion trap, *Phys. Rev. A* **91**, 033408 (2015).
9. K. Mølhave and M. Drewsen, Formation of translationally cold MgH^+ and MgD^+ molecules in an ion trap, *Phys. Rev. A* **62**, 011401(R) (2000).
10. K. Hojbjerre *et al.*, Consecutive photodissociation of a single complex molecular ion, *Phys. Rev. A* **77**, 030702 (2008).
11. A. Ostendorf *et al.*, Sympathetic cooling of complex molecular ions to millikelvin temperatures, *Phys. Rev. Lett.* **97**(24), 243005 (2006).
12. B. Roth *et al.*, Rovibrational spectroscopy of trapped molecular hydrogen ions at millikelvin temperatures, *Phys. Rev. A* **74**(4), 040501 (2006).
13. R. Otto *et al.*, How can a 22-pole ion trap exhibit 10 local minima in the effective potential?, *J. Phys. B* **42**, 154007 (2009).
14. D. Gerlich, Inhomogeneous RF fields: A versatile tool for the study of processes with slow ions, *Adv. Chem. Phys.* **82**, 1 (1992).
15. D. Gerlich, Ion-neutral collisions in a 22-pole trap at very low energies, *Phys. Scr.* **T59**, 256 (1995).
16. H. G. Dehmelt, Radiofrequency spectroscopy of stored ions I: Storage, *Adv. At. Mol. Phys.* **3**, 53 (1967).
17. O. Asvany and S. Schlemmer, Numerical simulations of kinetic ion temperature in a cryogenic linear multipole trap, *Int. J. Mass. Spectrom.* **279**, 147 (2009).
18. J. Mikosch *et al.*, Evaporation of trapped anions studied with a 22-pole ion trap in tandem time-of-flight configuration, *Phys. Rev. A* **78**, 023402 (2008).
19. T. Best *et al.*, Absolute photodetachment cross-section measurements for hydrocarbon chain anions, *Ap. J.* **742**, 63 (2011).
20. O. V. Boyarkin *et al.*, Electronic spectroscopy of cold, protonated tryptophan and tyrosine, *J. Am. Chem. Soc.* **128**(9), 2816 (2006).
21. J. P. Schiffer, Order in confined ions, *J. Phys. B* **36**(3), 511 (2003).
22. A. Bertelsen *et al.*, polar molecular ions in Coulomb crystals, *J. Phys. B* **39**, L83–L89 (2006).
23. R. Cote and A. Dalgarno, Ultracold atom-ion collisions, *Phys. Rev. A* **62**, 012709 (2000).
24. S. Schlemmer *et al.*, Laser excited N_2^+ in a 22-pole ion trap: Experimental studies of rotational relaxation processes, *Int. J. Mass Spectrom.* **185–187**, 589 (1999).
25. R. Otto *et al.*, Internal state thermometry of cold trapped molecular anions, *Phys. Chem. Chem. Phys.* **15**, 612 (2013).

26. Z. Amitay *et al.*, Rotational and vibrational lifetime of isotopically asymmetrized homonuclear diatomic molecular ions, *Phys. Rev. A.* **50**, 2304 (1994).
27. R. D. Levine, *Molecular Reaction Dynamics*, Chapter 3.2.5, p. 92. Cambridge, Cambridge University Press (2005).
28. D. Hauser *et al.*, Rotational state-changing cold collisions of hydroxyl ions with helium, *Nat. Phys.* **11**, 467 (2015).
29. A. K. Hansen *et al.*, Efficient rotational cooling of Coulomb-crystallized molecular ions by a helium buffer gas, *Nature* **508**, 76–79 (2014).
30. P. F. Staanum *et al.*, Rotational laser cooling of vibrationally and translationally cold molecular ions, *Nat. Phys.* **6**, 271 (2010).
31. T. Schneider *et al.*, All-optical preparation of molecular ions in the rovibrational ground state, *Nat. Phys.* **6**, 275 (2010).
32. X. Tong *et al.*, Sympathetic cooling of molecular ions in selected rotational and vibrational states produced by threshold photoionization, *Phys. Rev. Lett.* **105** (14), 143001 (2010).
33. P. Yzombard *et al.*, Laser cooling of molecular anions, *Phys. Rev. Lett.* **114**, 213001 (2015).

CHAPTER SEVENTEEN

PRECISE TESTS OF FUNDAMENTAL SYMMETRIES WITH TRAPPED IONS

S. Ulmer*, K. Blaum†, and W. Quint‡

*RIKEN, Ulmer Initiative Research Unit, Wako, Saitama 351-0198, Japan

†Max-Planck-Institut für Kernphysik, D-69117 Heidelberg, Germany

‡GSI Helmholtzzentrum für Schwerionenforschung, Planckstrasse 1, 64291 Darmstadt, Germany

1. Introduction

Precision measurements performed with single particles in Penning traps provide sensitive tests of the fundamental laws of nature. Using Penning traps, the properties of charged particles and their antiparticles were compared with ultrahigh precision [1–4], and thus provided stringent tests of the fundamental charge, parity time-reversal (CPT) symmetry [5]. Other Penning trap measurements which achieved fascinating precision include the determination of the magnetic moment of the bound electron [6–10], which provides the most stringent tests of bound state quantum electrodynamics in extreme fields, and based on this type of measurements the electron mass [11] has recently been determined with a fractional precision of 30 ppt. Furthermore, the most precise measurements of the magnetic moment of the electron, and thus, the fine structure constant [12], the most precise test of Einstein's famous equation $E = mc^2$ [13], the most accurate measurement of the proton mass [14], as well as the first direct high-precision measurement of the proton magnetic moment [15–18] are based on measurements performed with single particles in Penning traps. Other experiments carried-out with Penning traps focus on high-precision mass measurements of radioactive nuclides [19]. The results provide crucial impact parameters for astrophysics models and thus contribute, among

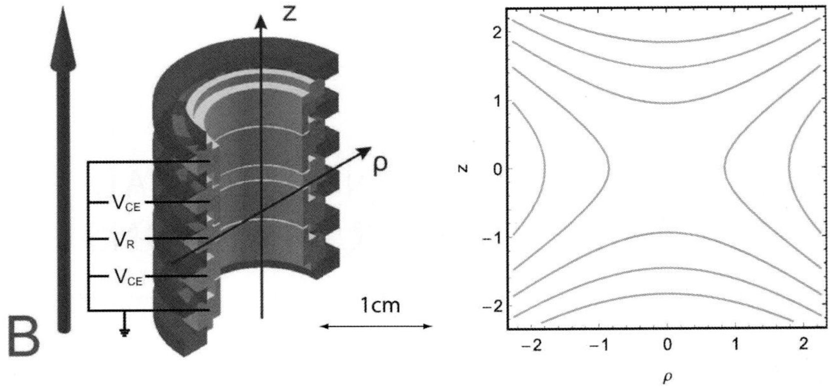

(a) (b)

Fig. 1. Left: Cylindrical Penning trap. Right: Electrostatic quadrupolar potential.

others, to our understanding of element abundance observed in our universe. Moreover, such measurements enable tests of fundamental physics such as unitarity tests of the CKM-matrix [20,21] or measurements to determine the nature of the neutrino [22,23] and its mass [24,25].

In this chapter, precision experiments using single particles in Penning traps are described. We start with a basic introduction to Penning traps and describe the methods typically used in high-precision Penning trap experiments. In the following chapters, Penning trap experiments with matter and antimatter particles, highly-charged ions and radioactive nuclides are discussed.

2. Basics of Penning Traps

In a Penning trap (see Figure 1(a)), a charged particle is stored in a combination of a homogeneous magnetic field B_0 and an electrostatic quadrupole potential (see Figure 1(b)). The magnetic field confines the particle in the plane perpendicular to the magnetic field lines, and the electrostatic potential in the direction parallel to the magnetic field lines. The three eigenmotions (Figure 2(a)) that result in such a combination of electromagnetic fields are the trap-modified cyclotron motion at

$$\nu_+ = \frac{\nu_c}{2} + \sqrt{\frac{\nu_c^2}{4} - \frac{\nu_z^2}{2}}, \tag{1}$$

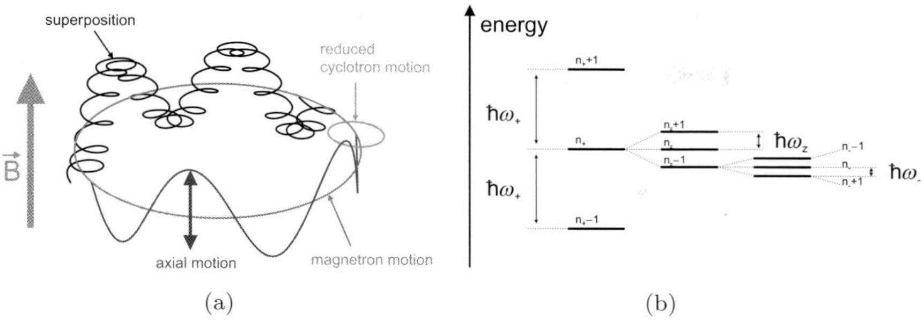

Fig. 2. (a) Trajectory of a single particle in a Penning trap. It is composed of three uncoupled harmonic oscillators. For further details see text. (b) Equivalent energy levels of a single particle in a Penning trap. Note that the magnetron energy decreases with increasing quantum number n_-.

where

$$\nu_c = \frac{1}{2\pi}\frac{q}{m}B_0, \tag{2}$$

is the free-space cyclotron frequency for a particle with charge-to-mass ratio q/m. The magnetron motion at

$$\nu_- = \frac{\nu_c}{2} - \sqrt{\frac{\nu_c^2}{4} - \frac{\nu_z^2}{2}} \tag{3}$$

is a circular $E \times B$ drift motion perpendicular to the magnetic field lines, and the axial motion oscillates along the magnetic field lines at

$$\nu_z = \frac{1}{2\pi}\sqrt{2C_2 V_R \frac{q}{m}}. \tag{4}$$

Here, V_R is the voltage applied to the central ring electrode of the trap to provide the quadrupolar trapping potential [26,27]

$$V(\rho, z) = V_R\, C_2(z^2 - \rho^2/2), \tag{5}$$

and $1/\sqrt{C_2}$ is a trap specific length.

The trajectory of a trapped particle is thus a composition of three decoupled harmonic oscillations, as shown in Figure 2. The free-space cyclotron frequency ν_c of a trapped ion can be determined from a combination of the trapped ion's three eigenfrequencies, either by using the sideband relation

$$\nu_c = \nu_+ + \nu_-, \tag{6}$$

or by means of the Brown Gabrielse invariance theorem [28]:

$$\nu_c^2 = \nu_+^2 + \nu_z^2 + \nu_-^2. \tag{7}$$

While Equation (6) is often used in on-line mass spectrometry experiments dealing with short-lived nuclei, the invariance theorem Equation (7) is used in ultrahigh precision measurements down to the sub-ppt level. In comparison to the sideband relation, the invariance theorem is robust with respect to typical first order trap imperfections as:

- a tilt of the magnetic axis of the trap with respect to the electrostatic potential, and
- slight ellipticities of the trapping potential.

All other systematic frequency shifts induced by trap imperfections such as a slightly inhomogeneous magnetic field or higher-order potential corrections have to be characterized by measurements [27].

3. Ingredients

All high-precision Penning trap experiments consist of similar basic ingredients. These are:

- a highly stable, very homogeneous superconducting magnet, with magnetic field strength B_0 in a typical range between 1 and 7 T;
- dc power supplies with high stability;
- a set of precisely machined trap electrodes of hyperbolic or cylindrical geometry with a typical inner diameter of 5–20 mm;
- Radiofrequency (RF) electronics; and
- in case of non-destructive detection, superconducting low-noise electronics.

Figure 3 shows two typical high-precision experiments, one in horizontal, the other one in vertical design. The central volume of a good magnet has a homogeneity on the order $B_1 < 10\,\mu\mathrm{T/m}$ and $B_2 < 100\,\mu\mathrm{T/m}^2$. Actively shielded devices show a temporal stability of $1/B \cdot \Delta B/\Delta t = 40\,\mathrm{ppt/h}$, the best magnet systems exceed these numbers by a factor of 10 [25]. Power supplies for the trap electrodes have fractional voltage stabilities on the order of 10^{-7}. The trap electrodes are typically machined out of oxygen-free high conductivity copper in some applications of silver [12]. To prevent oxidation, the electrodes, typically made with a machining precision $<$ $10\,\mu\mathrm{m}$, are gold-plated.

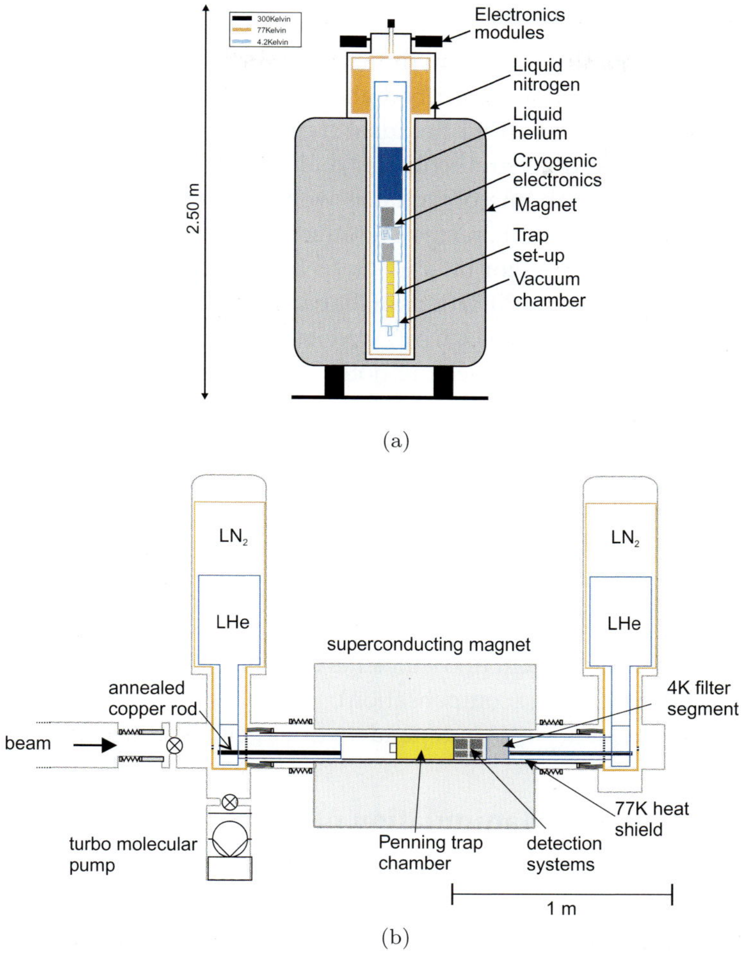

Fig. 3. (a) Penning trap experiment in vertical design (HCI experiment at University of Mainz [8]). (b) Penning trap experiment in horizontal design (BASE experiment at CERN [29]).

Most of the high-precision experiments are operated under cryogenic conditions. This reduces electronic noise and enables utilization of superconducting electronics, and thus, particle detection and cooling with high efficiency. In some applications, the trap system is mounted in a cryogenic vacuum chamber which is pumped, pinched-off and cooled to 4 K. In such trap-cans, pressures $< 10^{-17}$ mbar are achieved, which allows for particle storage times of years, even for antiprotons or highly-charged ions.

4. Trap Imperfections

All precision Penning trap experiments are designed in a way to meet the theoretical conditions described above, however, in each experimental assembly deviations from the ideal trap geometry are present. Leading order imperfections are octupolar and hexadecupolar modifications $C_4z^4 + C_6z^6$ of the trapping potential as well as a slightly inhomogeneous magnetic field. In addition, relativistic effects, frequency shifts induced by image charge- and detector interaction have to be considered [11, 18]. All imperfections lead to modifications of the oscillation frequencies ν_+, ν_-, and ν_z as a function of mode energies E_k. A detailed discussion of these effects is beyond the scope of this lecture-notes chapter, for further information we refer to [27].

A prominent trap design used in many high-precision Penning trap experiments is the so-called orthogonal, compensated cylindrical trap, which consists of five electrodes [30]. At given trap diameter the lengths of the ring electrode and two adjacent correction electrodes, as well as the voltage ratio $V_{\mathrm{CE}}/V_{\mathrm{R}}$, where V_{CE} is the voltage at the correction electrodes, are chosen in a way that:

- the higher order potential coefficients C_4 and C_6 vanish simultaneously for a certain $V_{\mathrm{CE}}/V_{\mathrm{R}}$ (compensation);
- the axial frequency ν_z is independent of $V_{\mathrm{CE}}/V_{\mathrm{R}}$ (orthogonality).

5. Detection and Manipulation of Charged Particles in High-Precision Penning Trap Experiments

All information about the trapped charged particles is obtained by various detection and excitation techniques. In this section, we describe the most prominent methods, time-of-flight detection as well as non-destructive image current detection. Furthermore, basic manipulation and measuring techniques are explained.

5.1. *Time-of-flight detection technique*

In precision Penning trap mass spectrometry with short-lived exotic ions, the time-of-flight–ion-cyclotron resonance (ToF–ICR) detection technique [31] is the method of choice to determine the ions' cyclotron frequency. To this end, the ions are first prepared at a well-defined radius of the magnetron motion, typically at 0.7–1.0 mm. By application of a resonant quadrupolar excitation of a properly chosen amplitude and excitation time

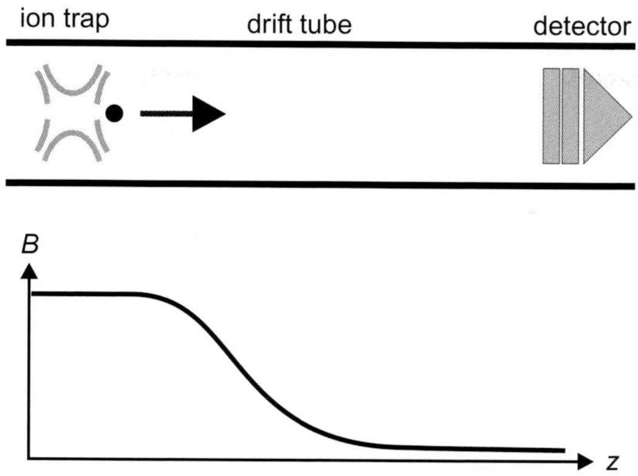

Fig. 4. Principle of the time-of-flight ion cyclotron resonance detection technique [31]. The upper panel shows the experimental configuration, the lower panel the magnetic field strength along the ion trajectory.

and with frequency ν_{RF}, the magnetron motion is completely converted into the (modified) cyclotron motion. After one full conversion, when the final cyclotron radius is identical to the initial magnetron radius, the ions are ejected from the trap and sent towards a particle detector (see Figure 4, top) by lowering the trapping potential of the downstream endcap electrode. Due to the radial energy and hence the associated radial magnetic moment the ions have in the trap, they experience an accelerating force while passing through the magnetic field gradient (see Figure 4, bottom) due to the gradient force. Thus, the velocity of the ions increases and those with highest radial energy have the shortest time of flight to the detector.

After each reloading of the trap with the same ion species, different quadrupolar excitation frequencies ν_{RF} are applied resulting in different degrees of conversion from magnetron to cyclotron motion and thus in different radial energies and magnetic moments. After ejection, the resonantly excited ions arrive earlier at the detector than those that have been excited non-resonantly. The start and stop signal for the measurement of the ions' time-of-flight from the trap to the detector are the ejection pulse to lower the voltage of the upper endcap electrode and the ions' arrival at the detector, respectively.

A variation of the quadrupolar excitation frequency ν_{RF} results in a characteristic time-of-flight ion cyclotron resonance curve, as shown in the left part of Figure 5. The solid line is a fit of the theoretically expected

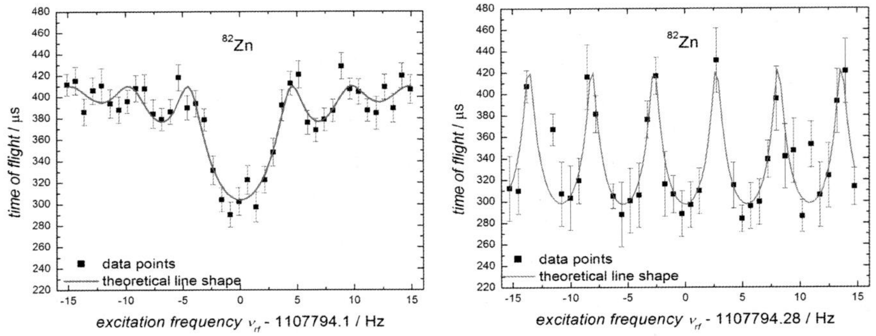

(a) (b)

Fig. 5. ToF–ICR resonance curves of the short-lived nuclide $^{82}Zn^{+}$ using the standard continuous (a) and the Ramsey-type (b) quadrupolar excitation technique. The solid lines are fits of the theoretically expected line shapes to the data (Ref. [32]). For the conventional ToF-ICR measurement a 200 ms RF-excitation time was chosen, for the Ramsey-type ToF-ICR resonance an excitation-waiting-excitation scheme of 20–160–20 ms was applied.

line shape and is mainly determined by the Fourier transformation of the rectangular time profile of the quadrupolar excitation [32]. The centroid of the resonance yields the searched for free cyclotron frequency ν_c of the stored ions. The width of the ToF–ICR $\Delta\nu$, and thus the resolving power $\nu/\Delta\nu$, is given by the Fourier limit $\Delta\nu = 1/T_{\rm RF}$ where $T_{\rm RF}$ is the duration of the quadrupolar excitation.

Instead of a continuous RF-excitation for the conversion from magnetron to cyclotron motion, a Ramsey-type excitation, i.e., time-separated oscillatory fields can be applied (see Figure 5(b)). Using Ramsey's method in Penning trap mass spectrometry a statistical uncertainty similar to that obtained by the conventional ToF-ICR technique can be achieved 10 times faster [33].

Most recently, a novel phase-imaging technique for cyclotron-frequency measurements, called PI-ICR, was developed [34]. It is based on the projection of the radial ion motion in a Penning trap onto a position-sensitive delay-line detector. Thus, in addition to the time of flight also the x–y-position of the ion hit on the detector can be measured and analyzed, allowing for the determination of the motional phases of the ion in the trap prior ejection. Compared to the conventional ToF–ICR technique, the PI-ICR method is 25-times faster and provides a 40-fold gain in resolving power. By using this technique, mass measurements with relative uncertainties of a few times 10^{-10} were performed [35].

5.2. *Non-destructive detection*

A charged particle oscillating in a Penning trap induces image currents $I_p = 2\pi \cdot (q/D) \cdot \nu_k x_k$ in the trap electrodes, where ν_k and x_k are the frequencies and coordinates of an individual mode $k = +, -, z$, respectively. The parameter D represents a trap specific length, typically between 5 mm to 50 mm. Although the induced currents I_p are only on the order of fA, detection by means of highly sensitive resonant pick-up systems is possible. To this end, an inductor L is connected to the trap. Together with the trap capacitance C_0, a parallel tuned circuit with resonance frequency $\nu_0 = (2\pi\sqrt{LC_0})^{-1}$ is formed. At resonance ν_0, the inductance L compensates the trap capacitance, and the circuit appears as an effective resistance $R_p = 2\pi\nu_0 QL$, where Q is the quality-factor of the tank circuit, which is a measure of energy loss per oscillation cycle. By using type II superconducting inductors, quality factors on the order of 10,000–100,000 can be achieved, leading at resonance frequencies of about 1 MHz and inductances of a few mH to effective parallel resistances of typically 10–100 MΩ. Once the particles' resonance frequency ν_k is tuned to resonance ν_0 with the detector, the fA currents are converted to voltage drops of several 10 nA, which are amplified by cryogenic ultralow noise amplifiers and processed with a fast Fourier transform (FFT) spectrum analyzer. Figure 6(a) shows the FFT spectrum of a single excited antiproton at resonance with the detection system. The sharp peak is the signal induced by the particle, the broad resonance is due to resistive Johnson noise $u_n = \sqrt{4k_B T \mathrm{Re}(Z(\nu))}$ of the detector's effective impedance

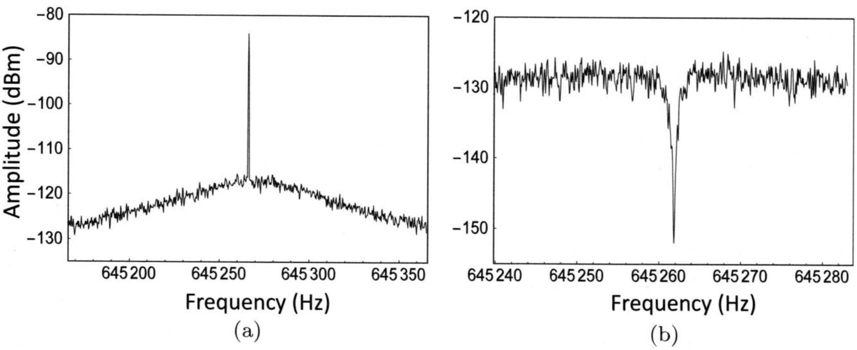

Fig. 6. (a) Peak detection: Single excited antiproton tuned to resonance with the image-current detection system. (b) Dip detection: Resistively cooled antiproton tuned to resonance with the detection system.

with $\mathrm{Re}(Z(\nu_0)) = R_p$. Here, k_B is the Boltzmann constant and T the temperature of the detection system.

The interaction with the resistor R_p cools the particle with mass m resistively with cooling time constant

$$\tau = \frac{m}{R_p}\frac{D^2}{q^2} . \tag{8}$$

Once cooled to thermal equilibrium with the detector, the particle acts as a serial tuned circuit which shorts at its resonance frequency ν_k all signals in parallel to ground. Consequently, a dip appears in the FFT-spectrum of the detectors transient noise, which is shown in Figure 6(b) [36]. A best fit of a resonance curve to such a spectrum allows extraction of ν_k in thermal equilibrium, typically at 4 K. At such low temperatures (corresponding to $E = 350\,\mu\mathrm{eV}$), systematic frequency shifts induced by trap anharmonicities are small. Thus, single particle frequency measurements by noise dip detection constitute a strong tool in high-precision experiments.

5.3. *Trap loading*

To load a Penning trap with ions, different methods can be applied depending on experimental constraints and applications. Many online Penning trap experiments are supplied by external ion sources or accelerators, and the particles are guided to the trap by means of magnetic or electrostatic transfer-lines. Antiproton experiments use in addition degrader-foils for the deceleration of MeV particles to keV energies which can be handled by the typical trap assemblies. In all these cases, trapping is achieved by adequate timing of high-voltage pulses applied to the trap electrodes.

Next, we describe loading of a trap-system which is enclosed in a sealed vacuum housing. First, a trapping potential is applied to the electrodes and an electron beam is turned on for several seconds to evaporate atoms from a target placed close to the trap. A fraction of these atoms is electron-impact ionized in the center of the trap and the created ions are stored. To analyze the trap content, a voltage ramp $V(t) = V_0 \pm \Delta V/\Delta t \cdot t$ where $t \in [0, \Delta t]$, is applied to the electrodes. Thus, different ion species at different m/q-ratios are tuned to resonance with the sensitive particle detection systems. Particles on resonance dissipate energy leading to a peak in the power-spectrum of an attached spectrum analyzer. Results of such a *mass-spectrum* are shown in Figure 7(a). The trap content shows the typical composition of frozen air. To reduce this ion-composition, e.g. to a pure cloud of trapped

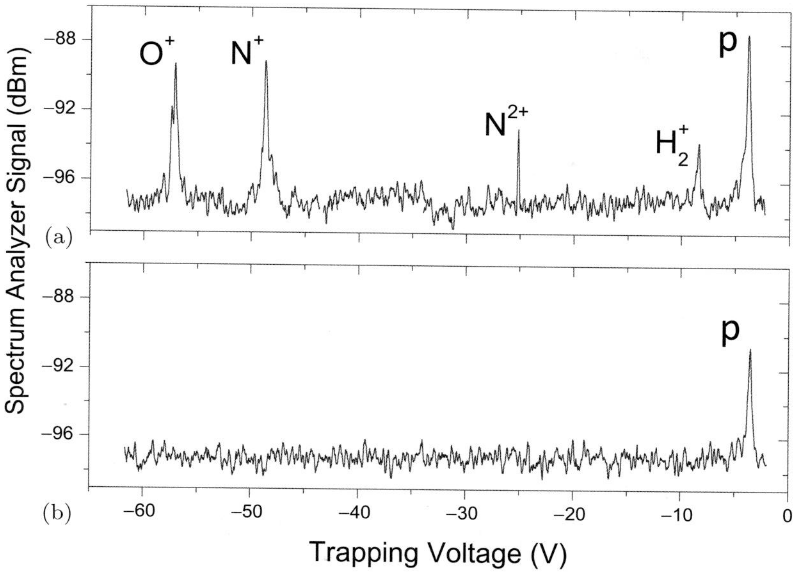

Fig. 7. (a) Trap content after particle loading. (b) Trap content after the trap-cleaning procedure described in the text. In this case all particles except of protons were removed from the trap.

protons, strong noise drives are applied to the trap while the protons are tuned to a notch filter. Subsequently, the trap potential is lowered to evaporate the heated contaminants. A mass spectrum recorded after such a cleaning procedure is shown in Figure 7(b), in this case it contains a pure proton-cloud.

5.4. *Sideband Coupling*

An important technique applied in numerous high-precision Penning trap experiments is *sideband coupling* [37]. The technique is used for measurements of the radial frequencies, mode cooling, temperature measurements and mode-temperature calibration, manipulation, and preparation. By applying RF-drives with frequency $\omega_{\rm RF}$ and a field amplitude E_0 to the trap electrodes, which couple the coordinates

$$\vec{E}\,(x_i, x_k) = \mathrm{Re}\left(E_0 \exp\left(i\omega_{\rm RF} t\right)\right)(x_i \vec{e}_k + x_k \vec{e}_i), \tag{9}$$

at the sum and the difference frequency $\omega_{\rm RF} = \omega_i \pm \omega_k$ of two modes described by the coordinates $x_{i,k}$ and frequencies $\omega_{i,k}$, energy can be transferred from one mode i into the other k. The system of differential equations describing the related dynamics is given by

$$\ddot{x}_i + \omega_i^2 x_i = \frac{qE_0}{m} \exp(i\omega_{\text{RF}} t)\, x_k, \tag{10}$$

$$\ddot{x}_k + \omega_k^2 x_k = \frac{qE_0}{m} \exp(i\omega_{\text{RF}} t)\, x_i. \tag{11}$$

Such systems are typically solved either by:

(1) a transformation to a system in which the dynamical matrix has only non-diagonal terms, or
(2) a transformation to a system in which the dynamical matrix is diagonal.

The two treatments focus on different aspects of the coupling. While in the non-diagonal form a "time-like" interpretation of the dynamics is given, the diagonal form is "energy-like" describing effective shifts of the mode energy levels due to the superimposed coupling field. By assuming that the field amplitude of the RF-drive is small compared to the field strengths of the trap, being valid for typical experimental conditions, the transformation

$$x_i \rightarrow \frac{X_i(t)}{\sqrt{\pi m \omega_i}} \exp(i\omega_i t), \tag{12}$$

$$x_k \rightarrow \frac{X_k(t)}{\sqrt{\pi m \omega_k}} \exp(i\omega_k t), \tag{13}$$

leads to a non-diagonal system matrix with vanishing trace and complex eigenvalues, which is the definition of an oscillator. The transfer rate is defined by the strength E_0 of the drive and can be expressed in terms of a "Rabi frequency"

$$\Omega_0 = \frac{qE_0}{2m\sqrt{\omega_i \omega_k}}. \tag{14}$$

This aspect is shown in Figure 8, where the magnetron mode was excited, a resonant sideband drive was applied for a certain coupling time, and the axial amplitude was measured. In the following, we concentrate on the coupling of the magnetron mode to the axial mode. Assume that the particle has initially zero axial amplitude and non-vanishing radial amplitude, and a resonant coupling drive $\omega_{\text{RF}} - (\omega_z + \omega_-) = \delta = 0$ is turned on. Due to the

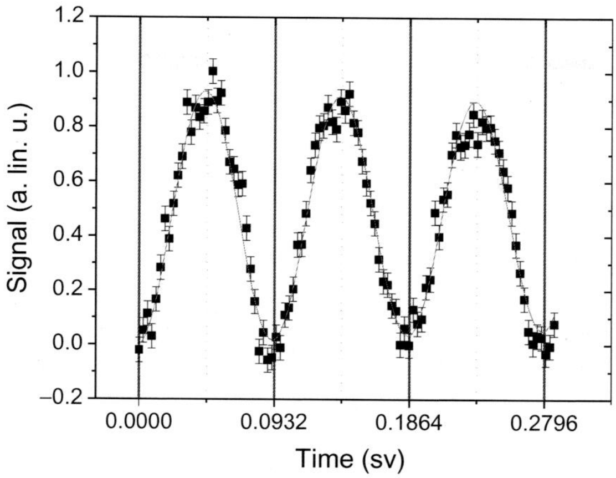

Fig. 8. "Classical" Rabi oscillations in a Penning trap. In this measurement the magnetron mode was excited, subsequently resonant sideband drives at variable coupling time t were applied and the axial amplitude was measured.

energy transfer, the mode trajectories can be rewritten as

$$z(t) = z_0 \sin\left(\frac{\Omega_0}{2}t\right) \sin(\omega_z t + \phi_z), \tag{15}$$

$$\rho_-(t) = \rho_{-,0} \cos\left(\frac{\Omega_0}{2}t\right) \sin(\omega_- t + \phi_-), \tag{16}$$

$\phi_{z,-}$ being arbitrary phases. The mode amplitudes z and ρ_- are modulated with the frequency $\Omega_0/2$. A frequency analysis of Equation (16) gives modified eigenfrequencies at $\omega_{l,r} = \omega_z \mp \Omega_0/2$. This is shown in Figure 9(a) for coupling of the magnetron mode to the axial mode by a coupling field with $\omega_{\mathrm{RF}} = \omega_z + \omega_-$. For resonant coupling $\omega_{\mathrm{RF}} - (\omega_z + \omega_-) = \delta = 0$ the separation of the two dips in the frequency spectrum is exactly the resonant Rabi frequency Ω_0. For non-resonant coupling $\delta \neq 0$ the system oscillates at the modified Rabi frequency $\Omega = \sqrt{\Omega_0^2 + \delta^2}$ and energy is not fully transferred between the modes. To investigate how non-resonant coupling affects the new eigenfrequencies ω_l and ω_r, the system is diagonalized by the assumption that the axial mode oscillates at $\omega = \omega_z + \epsilon$ and the magnetron mode at $\omega - \omega_p$, where $\omega_p = \delta + \epsilon + \omega_- - \omega$ [37]. By inserting this ansatz into the system, Equation (13), we find for the frequency values ω_l and ω_r of the

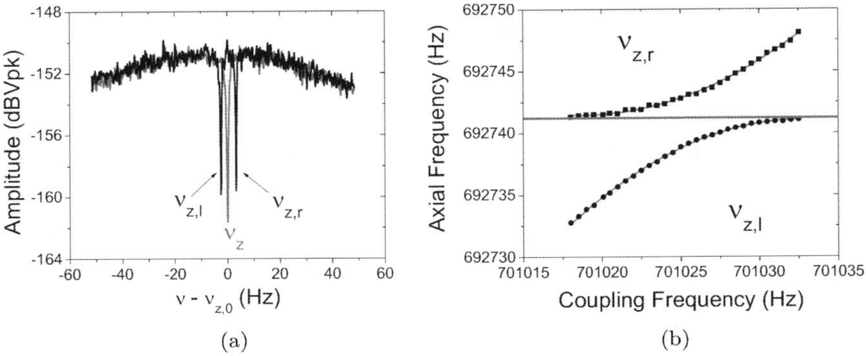

Fig. 9. (a) Single- and double-dip in the noise spectrum of the axial detector. The double-dip is due to an irradiated coupling drive with frequency $\nu_{\mathrm{RF}} \approx \nu_z + \nu_-$. Such a drive transfers energy between the axial and the magnetron mode, leading to an amplitude modulation with the Rabi frequency $\Omega/4\pi$ and consequently to frequencies $\nu_l = \nu_z - \Omega/4\pi$ and $\nu_r = \nu_z + \Omega/4\pi$ in the noise spectrum of the axial resonator. (b) "Classical avoided level crossing" recorded by a coupling of the magnetron mode to the axial mode. The frequency ν_{RF} of the coupling drive is tuned in steps over the resonance $\nu_z + \nu_-$ and the frequencies ν_l and ν_r of the respective dips are measured. For further details see text.

dips $\omega_{l,r} = \omega_z + \epsilon_{l,r}$, where

$$\epsilon_{l,r} = -\frac{1}{2}(\delta \pm \Omega) = -\frac{1}{2}\left(\delta \pm \sqrt{\Omega_0^2 + \delta^2}\right). \tag{17}$$

The result of a measurement where the coupling frequency was detuned from resonance is shown in Figure 9(b). The filled circles represent the measured frequency values of ν_r while the filled squares are the frequencies ν_r, being called a "classical avoided level crossing". By measuring ν_l, ν_r, and ν_z at known ν_{RF} and using the above equations, the radial frequencies can be extracted:

$$\nu_\pm = \nu_l + \nu_r - \nu_z \pm \nu_{\mathrm{RF}}. \tag{18}$$

5.5. *Particle Temperature*

In the thermodynamic limit, the radial mode is "thermalized". Once the particle is initially in a state (n_z, n_-), n_k being the quantum numbers of the respective harmonic oscillator $(z, -)$, and interacts with an RF-photon with energy $\hbar(\omega_z + \omega_-)$, transitions to states $(n_z + 1, n_- - 1)$ and $(n_z - 1, n_- + 1)$ are possible. The matrix element $(n_z, n_-) \rightarrow (n_z + 1, n_- - 1)$ "heats" the magnetron mode and scales with $(n_z + 1)n_-$ while the process

$(n_z, n_-) \rightarrow (n_z - 1, n_- + 1)$ "cools" the magnetron mode with proportionality $\propto n_z(n_- + 1)$. Thus, as long as $n_- > n_z$ the cooling transition dominates, until the equilibrium state characterized by equal quantum numbers of the modes $n_z = n_-$ is reached. For the limit temperature, the relation

$$T_- = \frac{\nu_-}{\nu_z} T_z \tag{19}$$

is found. In case of the modified cyclotron frequency ν_+, the equilibrium cyclotron temperature is

$$T_+ = \frac{\nu_+}{\nu_z} T_z \tag{20}$$

being a factor of ν_+/ν_z larger than the temperature achieved by direct resistive mode-cooling.

The thermal amplitude of the axial mode is about $20\,\mu\text{m/K}^{0.5} \cdot \sqrt{T_z}$, the magnetron as well as the cyclotron mode amplitudes are in the range of a few $\mu\text{m/K}^{0.5} \cdot \sqrt{T_z}$. For such tiny particle-amplitudes, the relative eigenfrequency-shifts are typically below the ppb level.

5.6. *Spin detection*

Measurements of magnetic g-factors in Penning traps provide sensitive tests of fundamental physics such as CPT invariance or bound state quantum electrodynamics, and allow the precise determination of fundamental constants. The determination of a g-factor reduces to a measurement of a frequency ratio

$$g = 2\frac{\nu_L}{\nu_c}, \tag{21}$$

where ν_L is the spin-precession frequency, also called Larmor frequency. In case of measurement of the electron g-factor bound to highly-charged ions (see below), Equation (21) has to be multiplied by a factor $m_e/M_{\text{ion}} \cdot Q/e$, where M_{ion} and Q are the mass and charge of the highly-charged ion and m_e and e the mass and charge of the electron, respectively. In comparison to the image current detection described above, the determination of ν_L constitutes a considerable challenge. Spin precession is not accompanied by a shift of charge, thus hampering the direct measurement of ν_L. An elegant solution to determine ν_L in Penning traps is provided by the continuous Stern–Gerlach effect [38], which is illustrated in Figure 10. In this scheme, a magnetic-bottle inhomogeneity $B(z) = B_0 + B_2 z^2$ is superimposed on the Penning trap by introducing a ferromagnetic electrode.

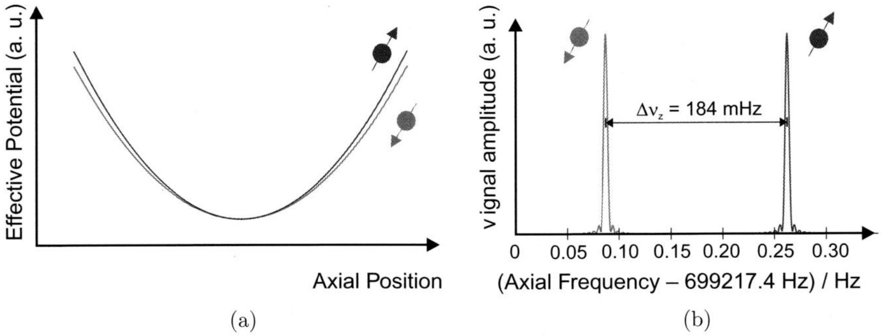

Fig. 10. Illustration of the continuous Stern–Gerlach effect. (a) Effective axial potential parabola for a "spin-up" antiproton (lower curve) and a "spin-down" antiproton (upper curve). (b) Representation of the left panel in frequency space.

Consider the energy E of a magnetic moment μ_z in such a magnetic field

$$E = -\mu_z \cdot (B_0 + B_2 z^2). \tag{22}$$

The magnetic bottle adds a spin dependent harmonic force $F = -\nabla(E) = 2\mu_z B_2 z$ to the electrostatic axial potential, and the axial frequency becomes a function of the spin state

$$\nu_z \approx \nu_{z,0}\left(1 \pm \frac{1}{4\pi^2}\frac{\mu_z B_2}{m\nu_{z,0}^2}\right). \tag{23}$$

Thus, in the presence of a magnetic bottle a measurement of the axial frequency allows for a quantum non-demolition detection of the particle's spin state. Note that the axial frequency shift scales are proportional to the strength B_2 of the magnetic bottle and the magnetic moment of the particle, as well as antiproportional to the particle's mass. Thus, compared to electrons, spin-flip measurements on e.g. protons are considerably more challenging since

$$\frac{\mu_p}{m_p}\frac{m_e}{\mu_e} \approx 10^{-6}. \tag{24}$$

Once non-destructive spin-flip detection is possible the Larmor frequency is determined by measuring the spin-flip probability as a function of the RF of an applied spin-flip drive. The result of such a measurement, carried out with a single proton [15], is shown in Figure 11. The resonance line is asymmetric due to particle-detector interaction. The contact of the particle with the thermal bath of the axial detector leads to a random walk of the

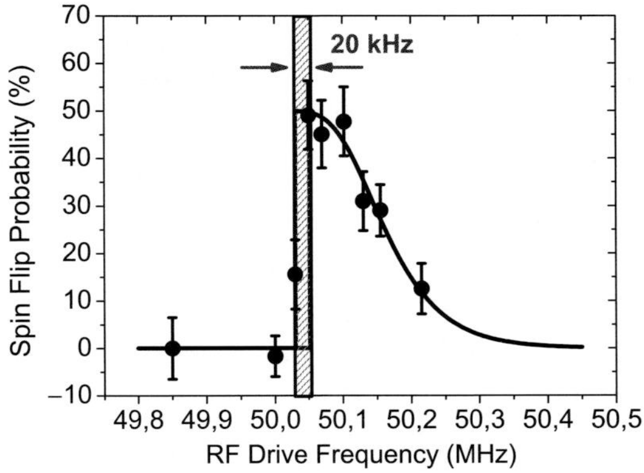

Fig. 11. Larmor resonance curve measured with a single trapped proton [15].

axial energy E_z. Thus, the resonance line is a convolution of the unperturbed spin-line and the thermal exponential distribution of the detector's thermal energy. The sharp cut-off corresponds to $E_z = 0$ and represents the Larmor frequency at vanishing axial energy.

5.7. *Phase sensitive measurements*

The precision of measurements of the modified cyclotron frequency ν_+ which are based on sideband methods, as described above, is limited by the stability of the trapping voltage. By measuring ν_+ directly, the influence of voltage variations during the sampling time of the axial oscillation can be dramatically reduced. To this end, phase sensitive measurement techniques as the pulse and phase (PNP) or the pulse and amplify (PNA) techniques have been developed. These methods rely on the fact that sideband pulses which transfer energy from one mode to the other are phase conserving. In the PNP measurement scheme [24], first the modified cyclotron mode is excited, after a certain waiting time a sideband pulse transfers the cyclotron energy to axial energy and the phase is read-out. Phase unwrapping is performed by repeating this scheme for different phase evolution times T_{evol}. By using this PNP technique, mass measurements at fractional precisions on the ppt level were demonstrated. An even more powerful tool is the so-called PNA method [9], which adapts the PNP scheme, however, the phase conserving pulse is driven by using the upper sideband $\nu_+ + \nu_z$. This transfers particle phase and simultaneously amplifies the axial signal. Thus, in the PNA scheme utilization of smaller cyclotron amplitudes is possible, making this method more robust with respect to trap errors. This method was applied very recently to measure the mass of the electron with a fractional precision of 30 ppt [11], further details are described in Section 6.2 of this chapter.

6. Fundamental Physics Studies

The techniques described above constitute the basic methods applied in high-precision Penning trap experiments to test fundamental symmetries. In the following sections, applications are described, such as high-precision tests of CPT invariance using leptons and baryons, tests of quantum electrodynamics with highly-charged ions, unitarity tests of the CKM matrix as well as neutrino-physics using short-lived radioactive ions.

6.1. *Tests of CPT invariance*

All relativistic quantum field theories involved in the Standard Model (SM) of particle physics are invariant with respect to CPT transformation, where C stands for charge conjugation, P for parity transformation and T for time reversal. Although it is the most fundamental cornerstone of the SM, high-precision tests of CPT invariance are rare. Comparisons of the fundamental properties of matter and antimatter equivalents, however, provide sensitive CPT tests. The masses of neutral K-mesons, for example, were compared at precisions of $\Delta m_K/m_K < 10^{-18}$, being one of the highest fractional uncertainties ever achieved in an experiment [39]. However, if e.g. a CPT violating cosmic background-field exists, its coupling will modify the SM Hamiltonian H_{SM} by introducing energy shifts ΔE to the system. Thus, fractional precision is not necessarily an appropriate measure to quantify the sensitivity of a CPT test [40]. With the mass of the neutral K-meson of $m_K = 497.6\,\mathrm{MeV}/c^2$, for example, the 10^{-18} measurement probes an energy scale on the order of 0.5 neV. Comparisons of electron/positron g-factors in Penning traps, on the other hand, compare particle/antiparticle anomaly frequencies ν_a of 160 MHz (0.66 μeV) with ppb precision [41] and probe thus energy scales at the level of 10^{-15} eV. Proton/antiproton mass comparisons at the level of 90 ppt were performed [2] probing even energy scales at 10^{-17} eV. Thus, high-precision Penning trap experiments comparing the fundamental properties of protons and antiprotons, or electrons and positrons, are an ideal tool to perform this type of test. For a detailed discussion of CPT and Lorentz tests in Penning traps, we refer to [42].

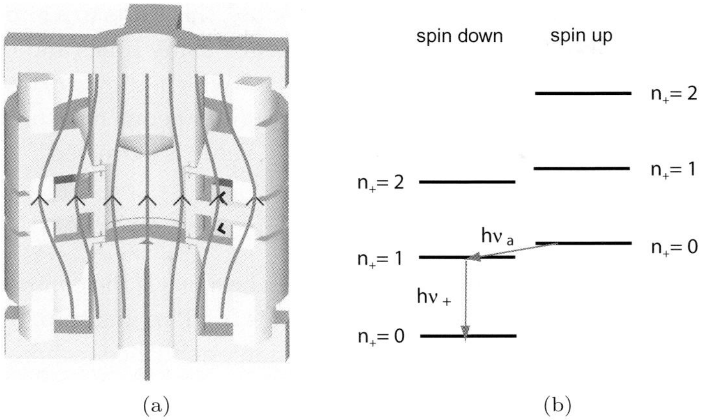

Fig. 12. Elements of the experiment to measure $g - 2$ of the electron. (a) Penning trap with superimposed magnetic bottle. (b) Level scheme of "spin down" and "spin up" states in the Penning trap to illustrate the measurement procedure used in the determination of the $g - 2$ value of the electron. For further details we refer to the text. Left Figure taken from [12].

6.1.1. *The magnetic moments of the electron and the positron*

The comparison of the $g - 2$ values of the electron and the positron constitutes the most precise test of CPT invariance in Penning traps. The dimensionless g-factor relates the magnetic moment

$$\mu_{e,\bar{e}} = g \cdot \frac{e_{e,\bar{e}}}{2m_{e,\bar{e}}} S \tag{25}$$

of the electron (positron) to the charge-to-mass ratio $(e_{e,\bar{e}})/(m_{e,\bar{e}})$ and the spin S of the particles. The measurement of the $g - 2$ value makes use of a measurement of the anomaly frequency (see Figure 12)

$$\nu_a = \frac{g-2}{2}\nu_c. \tag{26}$$

Here, we describe the experiment scheme developed to measure $g - 2$ of the electron [12] which is slightly more advanced than the original experiment [1]. Efforts are underway to apply this scheme as well to the positron. The experiment uses the continuous Stern–Gerlach effect, i.e. a magnetic bottle is superimposed on the trap, which is shown in Figure 12(a). The electron is prepared to the state $|0, 1/2\rangle$, as shown in Figure 12(b). Subsequently, the anomaly transition $|0, 1/2\rangle \rightarrow |1, -1/2\rangle$ is driven. Once successful, the particle cools to the ground state $|0, -1/2\rangle$ by means of cyclotron radiation. In the presence of the magnetic bottle, this leads to a jump of the axial frequency ν_z. By repeating this scheme for many times and different drive frequencies a resonance-line is obtained which allows extraction of the anomaly frequency ν_a. Together with a simultaneous measurement of the cyclotron frequency, eventually the $g-2$ value is extracted.

6.1.2. *Proton to Antiproton charge-to-mass ratio*

The most precise test of CPT symmetry with baryons is the comparison of the proton to antiproton charge-to-mass ratios in a Penning trap. By developing this experiment, the TRAP collaboration established techniques [45] to trap and cool MeV-antiprotons from the Low Energy Antiproton Ring (LEAR) at CERN, which are meanwhile used with great success in a wide variety of experiments dealing with low-energy antimatter. In the experiment, first, a proton is loaded into the trap and its cyclotron frequency $\nu_{c,p}$ is measured by direct non-destructive detection of the modified cyclotron frequency $\nu_{+,p}$ (see above). Together with a measurement of the axial frequency $\nu_{z,p}$ the cyclotron frequency $\nu_{c,p}$ is obtained. Subsequently, a single antiproton $\bar{p}$ is prepared and $\nu_{c,\bar{p}}$ is measured. The charge-to-mass ratio is obtained as

$$\frac{\nu_{c,p}}{\nu_{c,\bar{p}}} = \frac{(q/m)_p}{(q/m)_{\bar{p}}}. \tag{27}$$

In a sequence of experiments (see Figure 13), the precision was gradually increased from initially 50 ppb [46], measured with clouds of trapped particles, to 1.1 ppb, comparing single protons and antiprotons [47]. Here, the experimental precision was limited by polarity switching of the trapping voltage, which induces systematic errors. One of the most precise $p/\bar{p}$ charge-to-mass ratio comparisons has a fractional precision of 90 ppt [2]. It is based on the comparison of the cyclotron frequencies of a negative hydrogen ion H^- and an antiproton, which avoids polarity switching of the trapping voltage. Both particles were simultaneously trapped, one on a large orbit, the other one in the center of the trap, and alternate measurements of the respective cyclotron frequencies were carried out (see Figure 13(b)). Particle exchange was performed by resistive cooling and resonant excitations (see above). The antiproton to H^- charge-to-mass ratio is given as

$$R_{\mathrm{theo}} = \frac{m_{H^-}}{m_{\bar{p}}} = \frac{m_p}{m_{\bar{p}}}\left(1 + 2\frac{m_e}{m_p} + \frac{\alpha_{H^-}B^2}{m_p} - \frac{E_B}{m_p} - \frac{E_A}{m_p}\right), \tag{28}$$

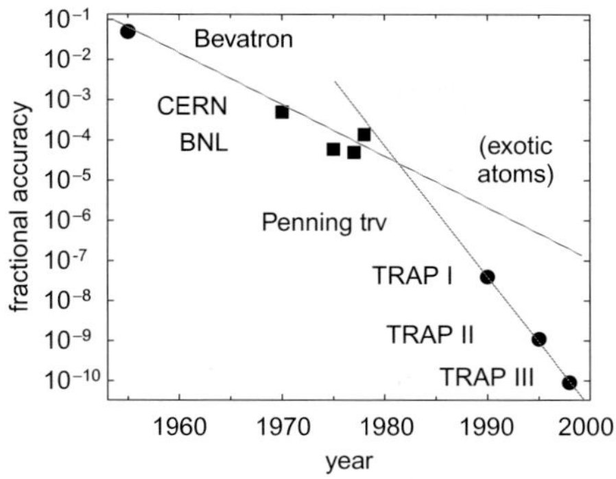

(a)

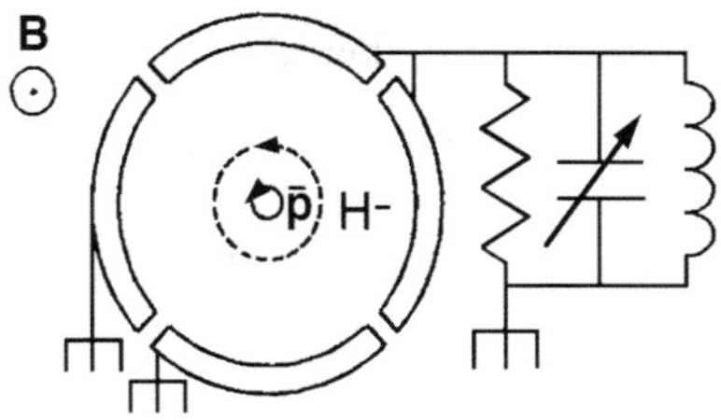

(b)

Fig. 13. Comparison of the proton-to-antiproton charge-to-mass ratios. (a) Achieved fractional precision as a function of time. Values up to 1980 are from accelerator and exotic atom experiments, the measurements afterwards are based on Penning trap spectroscopy. (b) Schematic of the most precise proton-to-antiproton charge-to-mass ratio comparison. The experiment was based on co-trapped antiproton/H^--ions. For details we refer to the text. Figures taken from [2].

with the electron-to-proton mass ratio m_e/m_p [11, 14], a polarizability shift $(\alpha_{H^-}B^2)/m_p$ [43, 44], binding energy E_B and the electron affinity E_A. The ratio R_{theo} is known with a precision on the ppt level, limited by the current knowledge of the proton mass [14]. Thus, at measuring precisions down to the ppt-level, the H^- ion serves as a perfect proxy for the proton, however, reducing systematic shifts.

By following the arguments of Holzscheiter and Hughes [48], this measurement can be interpreted as a test of the weak equivalence principle with antimatter. By assuming that CPT symmetry is exact, the particle and antiparticle cyclotron frequencies are, in the absence of a gravitational field, identical. However, if matter respects weak equivalence while antimatter experiences an anomalous coupling to the gravitational field, the cyclotron frequencies of the two particles will experience different gravitational red-shifts when moved to the surface of the earth. We assume that a gravitational anomaly acting on antimatter can be parameterized by α_g, which modifies the effective Newtonian gravitational potential U as $\alpha_g U$. This contributes a possible difference in the measured cyclotron frequencies

$$(\nu_{c,p} - \nu_{c,\bar{p}})/(\nu_{c,p}) = -3(\alpha_g - 1)U/c^2. \tag{29}$$

Thus, the above measurement sets an upper limit on $|\alpha_g - 1| < 10^{-6}$.

While this text-book was edited being the BASE collaboration at CERN reported on an antiproton-to-proton charge-to-mass ratio comparison with a fractional precision of 69 ppt. To date, this constitutes the most precise test of CPT invariance with baryons [3].

6.1.3. *The magnetic moments of the proton and the antiproton*

Among the numerous comparisons of different fundamental particle/antiparticle properties, one measurement has not yet been performed with high-precision: the comparison of the magnetic moments of the proton μ_p and the antiproton $\mu_{\bar{p}}$. Until 2014, the magnetic moment of the proton was known with a fractional accuracy of $8.6 \cdot 10^{-9}$. This value is based on hyperfine spectroscopy data of an atomic hydrogen maser in a magnetic field [49], from which the magnetic moment ratio of the proton and the electron bound in atomic hydrogen $\mu_{\mathrm{p}}(\mathrm{H})/\mu_{\mathrm{e}}(\mathrm{H})$ was extracted. The g-value of the free proton

$$g_{\mathrm{p}} = g_{\mathrm{e}} \cdot \frac{\mu_{\mathrm{p}}(\mathrm{H})}{\mu_{\mathrm{e}}(\mathrm{H})} \cdot \frac{g_{\mathrm{p}}}{g_{\mathrm{p}}(\mathrm{H})} \cdot \frac{g_{\mathrm{e}}(\mathrm{H})}{g_{\mathrm{e}}} \cdot \frac{m_{\mathrm{p}}}{m_{\mathrm{e}}} \tag{30}$$

is calculated, where the g-factor of the electron g_{e}, and the proton-to-electron mass ratio $m_{\mathrm{p}}/m_{\mathrm{e}}$ are known at a level of $2.8 \cdot 10^{-13}$ and $7.3 \cdot 10^{-10}$, respectively [11,12]. The theoretical corrections $g_{\mathrm{p}}/g_{\mathrm{p}}(\mathrm{H})$ and $g_{\mathrm{e}}(\mathrm{H})/g_{\mathrm{e}}$ are reviewed in [50] and are also known to the level $< 10^{-9}$, resulting in [51]

$$g_{\mathrm{p}} = 5.585\,694\,713\,(46), \tag{31}$$

limited by the experimental precision achieved in the hydrogen-maser experiment [49]. In contrast, the magnetic moment of the antiproton was, until 2013, only known with a fractional precision at the level of 0.1%, the values being based on exotic atom spectroscopy. A major step towards a direct high-precision measurement of the proton magnetic moment was achieved in 2011, when spin flips of a single trapped proton were detected for the first time [15] by using the methods described in Section 5.6. This led eventually to magnetic moment measurements at fractional precisions on the ppm level [52,53]. In 2013, the ATRAP collaboration at the antiproton decelerator of CERN applied these techniques to a single trapped antiproton and reported on a $4.4 \cdot 10^{-6}$ measurement [4].

The difficulty in proton/antiproton magnetic moment measurement is the tiny magnetic moment of the particle, which is 658 times smaller than that of the electron. Thus, to resolve (anti)proton spin transitions by means of the continuous Stern–Gerlach effect, large magnetic bottles are superimposed on the trap. Both collaborations use a bottle strength on the order of $B_2 = 300{,}000\,\text{T/m}^2$. This is a rather abstract number and means that once the particle is shifted by 1.5 mm from the center of the trap, the average magnetic field seen by the particle changes already by 1 T. Under these extreme magnetic conditions, a spin-flip shifts the axial frequency by 200 mHz, out of about 700 kHz axial frequency. The ppm measurements of the proton/antiproton magnetic moments were carried out in single Penning traps with the strong superimposed magnetic bottle. This broadens the width of the spin-line and ultimately limits experimental resolution to the achieved level.

An elegant solution to overcome this limitation is provided by the double Penning trap technique [54], which was developed at the University of Mainz in experiments to measure the magnetic moment of the electron bound to highly-charged ions (see Section 6.2). Here the spin-flip analysis and the high-precision frequency measurements are separated to two traps, an analysis trap (AT) for spin detection and a precision trap (PT) for precision frequency measurements. Such a double trap set-up is shown in Figure 14. The two traps are connected by transport electrodes. Voltage ramps applied to these electrodes are used to shuttle the particle between

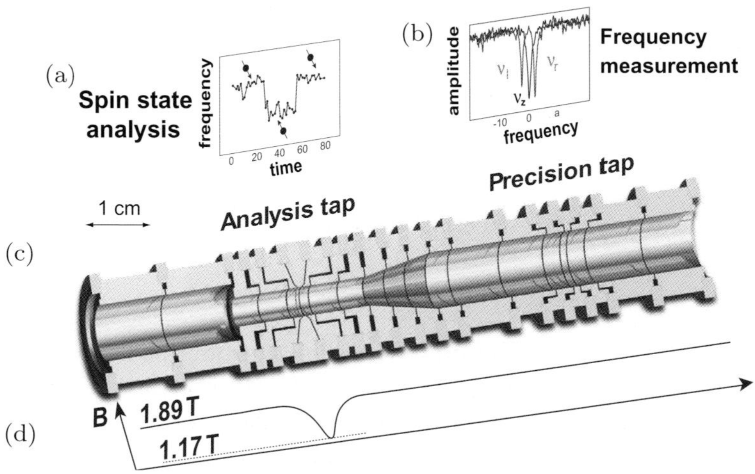

Fig. 14. Schematic of a double Penning trap set-up [15]. The system consists of two Penning traps, and AT and PT, which are connected by transport electrodes. The central ring electrode of the analysis trap is made out of ferromagnetic material. The distance between the trap centers is 45 mm. The lower graph shows the magnitude of the magnetic field along the z-axis. For further details see text.

the traps. A magnetic moment measurement starts with the determination of the spin state in the AT. Subsequently, the particle is transported to the PT, where the cyclotron frequency is measured, while a spin flip drive is injected to the trap. Afterwards, the particle is shuttled back to the AT and the spin state is analyzed again. The major difference to single trap experiments is that spin flips are driven in the PT, and thus, in a magnetic field which is about a factor of 100,000 more homogeneous than in the AT. This dramatically reduces the line-width and boosts experimental precision [18].

The first demonstration of the double Penning trap technique with a single proton was reported by the BASE collaboration which also applied the scheme to perform the first direct high-precision measurement of the magnetic moment of a single trapped proton [18]. In these measurements, the proton magnetic moment was obtained with a fractional precision of 3.3 ppb, representing the most precise measurement of μ_p to date. Currently, the BASE collaboration is working on the implementation to apply this technique to a single trapped antiproton. This will eventually provide one of the most stringent tests of CPT invariance in the baryon-sector.

6.2. *Tests of quantum electrodynamics with highly-charged ions*

The g-factor of the electron relates its magnetic moment μ, in units of the Bohr magneton μ_B, to its spin angular momentum s, in units of Planck's constant $\hbar$.

$$\frac{|\mu|}{\mu_B} = g\frac{|s|}{\hbar}. \tag{32}$$

In the Dirac theory, the g-factor of the free electron is

$$g_{\text{Dirac}} = 2. \tag{33}$$

The g-factor of the free electron differs slightly from this Dirac value due to the presence of the virtual radiation field. The g-factor of the free electron was measured by Van Dyck *et al.* to a relative uncertainty of $4 \cdot 10^{-12}$ in 1987 and by Gabrielse *et al.* to a relative uncertainty of $2.8 \cdot 10^{-13}$ in 2008 [12] (see also Section 6.1.1). The value obtained from calculations within the theory of quantum electrodynamics (QED) is in very good agreement with the experiment. Thus, investigations on the magnetic moment anomaly of the electron represent the most stringent test of QED for a free particle.

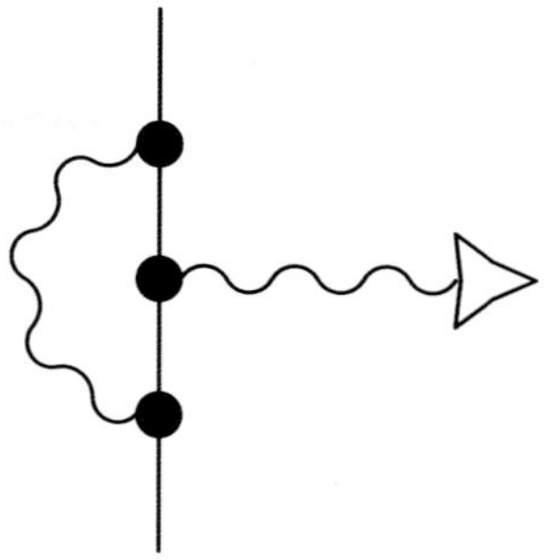

Fig. 15. Feynman diagram describing the QED contribution to the g-factor of the free electron of order α/π (Schwinger term). The straight line is the propagator of the free electron, the wavy line is the photon propagator, and the triangle denotes the magnetic field.

6.2.1. *Quantum electrodynamics of the free electron*

The first calculation of a radiative correction to the g-factor of the free electron was done by Schwinger [55]. The Schwinger term α/π describes the virtual emission and absorption of a photon by the electron, where $\alpha \approx 1/137$ is the fine structure constant. A Feynman diagram of this correction is shown in Figure 15. The higher-order QED terms account for the virtual emission and absorption of several photons and for the vacuum polarization, i.e. virtual particle–antiparticle pairs. Meanwhile, the radiative corrections have been calculated up to the fifth order in α [56].

$$g_{\text{free}} = 2 + C_1\left(\frac{\alpha}{\pi}\right) + C_2\left(\frac{\alpha}{\pi}\right)^2 + C_3\left(\frac{\alpha}{\pi}\right)^3 + C_4\left(\frac{\alpha}{\pi}\right)^4 + C_5\left(\frac{\alpha}{\pi}\right)^5 + 0\left(\frac{\alpha}{\pi}\right)^6. \tag{34}$$

The precision of the quantum electrodynamical calculations of the g-factor of the free electron is limited by our knowledge of the fine-structure constant α. In turn, the theoretical value for the g-factor of the free electron can be combined with the experimentally determined value to extract the fine-structure constant α with the highest precision up to date [12].

6.2.2. *Stringent tests of bound state QED*

The experimental and theoretical investigation of highly-charged ions provides unique tests of the theory of quantum electrodynamics in extremely strong electric and magnetic fields which are not accessible otherwise. For example, very precise measurements and calculations have been performed on the Lamb shift in hydrogen-like and lithium-like heavy ions and also on the hyperfine splitting (HFS) in highly-charged ions [57]. Another quantity suitable for testing QED in strong fields is the g-factor of the electron bound in a highly-charged ion [6–8, 58, 59].

The different contributions to the g-factor of the bound electron in hydrogen-like ions are the relativistic correction, radiative corrections (QED), and nuclear corrections.

6.2.3. *Bound-electron g-factor measurements on highly-charged ions*

Also, the g-factor measurements on highly charged ions [6–10] are performed in cryogenic Penning traps. The highly-charged ions are created by electron impact ionization of neutral atoms or molecules inside the trap. An electron beam with an energy of a few keV and a current of some nA is emitted from a tungsten field emission point close to the trap electrodes. Unwanted ion species are removed and single particles are prepared as described in Section 5.3. Once a single ion is prepared, the g-factor is measured by applying the double Penning trap method described in Section 6.1.3. The oscillation frequencies ν_+, ν_z and ν_- of the single trapped highly charged ion are measured non-destructively with the electronic detection method through the image currents induced in the trap electrodes by the particle motion (see Section 5.2). The quantum state of the hydrogen-like ion, i.e. the magnetic quantum number m_s of the bound electron in the $1s_{1/2}$ ground state, can be monitored non-destructively by the continuous Stern–Gerlach effect in the analysis trap in repeated measurements of the axial frequency of the trapped ion. The technique is similar as described in Section 5.6 for protons and antiprotons, however, the magnetic bottle strengths used in these experiments are typically about a factor of 30 smaller, which is possible due to the large electron magnetic moment which is on the level of the Bohr magneton. Transitions between the two spin states $m_s = \pm 1/2$ are induced by a microwave field (at typically 100 GHz) resonant with the Larmor precession frequency ω_L of the bound electron.

$$\hbar\omega_L = g\frac{e\hbar}{2m_e}B = g\mu_B B. \tag{35}$$

Here, g is the g-factor of the bound electron and $\mu_B = e\hbar/2m_e$ is the Bohr magneton. The spin-flip transitions are observed as discrete changes of the ion's axial frequency. The measured axial frequency shift for a transition between the two quantum levels amounts to a few 100 mHz out of $\approx$ 500 kHz. The observation of the continuous Stern–Gerlach effect on a hydrogen-like ion makes it possible to measure its electronic g-factor to high accuracy. Using the cyclotron frequency ω_c of the ion for the calibration of the magnetic field B, the g-factor of the bound electron can be expressed as the ratio of the Larmor precession frequency ω_L of the electron and the cyclotron frequency ω_c of the $^{12}C^{5+}$ ion.

$$g = 2 \cdot \frac{\omega_L}{\omega_c} \cdot \frac{Q/M_{\text{ion}}}{e/m_e}. \tag{36}$$

The ratio of charge-to-mass ratios of the hydrogen-like ion (Q/M) and of the electron (e/m_e) is an external input parameter in the determination of the bound-electron g-factor [60]. A resonance spectrum of the Larmor precession frequency ω_L of the bound electron is obtained in a similar way as in the proton–antiproton experiments described above. Our measurements of the bound-electron g-factor in hydrogen-like carbon $^{12}C^{5+}$ [6,11], oxygen $^{16}O^{7+}$ [7], and $^{28}Si^{13+}$ [7] are in excellent agreement with theoretical QED calculations. Together, experiment and theory test the bound-state QED contributions to the g-factor of the bound electron with high sensitivity. We also performed measurements of the g-factor of the bound electron in the 2s-state in lithium-like ions [10]. These investigations test the electron–electron correlation effects and reveal the direct influence of the negative-energy continuum within Dirac theory on atomic properties.

6.2.4. *Determination of the electron mass*

In the determination of the g-factor of the bound electron in highly charged ions, see Equation (36), the mass of the electron in relation to the mass of the atomic ion is used as an external input parameter. During the course of the years, the accuracy of the Penning trap experiments as well as the theoretical QED calculations of the bound-electron g-factor has steadily improved. At some point, both experiment and theory became more accurate than our knowledge of the electron mass [61]. Under these conditions, the experimental measurements of the Larmor and cyclotron frequencies in combination with the theoretical value of the bound-electron g-factor can be used to yield the electron mass in atomic mass units. Equation (36) is then modified such that the electron mass is determined from experiment and theory.

$$m_e = \frac{g}{2}\frac{e}{q}\frac{\omega_c}{\omega_L}M_{\text{ion}}. \tag{37}$$

Note that in this equation there is essentially no uncertainty in the atomic mass of the ion (except for the binding energies of the missing electrons), when the measurement is performed on hydrogen-like carbon $^{12}C^{5+}$, since the atomic mass unit is based on the neutral carbon atom ^{12}C. By recent g-factor measurements on carbon $^{12}C^{5+}$ together with QED theory, the atomic mass of the electron was determined with a fractional accuracy of $3 \cdot 10^{-11}$ [11], which is an improvement by about two orders of magnitude compared to the determination of the electron mass by direct cyclotron frequency measurements of the carbon ion and the electron [60].

The electron mass in atomic mass units is an important fundamental constant in physics and chemistry. The improved value of the electron mass, combined with the Rydberg constant [63], the atomic mass of rubidium [64] and an atom interferometric measurement of h/m_{Rb} [62], yields a value for the fine-structure constant α. By inserting this value into the Kinoshita theory [56] for the g-factor of the free electron, it is possible to test the SM through the Gabrielse experiment [12] on the g-factor of the electron.

6.3. *Fundamental tests with radioactive species*

Short-lived ions are ideal probes for fundamental studies of weak interaction and of the SM in general. High-precision mass measurements on radioactive ions provide key input data for, among others, a stringent test of the unitarity of the Cabibbo–Kobayashi–Maskawa (CKM) quark-mixing matrix and for nuclear astrophysics in order to gain information on the nucleo-synthesis paths. Precision nuclear masses are also of utmost importance for neutrino physics, e.g. for the search for resonant enhancement of neutrinoless double-electron capture. Many high-precision Penning trap mass spectrometers have contributed to this kind of research. The first of its type installed at a radioactive ion beam facility in 1986 is the ISOLTRAP experiment at ISOLDE/CERN, shown in Figure 16. In the following, two of the mentioned applications will be addressed in more detail.

6.3.1. *Nuclear masses and a test of the unitarity of the quark-mixing matrix*

Precision measurements of masses, half-lives and branching ratios of super-allowed β-emitters allow in combination with nuclear theory a precise determination of the first (V_{ud}) element of the CKM quark-mixing matrix, which relates the quark weak-interaction eigenstates to the quark mass eigenstates assuming three quark generations. Taking V_{us} and V_{ub} from the Particle Physics Data Group (PDG), a stringent top-row unitarity test of the CKM matrix can be performed [20]:

$$\sum_j |V_{uj}|^2 = |V_{ud}|^2 + |V_{us}|^2 + |V_{ub}|^2 = 1. \tag{38}$$

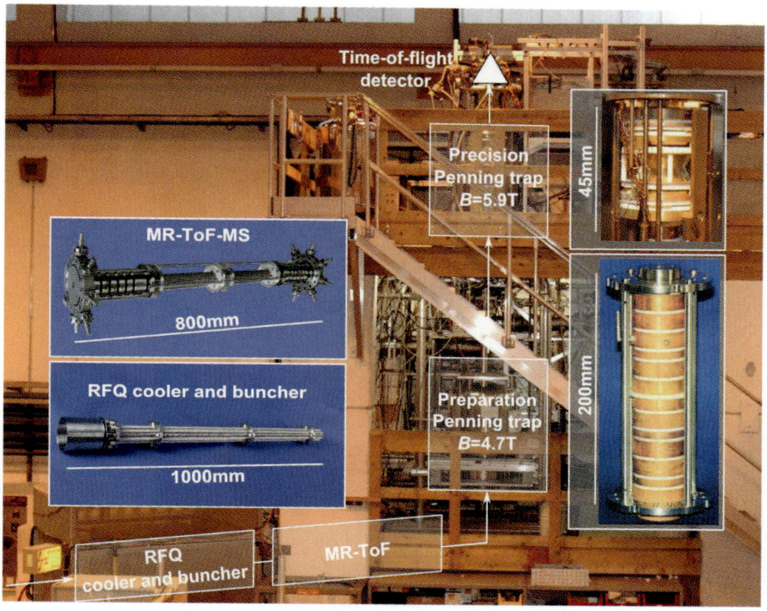

Fig. 16. Present set-up of the ISOLTRAP Penning trap mass spectrometer at ISOLDE for high-precision mass measurements on short-lived nuclides. The insets show the different trapping devices at ISOLTRAP.

Any deviation from 1 can be related to concepts beyond the SM such as the existence of an additional Z-boson or the existence of right-handed currents in the weak-interaction. V_{ud} can be determined from the fundamental vector coupling constant G_V and the well-known weak-interaction constant G_F of purely leptonic muon decay: $V_{ud} = G_V/G_F$, where G_V in turn can be derived from the corrected strengths (Ft-value) of superallowed β-transitions, which are a function of the experimental parameters: β-decay Q-value, half-life $T_{1/2}$, and branching ratio b, as well as of different correction terms including isospin-symmetry-breaking and radiative correction. The uncorrected ft-values can be derived purely from nuclear physics experiments, namely from mass, half-life and branching ratio measurements of superallowed β-transitions.

In the past years, tremendous effort has been put in by many online Penning trap mass spectrometers in order to measure the masses of almost all isotopes of interest for this kind of study with a relative mass uncertainty of 10^{-8} and below, despite the fact that many of these nuclides have minute production rates of only a few ten ions per second, see Figure 17. In combination with half-life and branching ratio measurements they provide

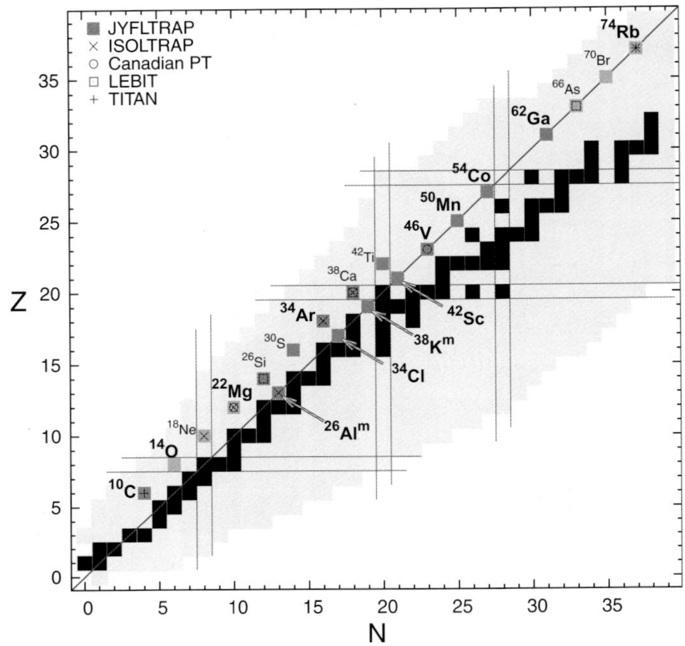

Fig. 17. Within this nuclear chart all superallowed-beta decaying nuclides that have so-far been studied by Penning trap mass spectrometry are given. The 13 nuclides named in bold are those contributing to the to-date best average Ft-value in order to test the conserved vector current hypothesis. All stable nuclides are indicated as dark boxes. Figure updated from Ref. [65].

the most accurate V_{ud} value to date of $|V_{ud}| = 0.974\,17(21)$ [21]. Taking V_{us} and V_{ub} from PDG, one obtains the result:

$$|V_{ud}|^2 + |V_{us}|^2 + |V_{ub}|^2 = 0.999\,78(55), \tag{39}$$

i.e. the unitarity is fully satisfied to a precision of 0.06%.

Another pillar of the SM is the conserved-vector-current (CVC) hypothesis, stating that the vector part of the weak interaction is not influenced by the strong interaction [21]. Thus, *Ft* should be constant for all super-allowed transitions. Taking all presently available data results in an amazing consistency at the 0.03% precision level [21].

6.3.2. *Nuclear masses for neutrino physics research*

Penning trap mass spectrometry can provide a significant contribution to neutrino physics. Since neutrinos are emitted in some nuclear decays, some of their properties can be determined by measuring the decay energies (Q-values) of these processes, i.e. mass differences of the decay mother and daughter nuclides.

The required uncertainty of the determination of the Q-values ranges from sub-eV to hundreds of eV depending on the neutrino property which is addressed in a particular experiment:

- The determination of the absolute neutrino mass requires the determination of the Q-values of certain β transitions with an uncertainty on the level of at most 1 eV.
- For the search for neutrinoless double-electron capture, it is sufficient to determine the Q-values on the level of approximately 100 eV. This is the typical scale of the values for the widths of the intermediate levels in neutrinoless double-electron capture, which govern the resonance enhancement of the process.
- In the search for heavy sterile neutrinos, the ratio of the capture probabilities from different electron orbits in electron capture is measured. This ratio contains the Q-value of the process, which must be determined with an uncertainty of better than a few 10 eV.

6.3.2.1. Electron neutrino mass

As neutrinos oscillate, i.e. change their flavor, they should be massive. To date, only the upper limit of about 2 eV for the absolute antineutrino mass has been obtained from the tritium β-decay [22,23], whereas for the neutrino mass the limit is stuck at the level of 225 eV from the measurements of ^{163}Ho inner bremsstrahlung spectrum [67]. At present, there are several experiments under construction with the goal to measure the electron (anti)neutrino mass with an uncertainty of well below 1 eV [68–71]. In these experiments the (anti)neutrino mass value will be determined by analyzing the atomic de-excitation spectrum of electron capture in ^{163}Ho or the electron energy spectrum of β-decay of tritium and ^{187}Re. Regardless of the decay, the analysis requires the knowledge of the Q-value of the decay under investigation at least on an eV level.

The most stringent limit on the antineutrino mass has been obtained in the Mainz/Troitsk experiments by investigating the end-point of the β-decay spectrum of tritium [22,23]. Here, a comparison of the Q-value determined from the fit with that measured independently by Penning traps is of importance in order to assess the level of the systematic effects in these very high-precision end-point experiments. So far, the most precise Q-value of

18.592.01(7) eV has been obtained with the FSU-trap at the Florida State University [24]. The next-generation KATRIN experiment requires in the long term a Penning trap measurement of the Q-value of tritium-decay with an uncertainty of at most 20 meV. This is the goal of the Penning trap mass spectrometer THe-trap [25].

The other experiments are being set-up to determine the (anti)neutrino mass from the analysis of electron capture in ^{163}Ho and β-decay of ^{187}Re. These experiments require independent Q-value measurements of the electron capture in ^{163}Ho and β-decay of ^{187}Re on an eV level. This task is planned to be accomplished in the near future by the novel Penning trap mass spectrometer PENTATRAP, which is being built at the Max-Planck Institute for Nuclear Physics [72].

6.3.2.2. Search for new candidates for absolute neutrino mass measurements

The most suitable decay process for the determination of the (anti)neutrino mass must have the smallest possible decay energy. In the β-decay sector, ^{3}H and ^{187}Re are the only relevant nuclides.

Meanwhile, in the orbital-electron-capture sector the variety of possibilities can be much bigger because the energy of the emitted monoenergetic neutrino depends on the difference $Q_\nu = Q_{EC} - B_i$, where B_i is the binding energy of the captured orbital electron (nuclear recoil energy is ignored). This difference can be very small for one of the electron orbits in the atom. This results in a very small neutrino energy and hence increases the contribution of the neutrino rest mass to the spectrum. Thus, the range of possible candidates is reduced to the electron-capture processes with $Q_{EC} \leq 100$ keV (see Figure 18).

As can be seen, some of the nuclides have a rather big Q_{EC}-uncertainty, which does not allow the assessment of their suitability to the neutrino-mass determination. Recently, a Q_{EC}-measurement campaign has been initiated at ISOLTRAP [73] and JYFLTRAP [74] to search for the most suitable electron-capture candidate for the determination of the neutrino mass. An uncertainty of few keV is sufficient, and thus, online Penning traps for radioactive nuclides are the best tool for this [19]. The first candidate addressed is the electron capture in ^{194}Hg, whose Q_{EC}-value has been determined with ISOLTRAP with an accuracy of few keV [73]. The obtained value of $Q_{EC} = 29(4)$ keV [73] strongly deviates from that of 69(14) keV [75] adopted before the ISOLTRAP-measurement.

It is worthwhile to note that finally the suitability of a certain low-energy decay candidate for determination of the neutrino mass is imposed

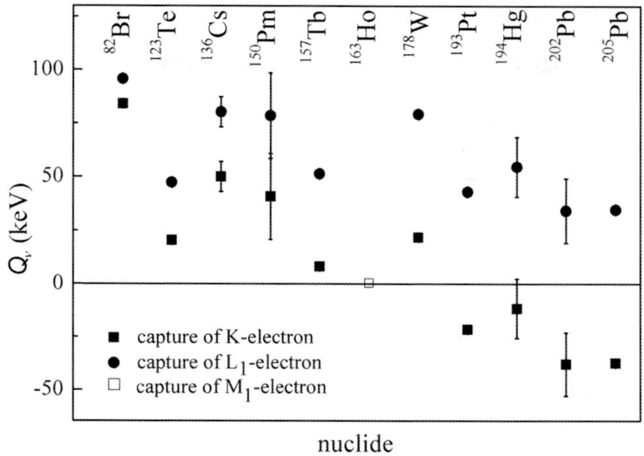

Fig. 18. (From [73]) Total energies of the neutrino $Q_\nu = Q_{EC} - B_i$ emitted in the capture of the K-shell electron (filled squares) and of the L-shell electron (filled circles) as expected for nuclides with $Q_{EC} \leq 100$ keV. B_i is the binding energy of the captured electron (i=K and L for nuclides in the figure). In ^{163}Ho the electron is captured from the M_1 atomic shell (empty square).

by the plannned microcalorimetric experiments. These will be used to measure the energy release from all atomic de-excitations following the emission of neutrino in the electron capture process.

6.3.2.3. Neutrinoless double-beta transitions

The fact of massiveness of neutrinos raises the question whether neutrinos and antineutrinos are different (Dirac) or identical (Majorana) particles. At present, the only practical way to unambiguously answer this question consists in the observation of the neutrinoless double-beta transformations: (1) double-β^- emission ($0\nu\beta^-\beta^-$), (2) double-positron emission ($0\nu\beta^+\beta^+$), (3) one electron capture with one-positron emission ($0\nu\epsilon\beta^+$), or (4) double-electron capture ($0\nu\epsilon\epsilon$). These neutrinoless transformations are possible only if neutrinos are Majorana particles that in turn implies a violation of the total-lepton-number conservation. Since these neutrinoless processes are not allowed in the SM, their observation will thus manifest new physics beyond this fundamental paradigm.

The most probable process among all neutrinoless transformations was thought to be neutrinoless double-β^- decay ($0\nu\beta^-\beta^-$) with an emission of two electrons. Over the last decades, about 20 large-scale projects [76] have been proposed to search for this phenomenon. In these experiments

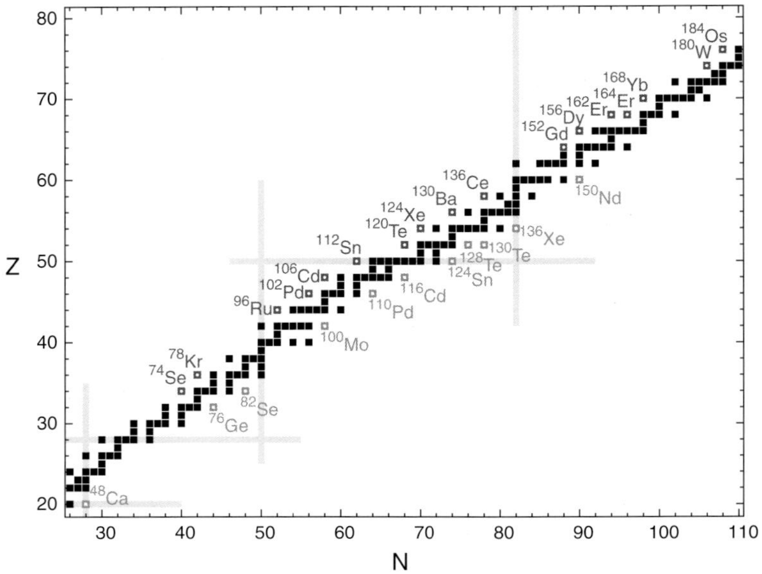

Fig. 19. Double-β decay (red) and double-electron capture (blue) nuclei that have been addressed by high-precision Penning trap mass spectrometry. Figure updated from Ref. [65].

[77], a monoenergetic peak is searched for in the sum-kinetic-energy spectrum of the two emitted electrons at the location which corresponds to the Q-value of the transition. Penning trap mass-spectrometry has provided these experiments with precise measurements of the Q-values of the used double-β^--decay transitions, see Figure 19. The complexity of these projects is conditioned by the required extraordinary sensitivity to neutrinoless double-β^- decay, whose rate is expected to be on the level of a few decay events/(ton yr) [78]. This demands a source/detector of a very large size placed underground as deeply as possible. Though there is still some room for improvements in sensitivity by current methods, a further breakthrough can be made only by invention of new alternative methods.

The inverse process, neutrinoless double-electron capture [79], can be considered such an alternative. This process was long kept in the shadow because of its expected smaller transition probability. But in some cases the probability of this process can be resonantly enhanced by many orders of magnitude and hence becomes comparable to that of neutrinoless double-beta decay. Although the possibility for a resonant enhancement of the process was already known long ago [80–82], the search for a resonantly enhanced transition was hampered by not having sufficiently precise knowledge of the $Q_{\epsilon\epsilon}$-values of possible candidate-transitions [83]. Tremendous progress in high-precision Penning trap mass spectrometry in the last decade [19] has provided a necessary base for the determination of atomic masses and mass differences with sufficient accuracy and thus stimulated an experimental campaign for a search for resonantly enhanced neutrinoless double-electron-capture transitions.

Five groups have contributed to the measurements of the Q-values of potentially resonantly enhanced transitions: SHIPTRAP, JYFLTRAP, TRIGATRAP, the FSU Penning trap, and LEBIT. Among the addressed transitions two have been found resonantly enhanced: (a) ^{152}Gd $\rightarrow$ ^{152}Sm and (b) ^{156}Dy $\rightarrow$ ^{156}Gd. In the latter transition, the possibility for the multi-resonance phenomenon has been discovered.

Figure 20 summarizes all double β-transitions, whose Q-values have been determined with high-precision Penning trap mass spectrometry.

6.3.2.4. Search for heavy sterile neutrinos

A possible existence of keV-sterile neutrinos, which would be good candidates for warm dark matter particles, is under discussion (see Ref. [84] and references therein). If the Q-value of a certain electron-capture process ranges from keVs to tens of keV, then the existence of keV-sterile neutrinos can be seen in the spectrum of emitted neutrinos as attenuation in the shape of the calorimetric spectrum [69] of the atomic de-excitation which accompanies the electron-capture. A merit of this attenuation can be the precise knowledge of Q-value, which gives information on the unperturbed spectrum, e.g. on the capture ratios from different atomic orbits which are expected without the sterile neutrino contribution. Our estimations show that if the contribution of sterile neutrinos in the mixing matrix is on the level of 10^{-3}, the uncertainty in the mass difference for the capture, e.g. in ^{123}Te should be better than 10 eV for the sterile neutrino mass of about 22 keV [85]. The higher the mass accuracy, the lower is the limit of the contribution which can be determined. A list of relevant candidates contains electron-capture transitions in ^{123}Te, ^{157}Tb, ^{163}Ho, ^{179}Ta, ^{193}Pt, ^{202}Pb, ^{205}Pb, and ^{235}Np [85]. Measurements of the Q-values with such a low uncertainty of the given electron-capture transitions required for the search for heavy sterile neutrinos will first become possible with the construction of the Penning trap mass spectrometer PENTATRAP [72].

7. Problems

Questions

(1) What is the minimum magnetic field required to balance the radial component of the applied electric field in a Penning trap?
(2) In high-precision mass spectrometry with ion traps only Penning traps are in use. Why?
(3) What is the mathematical reason for the side-bands in the destructive time-of-flight cyclotron resonance detection?
(4) In high-precision g-factor measurements, a frequency ratio is measured to cancel the magnetic field. What are the ultimate limitations in such Penning trap experiments?
(5) What are the amplitudes and typical quantum numbers of a particle at 4K with a certain q/m ratio which is trapped in a magnetic field of 5T, at an axial frequency of 1MHz?

Exercises

Continuous Stern–Gerlach Effect

Derive the shift of the axial frequency induced by a spin quantum jump in a magnetic bottle. Compare the spin quantum jump of different systems, e.g. an electron, a proton and an electron bound to a hydrogen-like ion. Why are proton magnetic moment measurements specifically difficult?

Hint: Derive the contribution of the magnetic potential to the axial potential and perform a series expansion. A solution can be found in Ulmer et al., Phys. Rev. Lett. ***106****, 253001 (2011).*

Sympathetic Coupling

Two charged particles are trapped close to each other and interact by Coulomb interaction. Assuming the particles are tuned to the same resonance frequency, what is the Rabi frequency for the energy exchange?

Hint: Consider two harmonic oscillators coupled by Coulomb interaction. Write down the Hamiltonian. Separate the Hamiltonian into a static and a dynamic part. You may consider to introduce Harmonic oscillator creation and annihilation operators to replace coordinates. The solution can be found in K.R. Brown et al., Nature ***471****, 169 (2011).*

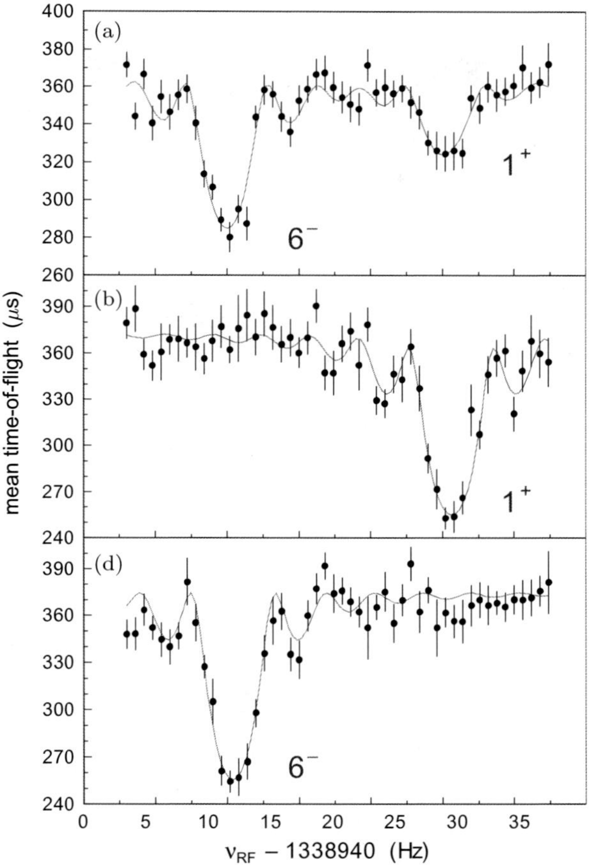

Fig. 20. Separation of ground state and isomeric state of ^{68}Cu measured at ISOLTRAP. (a) Mixture of both states; (b) and (c) isolated states.

Separation of Isomers

Figure 20 shows the separation of the ground and an isomeric state of ^{68}Cu, measured at ISOLTRAP.

(1) Which of the curves shown in (b) and (c) belong to the ground state and which to the excited state?
(2) What mass resolution was achieved?
(3) What quadrupole excitation time was chosen to achieve the observed line-width? (*Hint: The line-width reflects the excitation time.*)
(4) ^{85}Rb^{+} was chosen as reference ion for these measurements. The measured frequency ratio for the ground state is 0.800 000 818 (20) and

0.800 009 879 (19) for the isomeric state, respectively. Calculate the mass excesses $D = m - A \cdot u$ in keV.

(5) What is the excitation energy of the isomeric state?

(6) What would be the advantage of using highly charged ions (e.g. He-like ions) for these measurements under the same conditions, i.e. excitation time and isotope? (*Hint: How does relative precision scale with the charge-state?*)

References

1. R. Van Dyck Jr *et al.*, New high-precision comparison of electron and positron g factors, *Phys. Rev. Lett.* **59**, 26–29 (1987).
2. G. Gabrielse *et al.*, Precision mass spectroscopy of the antiproton and proton using simultaneously trapped particles, *Phys. Rev. Lett.* **82**, 3198–3201 (1999).
3. S. Ulmar *et al.*, High-precision comparison of the antiproton-to-proton charge-to-mass ratio, *Nature* **524**, 196 (2015).
4. J. DiSciacca *et al.*, One-particle measurement of the antiproton magnetic moment, *Phys. Rev. Lett.* **110**, 130801 (2013).
5. G. Lueders, Proof of the TCP theorem, *Ann. Phys.* **2**, 1 (1957).
6. H. Häffner *et al.*, High-accuracy measurement of the magnetic moment anomaly of the electron bound in hydrogenlike carbon, *Phys. Rev. Lett.* **85**, 5308 (2000).
7. J. Verdú *et al.*, Electronic g-factor of hydrogenlike oxygen $^{16}O^{7+}$, *Phys. Rev. Lett.* **92**, 093002 (2004).
8. S. Sturm *et al.*, g-factor of hydrogenlike $^{28}Si^{13+}$, *Phys. Rev. Lett.* **107**, 023002 (2011).
9. S. Sturm *et al.*, g-factor measurement of hydrogenlike $^{28}Si^{13+}$ as a challenge to QED calculations, *Phys. Rev. A* **87**, 030501(R) (2013).
10. A. Wagner *et al.*, g-factor of lithiumlike silicon $^{28}Si^{11+}$, *Phys. Rev. Lett.* **110**, 033003 (2013).
11. S. Sturm *et al.*, High-precision measurement of the atomic mass of the electron, *Nature* **506**, 467 (2014).
12. D. Hanneke *et al.*, New measurement of the electron magnetic moment and the fine structure constant, *Phys. Rev. Lett.* **100**, 120801 (2008).
13. S. Rainville *et al.*, A direct test of $E = mc^2$, *Nature* **438**, 1096 (2005).
14. R. S. Van Dyck Jr. *et al.*, High precision Penning trap mass spectroscopy and a new measurement of the protons atomic mass, *AIP Conf. Proc.* **457**, 101–110 (1999).
15. S. Ulmer *et al.*, Observation of spin flips with a single trapped proton, *Phys. Rev. Lett.* **106**, 253001 (2011).
16. S. Ulmer *et al.*, Direct measurement of the free cyclotron frequency of a single particle in a Penning trap, *Phys. Rev. Lett.* **107**, 103002 (2011).
17. A. Mooser *et al.*, Resolution of single spin flips with a single trapped proton, *Phys. Rev. Lett.* **110**, 140405 (2013).

18. A. Mooser *et al.*, High-precision measurement of the magnetic moment of the proton, *Nature* **509**, 596–599 (2014).
19. K. Blaum, High-accuracy mass spectrometry with stored ions, *Phys. Rep.* **425**(1), 1–78 (2006).
20. J. C. Hardy and I. S. Towner, CKM unitarity normalization tests, present and future, *Ann. Phys.* **525**(7), 443–451 (2013).
21. J. C. Hardy and I. S. Towner, Superallowed $0^+ \rightarrow 0^+$ nuclear β decays: 2014 critical survey, with precise results for V_{ud} and CKM unitarity, *Phys. Rev. C* **91**(2), 025501 (2015).
22. V. N. Aseev *et al.*, Upper limit on the electron antineutrino mass from the Troitsk experiment, *Phys. Rev. D* **84**(11), 112003 (2011).
23. Ch. Kraus *et al.*, Final results from phase II of the Mainz neutrino mass search in tritium β decay, *Eur. Phys. J. C* **40**(4), 447–468 (2005).
24. E. G. Myers *et al.*, Atomic Masses of Tritium and Helium-3, *Phys. Rev. Lett.* **114**(1), 013003 (2015).
25. S. Streubel *et al.*, Toward a more accurate Q value measurement of tritium: Status of THe-Trap, *Appl. Phys. B* **114**, 137–145 (2014).
26. H. Dehmelt, Experiments with an isolated subatomic particle at rest, *Rev. Mod. Phys.* **62**, 525 (1990).
27. L. S. Brown and G. Gabrielse, Geonium Theory: Physics of a single electron or ion in a Penning trap, *Rev. Mod. Phys.* **58**, 233 (1986).
28. L. S. Brown and G. Gabrielse, Precision spectroscopy of a charged particle in an imperfect Penning trap, *Phys. Rev. A* **25**, 2423–2426 (1982).
29. C. Smorra *et al.*, Towards a high-precision measurement of the antiproton magnetic moment, *Hyperfine Interact.* **221**, 38 (2014).
30. G. Gabrielse *et al.*, Open-endcap Penning traps for high precision experiments. *Int. J. Mass Spec.* **88**, 319–324 (1989).
31. G. Gräff *et al.*, A direct determination of the proton electron mass ratio, *Z. Phys. A* **297**(1), 35–39 (1980).
32. M. König *et al.*, Quadrupole excitation of stored ion motion at the true cyclotron frequency, *Int. J. Mass Spectr. Ion Process.* **142**, 95–116 (1995).
33. S. George *et al.*, Ramsey method of separated oscillatory fields for high-precision penning trap mass spectrometry, *Phys. Rev. Lett.* **98**(16), 162501 (2007).
34. S. Eliseev *et al.*, Phase-imaging ion-cyclotron-resonance measurements for short-lived nuclides, *Phys. Rev. Lett.* **110**(8), 082501 (2013).
35. D. A. Nesterenko *et al.*, Direct determination of the atomic mass difference of ^{187}Re and ^{187}Os for neutrino physics and cosmochronology, *Phys. Rev. C* **90**(4), 042501(R) (2014).
36. D. J. Wineland and H. G. Dehmelt, The stored ion calorimeter. *J. Appl. Phys.* **46**, 919 (1975).
37. E. A. Cornell *et al.*, Mode coupling in a Penning trap: π pulses and a classical avoided crossing, *Phys. Rev. A* **41**, 312 (1990).
38. H. Dehmelt and P. Ekström, Continuous Stern–Gerlach effect: Principle and idealized apparatus, *Bull. Am. Phys. Soc.* **18**, 72 (1973).
39. B. Schwingenheuer *et al.*, CPT tests in the neutral Kaon system, *Phys. Rev. Lett.* **74**, 4376–4379 (1995).

40. D. Colladay and V. A. Kostelecký, CPT violation and the standard model, *Phys. Rev. D* **55**, 6760–6774 (1997).
41. R. K. Mittleman *et al.*, Bound on CPT and Lorentz symmetry with a trapped electron, *Phys. Rev. Lett.* **83**, 2116–2119 (1999).
42. R. Bluhm *et al.*, CPT and Lorentz tests in Penning traps, *Phys. Rev. D* **57**, 3932–3943 (1998).
43. A. K. Bhatia and R. J. Drachmann, Polarizability of helium and the negative hydrogen ion, *J. Phys. B: At. Mol. Opl. Phys.* **27**, 1299–1302 (1994).
44. J. K. Thompson *et al.*, Cyclotron frequency shifts arising from polarization forces, *Nature* **430**, 58–61 (2004).
45. G. Gabrielse *et al.*, Cooling and slowing of trapped antiprotons below 100 meV, *Phys. Rev. Lett.* **63**, 1360 (1989).
46. G. Gabrielse *et al.*, First capture of antiprotons in a Penning trap: A kiloelectronvolt source, *Phys. Rev. Lett.* **57**, 2504 (1986).
47. G. Gabrielse *et al.*, Special relativity and the single antiproton: Fortyfold improved comparison of $\bar{\mathrm{p}}$ and p charge-to-mass ratios, *Phys. Rev. Lett.* **74**, 3544 (1995).
48. R. J. Hughes and M. H. Holzscheiter, Constraints on the gravitational properties of antiprotons and positrons from cyclotron-frequency measurements. *Phys. Rev. Lett.* **66**, 854–857 (1991).
49. P. F. Winkler *et al.*, Magnetic moment of the proton in Bohr Magnetons, *Phys. Rev. A* **5**, 83 (1972).
50. P. Mohr *et al.*, CODATA recommended values of the fundamental physical constants: 2008, *Rev. Mod. Phys.* **80**, 633 (2008).
51. S. G. Karshenboim and V. G. Ivanov, The g-factor of the proton, *Phys. Lett. B* **566**, 27 (2003).
52. C. C. Rodegheri *et al.*, An experiment for the high precision determination of the magnetic moment of the proton, *New J. Phys.* **14**, 063011 (2012).
53. J. DiSciacca and G. Gabrielse, Direct measurement of the proton magnetic moment, *Phys. Rev. Lett.* **108**, 153001 (2012).
54. H. Häffner *et al.*, Double Penning trap technique for precise g-factor determinations in highly charged ions, *Eur. Phys. J. D., At. Mol. Opt. Plas. Phys.* **22**, 163 (2003).
55. J. Schwinger, On Quantum-Electrodynamics and the Magnetic Moment of the Electron, *Phys. Rev.* **73**, 416 (1948).
56. T. Aoyama *et al.*, Tenth-order QED contribution to the electron $g2$ and an improved value of the fine structure constant, *Phys. Rev. Lett.* **109**, 111807 (2012).
57. V. M. Shabaev *et al.*, QED and nuclear effects in high-Z few-electron atoms, *Phys. Scr. T* **86**, 7 (2000).
58. W. Quint, The g_J Factor of Hydrogenic Ions, *Phys. Scr.* **T59**, 203 (1995).
59. T. Beier, The g_j factor of a bound electron and the hyperfine structure splitting in hydrogenlike ions, *Phys. Rep.* **339**, 79 (2000).
60. D. L. Farnham *et al.*, Determination of the Electrons Atomic Mass and the Proton/Electron Mass Ratio via Penning Trap Mass Spectroscopy, *Phys. Rev. Lett.* **75**, 3598 (1995).
61. T. Beier *et al.*, New determination of the electron's mass, *Phys. Rev. Lett.* **88**, 011603 (2002).

62. R. Bouchendira *et al.*, New Determination of the Fine Structure Constant and Test of the Quantum Electrodynamics, *Phys. Rev. Lett.* **106**, 080801 (2011).
63. P. J. Mohr *et al.*, CODATA recommended values of the fundamental physical constants:2012, *Rev. Mod. Phys.* **84**, 1527 (2012).
64. B. J. Mount *et al.*, Atomic masses of ^{6}Li,^{23} Na,^{39,41} K,^{85,87} Rb, and ^{133}Cs, *Phys. Rev. A* **82**, 042513 (2010).
65. K. Blaum *et al.*, Precision atomic physics techniques for nuclear physics with radioactive beams, *Phys. Scr.* T **152**, 014017 (2013).
66. E. G. Adelberger *et al.*, and the ISOLDE Collaboration, Positron–neutrino correlation in the $0^+ \rightarrow 0^+$ Decay of ^{32}Ar, *Phys. Rev. Lett.* **83**(7), 1299 (1999) and **83**(15), 3101 (1999).
67. P. T. Springer *et al.*, Measurement of the neutrino mass using the inner bremsstrahlung emitted in the electron-capture decay of ^{163}Ho, *Phys. Rev. A* **35**(2), 679 (1987).
68. G. Drexlin *et al.*, Current Direct neutrino mass experiments, *Adv. High Ener. Phys.* **2013**, 293986 (2013).
69. L. Gastaldo *et al.*, The electron capture ^{163}Ho experiment ECHo, *J. Low Temp. Phys.* **176**, 876–884 (2014).
70. B. Alpert *et al.*, HOLMES — The electron capture decay of ^{163}Ho to measure the electron neutrino mass with sub-eV sensitivity, *Eur. Phys. J. C* **75**, 112 (2015).
71. J. W. Engle *et al.*, Evaluation of ^{163}Ho production options for neutrino mass measurements with microcalorimeter detectors, *Nucl. Instr. Meth. B* **311**, 131–138 (2013).
72. J. Repp *et al.*, PENTATRAP: A novel cryogenic multi-Penning-trap experiment for high-precision mass measurements on highly charged ions, *Appl. Phys. B* **107**(4), 983–996 (2012).
73. S. Eliseev *et al.*, Direct mass measurements of ^{194}Hg and ^{194}Au: A new route to the neutrino mass determination?, *Phys. Lett. B* **693**(4), 426–429 (2010).
74. T. Eronen *et al.*, JYFLTRAP: A Penning trap for precision mass spectroscopy and isobaric purification, *Eur. Phys. J. A* **48**(4), 46 (2012).
75. G. Audi *et al.*, The Ame2003 atomic mass evaluation: (II). Tables, graphs and references, *Nucl. Phys. A* **729**(1), 337–676 (2003).
76. S. R. Elliott, Recent progress in double beta decay, *Mod. Phys. Lett. A* **27**(7), 1230009 (2012).
77. K. Zuber, Double beta decay experiments, *J. Phys. G: Nucl. Part. Phys.* **39**(12), 124009 (2012).
78. F. T. Avignone III *et al.*, Double beta decay, Majorana neutrinos, and neutrino mass, *Rev. Mod. Phys.* **80**(2), 481 (2008).
79. R. G. Winter, Double K capture and single K capture with positron emission, *Phys. Rev.* **100**(1), 142 (1955).
80. H. M. Georgi *et al.*, Unconventional model of neutrino masses, *Nucl. Phys. B* **193**(2), 297–316 (1981).
81. M. B. Voloshin *et al.*, Conversion of an atomic electron into a positron and double β^+ decay, *JETP Lett.* **35**(12), 656 (1982).
82. J. Bernabeu *et al.*, Neutrinoless double electron capture as a tool to measure the electron neutrino mass, *Nucl. Phys. B* **223**(1), 15–28 (1983).

83. V. I. Tretyak and Y. G. Zdesenko, Tables of double beta decay data — an update, *At. Data and Nucl. Data Tables* **80**(1), 83–116 (2002).
84. M. Lindner, Sterile neutrinos and dark matter, Presentation at the NOW-2012 workshop, September 9–16, Italy (2012).
85. P. E. Filianin *et al.*, On the keV sterile neutrino search in electron capture, *J. Phys. G: Nucl. Part. Phys.* **41**(9), 095004 (2014).

CHAPTER EIGHTEEN

TRAPPED-ION OPTICAL FREQUENCY STANDARDS

Piet O. Schmidt* and Ian D. Leroux

Physikalisch-Technische Bundesanstalt,
Bundesallee 100, 38116 Braunschweig, Germany and
Institut für Quantenoptik, Leibniz Universität Hannover,
Welfengarten 1, 30167 Hannover, Germany
**piet.schmidt@quantummetrology.de*

Optical frequency standards based on trapped atoms are the most accurate measurement devices we have available. They not only serve as superior time keepers but also lend themselves to a wide variety of applications ranging from tests of fundamental physics to the measurement of heights in relativistic geodesy. This chapter provides an introduction to the basics of optical frequency standards and clocks based on trapped ions and their applications.

1. Introduction

Clocks count periodic events provided by the regular oscillations of a frequency reference. Ideally, the oscillation frequency remains constant and does not depend on external perturbations such as ambient temperature, pressure, or humidity to provide a stable measurement of time. Historically, clocks were based on the rotation of the earth, the level of water or sand in periodically refilled containers, or the oscillating motion of a pendulum or a quartz crystal. Such (electro-)mechanical oscillators are prone to changes in their resonance frequency discrediting them for the most demanding time-keeping applications. A possible solution with many advantages was conceived by Maxwell in the 1870s and laid the foundation of modern atomic clocks: *"If, then, we wish to obtain standards of length, time, and mass which shall be absolutely permanent, we must seek them not in the dimensions, or the motion, or the mass of our planet, but in the wavelength, the period of vibration, and the absolute mass of these imperishable and unalterable and perfectly similar molecules."*

It is well known that the first successful attempt to establish an atomic clock was based on the 9.2 GHz hyperfine transition in neutral cesium atoms, implemented by Essen and Parry in 1955. The clockwork consisted of an atomic reference to which the frequency of an oscillator was stabilized through microwave spectroscopy. Counting the cycles of the oscillator turns such a frequency standard into a clock. These basic building blocks are shared by all atomic clocks. The two main benchmarks of clocks are (in)accuracy and (in)stability, typically given in fractional frequency units. While inaccuracy denotes the (estimated) deviation of the standard's frequency from the unperturbed transition frequency of an ideal standard, instability quantifies the statistical uncertainty of a frequency measurement after a certain integration time. The statistical uncertainty scales in the simplest case as the inverse of the square-root of the number of atoms and integration time. Cesium fountain clocks operated as primary standards currently achieve fractional frequency inaccuracies in the low 10^{-16} regime with a stability of 10^{-13} after 1 s integration time.

In a communication published directly after the report from Essen and Parry on the first cesium clock, Bullard from the National Physics Laboratory (NPL) raised the question of a redefinition of the second based on this atomic reference. His argument was that the atomic frequency standard provided much better accuracy and stability compared to Ephemeris Time, where the latter is derived from the rotation of the Earth on which the definition of the second was based at the time. Interestingly, 60 years later we face the same situation: optical frequency standards outperform cesium microwave clocks by more than an order of magnitude in accuracy and stability. As a result, the largest uncertainty in determining the frequency of the most advanced optical frequency standards lies in the realization of the unit Hz. It is very likely that the definition of the SI second will be redefined based on an optical transition in the foreseeable future [1,2].

Optical clocks are based on laser spectroscopy of narrow reference transitions between two metastable states. The challenge of counting the optical cycles was solved through the invention of the optical frequency comb by Hänsch and Hall around the turn of the century and will be discussed in Section 5. It marked the starting point of a remarkable development in optical frequency standards based either on a single reference ion in a Paul ion trap or thousands of neutral atoms trapped in an optical lattice. Both types of traps are based on oscillating electric fields exerting forces onto the contained atoms and thus leading to perturbations in their reference transition. For neutral atoms the frequency of the optical lattice can be chosen to be near the so-called "magic-wavelength" where the shift of both involved states is equal, resulting in a vanishing differential shift. However, the details of the light–atom interaction are involved and require the precise knowledge of many atomic parameters. For some ions, a similar "magic-frequency" operation of the trap allows cancelation of the electric field-induced shift, as detailed in Section 3. Owing to the large number of probe atoms, neutral atom lattice clocks provide superior stability, whereas trapped ion systems feature a relatively small number of systematic frequency shifts with small magnitude in selected systems. In the future, this may enable frequency standards with superior accuracy. Currently both types of optical frequency standards have achieved inaccuracies in the low 10^{-18} regime and instabilities at 1 s integration time ranging from few times 10^{-16}–10^{-15} for neutral atom and ion-based standards, respectively. Why have optical clocks superior stability and accuracy compared to microwave clocks? As we will see in Section 2, improved stability arises from an increase in the oscillation frequency by more than four orders of magnitude. The inaccuracy of a frequency standard is determined by estimating or measuring all conceivable effects modifying the measured transition frequency from its unperturbed value. Also here optical clocks win over microwave clocks in terms of fractional frequency uncertainty, since the magnitude of the shifts are similar in both cases. The evaluation of some shifts requires changing an experimental parameter and observing the resulting effect on the transition frequency at the 10^{-18} fractional frequency level. While this level of uncertainty would require averaging for hundreds of years in microwave clocks, it can be achieved within hours or days in optical frequency standards.

This chapter is intended as a textbook-like introduction into optical frequency standards based on trapped ions. However, many of the described concepts and applications are common to both types of clocks. Furthermore, the quest to isolate an atomic system from the environment is shared with quantum information processing and quantum simulations. The two fields have many aspects in common and provide mutual stimulation and progress. Several excellent recent reviews on optical clocks [3, 4] and textbooks [5, 6] on clocks in general can be consulted on the history of time keeping and timescales, more technical details of clocks and frequency measurements, and the current status of the field. We will closely follow the arguments and notation introduced in Ref. [4]. In Section 2, we will describe the basic measurement principles and how clock performance is quantified.

We will then discuss the three main components of atomic clocks. Section 3 addressed the choice of clock atom by discussing the dominant frequency shifts of the reference transition. The properties and requirements of the clock laser play an important role for the performance of the clock and will be discussed in Section 4. Techniques for counting optical cycles and transmitting and comparing optical frequencies will be discussed in Section 5. Section 6 provides a detailed description of the aluminium quantum logic optical clock. Selected applications of optical clocks and future trends will be the topics of Sections 7 and 8, respectively.

2. Basic Principles: Measuring the Transition Frequency

The aim of any atomic frequency standard is to produce a measurable signal at the unperturbed transition frequency between two states in an atomic system. "Unperturbed" means the ideal frequency that the transition would have if the atom were at rest, in vacuum and in the absence of any external fields or radiation. In these conditions, the transition frequency should depend only on atomic properties, which are presumed to be universal, and not on details of a particular experimental set-up. However, these conditions are never satisfied in real experiments. That would require keeping the atom and its surroundings at absolute zero and forbid the experimenter from interacting with the system. In building a frequency standard, the central task is then to minimize, understand and control the inevitable perturbations, so that the unperturbed transition frequency may be reconstructed.

To this end, most high-accuracy frequency standards since the Shortt double-pendulum clock [7] use two separate oscillators: a *reference* oscillator, which is as well-isolated as possible, and a *local* oscillator (commonly abbreviated LO), that continuously produces an observable signal. The role of the LO is to produce a strong, classical signal that can be measured without perturbing the reference, and — in the context of a clock — to produce this signal continuously, so as to keep track of time in the intervals when the reference oscillator is unavailable for observation. Since the LO is a macroscopic object interacting with the outside world, its frequency is subject to drifts and fluctuations which must be detected and corrected by regular comparisons to the frequency of the reference oscillator. A trapped-ion optical clock thus comprises the trapped ion (reference oscillator), a *clock laser* (LO) and a feedback controller that locks the laser frequency to the atomic

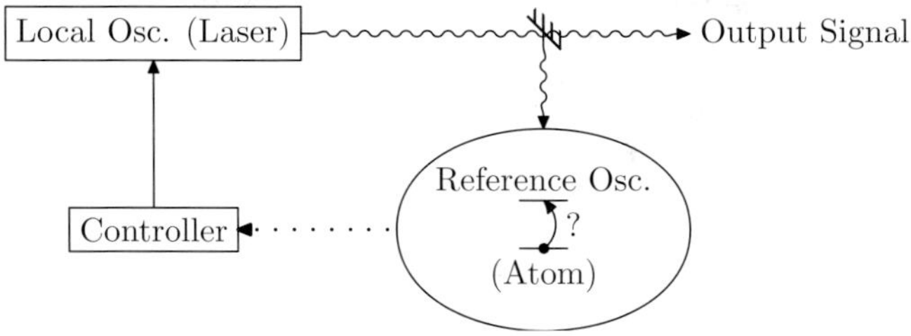

Fig. 1. Basic structure of modern frequency standard. An LO produces a strong periodic signal that serves as the standard's output. This signal is compared with the characteristic oscillation frequency of a well-isolated reference oscillator, in order to detect deviations of the output frequency from the target frequency (typically an atomic transition frequency). The detected deviations are used by a feedback controller to steer the LO back to the target frequency.

transition frequency, as illustrated schematically in Figure 1. The operation of such a clock follows a cycle, in which the ion is first prepared in a known initial state. The laser is then used to *interrogate* the ion by illuminating it with one or more pulses of light near the atomic transition frequency, after which the state of the ion (ground or excited) is measured. The feedback controller uses the measurement result to update its estimate of the laser frequency error. The laser frequency is adjusted and the cycle repeats.

The interrogation step generally uses either the Rabi or the Ramsey scheme. In Rabi spectroscopy, the interrogation consists of a single long pulse from the clock laser, whose intensity and duration are chosen so that it would, if the laser were on atomic resonance, reliably drive the reference atom from the ground state to the excited state. In the Bloch sphere picture (Figure 2), we say that the pulse parameters are chosen to drive a π pulse on atomic resonance. The laser is, however, deliberately detuned so that the excitation probability is only 50%, switching back and forth between the red and blue sides of the resonance. An error in the laser detuning can be detected as an imbalance in the excitation probability between the two cases. Ramsey spectroscopy, on the other hand, is carried out with two brief, intense pulses, each corresponding to a $\pi/2$ rotation on the clock transition, separated by a long interval of free evolution. If the laser is on atomic resonance, it will accumulate precisely the same phase in this free evolution period as does the ionic superposition state, and the two $\pi/2$ pulses will combine to form a π pulse and drive the ion to the excited state. If, however, the laser phase evolution differs from that of the ion, the second $\pi/2$ pulse will be about a different axis than the first and the ion will

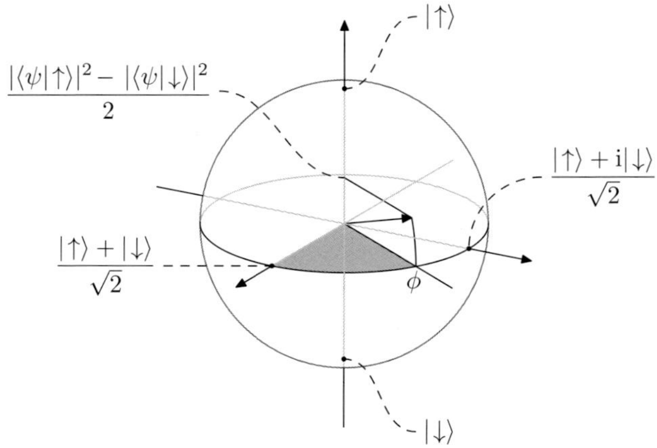

Fig. 2. Bloch sphere representation of a single two-level atom. The North and South poles of the sphere represent the two energy eigenstates of the atom $|\uparrow\rangle$ and $|\downarrow\rangle$, and all other points represent superpositions of these two. The vertical coordinate of a point represents the population difference between the two-levels, while the azimuthal angle represents the phase between them. Laser pulses at the atomic transition frequency drive rotations about an axis in the equatorial plane, with the orientation of that axis depending on the relative phase between laser and atom. For off-resonance laser pulses, the rotation axis lies outside the equatorial plane.

be incompletely excited. Again, the laser frequency error can be inferred by comparing excitation probabilities on either side of the resonance. Of the two schemes, Rabi interrogation is simpler to implement and, since it uses a single long laser pulse, is less sensitive to high-frequency laser noise. Ramsey spectroscopy is conceptually cleaner, since the ion evolution is unperturbed for most of the interrogation. In particular, Ramsey spectroscopy suffers much less than Rabi spectroscopy from light-shifts of the ion's transition frequency by the clock laser, an advantage that can be further enhanced by a three-pulse "hyper-Ramsey" interrogation sequence [8]. Ramsey interrogation also produces a narrower excitation fringe for a given interrogation time than does Rabi interrogation, allowing the detection and correction of smaller laser frequency errors.

In discussing the performance of a frequency standard, one must distinguish between two different concepts: instability and inaccuracy. Instability refers to observable fluctuations of the output frequency around its average value. To be observable, these fluctuations must have a correlation time substantially shorter than the total duration of a typical measurement campaign, so that their statistical properties can be estimated from several independent measurement intervals. From these observed properties one can derive a statistical or type-A uncertainty on the average frequency of the standard during the measurement campaign. Inaccuracy, on the other hand, refers to perturbations that change slowly or not at all during a measurement. They shift the average frequency of the standard but cannot be observed directly: even if two standards consistently produce the same frequency we can never be sure that they are both reproducing the unperturbed transition frequency. They might both be wrong by the same amount. Inaccuracy cannot be measured, it can only be estimated, based on our best understanding of the possible perturbations in a standard. This best understanding is reflected in a systematic or type-B uncertainty on the frequency of the standard. Note that the division between type-A and type-B uncertainties depends on the duration of the measurements and can in some cases be controversial. We reserve the terms instability, statistical and type-A uncertainty for fluctuations whose statistical properties can be directly extracted from data, and consign all those perturbations that can only be modeled to inaccuracy, systematic or type-B uncertainty.

Although it is less often discussed, it is sometimes useful to distinguish reproducibility, a third concept, from the related ideas of stability and accuracy. A reproducible standard is one whose average frequency stays the same from run to run, whether or not that frequency accurately reflects the unperturbed atomic transition frequency. Reproducibility thus distinguishes between perturbations that drift slowly and perturbations that are known not to drift at all. For instance, consider the perturbation of the atomic transition frequency by blackbody radiation. The size of the associated frequency shift could be uncertain because the temperature of the environment, and thus the intensity of the radiation, is imperfectly known. This would lead, at some level, to both inaccuracy and irreproducibility in the frequency of the standard, since the temperature could differ from measurement to measurement or from set-up to set-up. But the shift could also be uncertain because the atomic polarizability is unknown. In that case the standard would suffer from inaccuracy, since thermal radiation would shift its frequency away from the unperturbed transition frequency by an unknown amount, but its frequency would still be reproducible, since the atomic polarizability is presumably the same for all atoms of the same species in every experiment. Typically, we are interested in the accuracy of frequency standards, but for some practical applications it suffices that a frequency standard's output be stable and reproducible.

As the output frequency of the standard fluctuates, it is not a single uncertain parameter but rather a function of time, whose statistical properties depend on how and for how long it is observed. Discussions of clock instability therefore require a convention that specifies how the clock's frequency fluctuations are to be measured, and the most common convention is the Allan deviation, which is defined as follows. Consider a sequence $\{y_k\}$ of observations of some fluctuating quantity, such as the fractional frequency difference between two frequency standards being compared. Each observation y_k corresponds to the uniformly-weighted average of the quantity over a time interval $[k\tau, (k+1)\tau)$ of duration τ, where the intervals are contiguous but non-overlapping. Then the Allan deviation at time τ is

$$\sigma_y(\tau) = \sqrt{\frac{1}{2}\left\langle (y_{k+1} - y_k)^2 \right\rangle} \approx \sqrt{\frac{1}{2N}\sum_{k=0}^{N-1} (y_{k+1} - y_k)^2}. \tag{1}$$

In the second equality, we have shown how to estimate $\sigma_y(\tau)$ given a string of $N + 1$ observations. Given such a measurement record, we can combine groups of successive observations together to obtain averages over longer and longer time intervals. The resulting plots of σ versus τ show different characteristic scaling behaviors for different noise types [6]. For white (frequency) noise that is uncorrelated from observation to observation, $\sigma_y(\tau) \propto 1/\sqrt{\tau}$. In this case, the Allan deviation is just the standard deviation of the white-noise fluctuations. The instability of trapped-ion frequency standards typically show such $1/\sqrt{\tau}$ scaling at timescales of minutes to hours, when it is dominated by the noise of the ion state readout, which is uncorrelated from one interrogation of the ion to the next. The so-called flicker-frequency or $1/f$ noise leads to an Allan deviation σ_y that is independent of time. Clock lasers exhibit such a τ-independent "flicker floor" due to thermal fluctuations of the reference cavity to which they are locked. Certain types of environmental fluctuations can lead to random walk noise, with $\sigma_y \propto \sqrt{\tau}$, while a drift at a stable rate produces a linear increase in the Allan deviation $\sigma_y \propto \tau$. In the special case where the phase of an oscillator can be tracked continuously for a time τ, without missing any cycles, and is then measured with a τ-independent phase error, the resulting frequency instability scales as $\sigma_y \propto 1/\tau$. This is the scaling seen within a single interrogation of the ion, since the ion's phase evolves continuously within one interrogation. From interrogation to interrogation, however, the ion's phase evolution is interrupted and reinitialized, so that the clock must average independent frequency readings and the scaling returns to $\sigma_y(\tau) \propto 1/\sqrt{\tau}$.

In the absence of all technical noise, this interruption and reinitialization of the ion's phase evolution leads to a fundamental limit for the stability of a single-ion standard known as the quantum projection noise (QPN) limit

$$\sigma_y(\tau) = \frac{1}{\omega T}\sqrt{\frac{T_c}{\tau}}. \tag{2}$$

Examining this limit, we see that for a given atomic transition frequency ω and averaging time τ, clock stability can be improved by extending the interrogation time T. What limits this time? Ultimately, the excited-state lifetime imposes a fundamental limit on the interrogation time, and thus on the clock stability. In practise, however, the interrogation time must be kept shorter than the phase coherence time of the clock laser, to be sure that the laser frequency stays on the slope of the Rabi resonance or Ramsey fringe. With current laser technology, this requirement limits interrogation times to a few hundred milliseconds. As we will see in the next section, the ionic transitions used as references typically have much longer excited-state lifetimes, ranging from seconds to years, so it is generally the laser performance that sets the current practical limit to clock stability.

3. The Atomic Reference

3.1. *Candidates*

The ideal reference atom would have a narrow optical clock transition for high stability that is immune to electric and magnetic fields for high accuracy, a fast cycling transition for laser cooling and internal state detection, and it should be heavy to minimize relativistic shifts arising from the residual motion of the atom in the trap. Unfortunately, such an atom does not exist. Therefore, the choice of reference will always be a compromise between several aspects, which are weighted according to the application of the clock. An informed choice is also not possible in all cases, since many of the atomic parameters relevant to assessing the sensitivity to external perturbations may not be accurately known. This is the reason why many different clock species are being investigated in laboratories around the world. In this section, we will discuss the most relevant aspects for choosing an atom, with special emphasis on possible shifts of the atomic resonance. For many of the discussed shifts, the two clock levels will be shifted by different amounts. Relevant for the accuracy of the clock is only the differential shift between the two-levels, but not the magnitude of the individual level shift.

3.2. *Spectroscopy of trapped atoms*

There are several advantages to performing spectroscopy on trapped atoms in contrast to freely moving atoms. We have seen in Section 2 that the stability of a clock improves linearly with the inverse of the interrogation time (Equation (2)). In fountain or beam clocks, the practical size of the apparatus puts a limit to the longest achievable interrogation time. Ion traps with their hour- to month-long uninterrupted storage capability of single ions provide essentially lifetime- or coherence time limited interrogation capabilities. Another important systematic effect in beam standards is the linear Doppler effect given by $\Delta\nu_{\mathrm{Dop}} = kv_{\|}$ for atoms moving with a residual velocity $v_{\|}$ in the direction of the spectroscopy laser. It can amount to several MHz for typical Doppler cooling temperatures. In a trap the linear Doppler shift creates sidebands at the oscillation frequency ω_z of the ion in the trap. The unshifted carrier can be spectrally resolved from the sidebands if the transition line-width $\Gamma \ll \omega_z$, thus eliminating the linear Doppler shift from the ion's motion. However, slow drifts between the laser's reference frame and the trap, e.g. from thermal expansion, can result in significant linear Doppler shifts and have to be accounted for. This can be done by using techniques similar to the fiber length stabilization discussed in Section 5.

Energy and momentum conservation demand that absorption and emission of photons by an unbound atom is associated with photon recoil, resulting in an energy shift $E_{\mathrm{rec}} = \frac{\hbar^2 k^2}{2m} = \hbar\omega_{\mathrm{rec}}$ of the observed line, where $k = 2\pi/\lambda$ is the wavenumber of the light with wavelength λ and m is the mass of the atom. This shift is typically on the order of a few to 10s of kHz for optical transitions. For a trapped atom, this shift is strongly suppressed if the harmonic oscillation frequency of the ion in the trap ω_z is much larger than the recoil frequency ω_{rec}. In this case, the additional kinetic energy associated with the absorption or emission of photons is not sufficient to excite a quantum of motion of the ion in the trap. To formulate this criterion more rigorously, we have to consider photon absorption by a trapped ion in more detail. There are three energy scales in the problem: electronic transition line-width Γ, trap frequency ω_z, and recoil frequency ω_{rec}. The interaction strength is given by the product of two matrix elements. The first is the electronic transition matrix element, characterized by the Rabi frequency. In the absence of saturation effects it has a Lorentzian lineshape with width Γ as a function of laser–atom detuning. The second matrix element concerns a possible change in the motional state from state $|\psi_m\rangle$ to state $|\psi'_m\rangle$ and is given by

$$\langle \psi'_m | e^{ik\hat{z}} | \psi_m \rangle = \langle \psi'_m | e^{i\eta(\hat{a}+\hat{a}^\dagger)} | \psi_m \rangle. \tag{3}$$

In a simple picture, the spatial gradient of the laser's electric field along its propagation direction interacts with the motional wavepacket of the ion in the trap (characterized by its ground state size $z_0 = \sqrt{\hbar/2m\omega_z}$). The parameter describing the strength of the interaction is the so-called Lamb–Dicke parameter $\eta = kz_0 = \sqrt{\omega_{\text{rec}}/\omega_z}$. We can define an effective Lamb–Dicke factor taking into account the increase in size of e.g. a thermal motional state by defining $\tilde{\eta} = \sqrt{\langle \psi_m | k^2\hat{z}^2 | \psi_m \rangle}$. Expanding the exponential in Equation (3), we see that in the resolved sideband regime ($\Gamma < \omega_z$) the spectrum contains an unshifted carrier and sideband transitions involving changes in the motional state. If we have in addition $\tilde{\eta} < 1$, most of the transition strength is concentrated in the carrier and we can truncate the expansion after the linear term. This regime is called the Lamb–Dicke regime and is reminiscent of the Mößbauer effect in nuclear spectroscopy. Further details on the transitions involving changes in the motional and electronic levels can be found in Chapter 6 of this book.

3.3. *External field shifts*

In the following, we will discuss possible shifts of atomic levels by external electric and magnetic fields [9]. Orders of magnitude for the shifts will be given for typical ion clock representatives. Furthermore, cancelation schemes and mitigation strategies will be discussed.

3.3.1. *Magnetic field shifts*

Magnetic moments of the atom interact with an external magnetic field. The magnetic moments arise from three different sources: (i) orbital angular momentum of the electrons, (ii) electron spin, and (iii) nuclear spin. The first two result in strong magnetic field coupling characterized by Bohr's magneton $\mu_B = \frac{e\hbar}{2m_e} \approx 14\,\text{MHz/mT}/h$, whereas the nuclear magnetic moments are characterized by the much smaller nuclear magneton $\mu_N = \frac{e\hbar}{2m_p} \approx 7.6$ kHz/mT/h. The Hamiltonian for an external magnetic field $\vec{B} = B\hat{n}_B$ interacting with these moments can be written as

$$H_B = hA\vec{I} \cdot \vec{J} + g_J\mu_B\vec{J} \cdot \vec{B} + g_I\mu_N\vec{I} \cdot \vec{B}, \tag{4}$$

where A is the hyperfine interaction constant, and g_J and g_I are the electronic and nuclear g-factors. Depending on the electronic and nuclear properties of the atom, some of these terms may vanish. The energy level shifts can be quite complex to calculate, since they depend on the strength of the external magnetic field and the internal couplings. Relevant in the context of clocks is the *relative* shift between the two clock level. It can be approximated by a Taylor expansion:

$$f - f_0 = \Delta f_M = C_{M1}B + C_{M2}B^2 + C_{M3}B^3 + \cdots, \tag{5}$$

where it is sufficient to consider only the first two terms for the small magnetic fields of a few 100 μT usually applied to provide a quantization axis for laser cooling and optical pumping. The linear Zeeman effect shifts each level according to $gm\mu_m/h$, where g and m are Landé's g-factor and the magnetic quantum number, respectively. The values of g-factors have to be calculated or measured with high precision. Depending on the electronic structure, μ_m is either given by Bohr's magneton ($J \neq 0$, e.g. Ca^+, Sr^+) or the nuclear magneton ($J = 0$, e.g. Al^+, In^+). The linear Zeeman effect vanishes for a clock transition based on a $m = 0 \to m' = 0$ transition (e.g. $^{171}Yb^+$ and $^{199}Hg^+$). If such a transition is not available, one can create a "virtual" transition with the same feature by averaging two (or more) transitions with equal, but opposite shifts. However, one needs to ensure that the magnetic field does not change between probing the components of the virtual transition.

After eliminating the linear Zeeman effect the quadratic dependence on the magnetic field is the next largest contribution. For atoms with non-vanishing electronic angular momentum and hyperfine structure, it arises from the small coupling of the magnetic field to the nuclear spin. It mixes states with different F quantum number and can be treated in first-order perturbation theory. The associated additional shift is proportional to the difference between nuclear and electronic magnetic moments and inversely proportional to the energy difference between the mixed hyperfine states, characterized by the hyperfine constant A: $(g_J\mu_B - g_I\mu_N)B^2/hA$. The magnitude of the corresponding C_{M2} coefficient for the clock transition is on the order of a few to a few ten kHz/mT^2 for the Yb^+ E3 and the Yb^+ and Hg^+ E2 transitions, respectively. Its magnitude is reduced by three orders of magnitude for $J = 0$ clock states where only levels with a small linear Zeeman shift get mixed, as is the case for Al^+ and In^+. Shifts of similarly small magnitude are found in Ca^+ and Sr^+ that do not have hyperfine structure, but in which the magnetic field couples different fine-structure components, that are typically separated by several THz. To evaluate the quadratic Zeeman effect, a precise knowledge of the magnetic field is required. This can either be provided by a transition with large C_{M1} coefficient, or by evaluating the difference of two transitions with opposite magnetic field shift used to design the virtual transition free of the linear Zeeman effect. Since the magnetic field can drift on timescales much longer than a few clock interrogation cycles, usually an additional servo keeps track of its current value.

Fast harmonic oscillations of the magnetic field B around its nominal value B_0, e.g. arising from 50 or 60 Hz fields or currents from the Radiofrequency (RF) drive of the Paul trap will average to zero and therefore not cause a linear shift. However, the quadratic time-averaged shift $\Delta f_{M2} = C_{M2}\langle (B - B_0)^2 \rangle$ may be significant. For slow oscillations, the modulation index may be large enough to measure and calibrate the magnitude of this AC component of the magnetic field from sideband spectroscopy on a transition with a large C_{M2} coefficient. This may not be possible for the small magnetic fields induced at the large RF trap drive frequencies of typically 10 ... 100 MHz. In this case, the shift needs to be measured for different RF drive powers and extrapolated to zero. Oscillating magnetic fields coupling the clock states to other internal states can also significantly shift the transition frequency and need to be detected.

3.3.2. *Electric field shifts*

Static electric fields move the ion to a new equilibrium position, where the electrical forces on the ion vanish. This typically induces micromotion and corresponding micromotion-related shifts as discussed in Section 3.5. The two dominant electric field shifts arise from oscillating electric fields leading to a quadratic electric field interaction (ac-Stark effect) and coupling of electric field gradients to an electric quadrupole moment of the clock states.

Significant sources for an ac-Stark effect are from thermal blackbody radiation (BBR) of the trap and surrounding vacuum system and from laser interaction, either from the clock laser itself or a simultaneously applied cooling laser in the case of the Al^+ quantum logic clock. Both sources can be treated on an equal footing by treating the quadratic Stark effect as a small perturbation of the linear Zeeman effect. The energy shift of an atomic level $|\,\gamma J\,\rangle$ with $J \leq 1/2$ is given by

$$h\Delta f_S(\gamma, J, \vec{E}) = -\alpha_S(\gamma, J)\frac{\left|\vec{E}\right|^2}{2}. \tag{6}$$

The Stark effect consists of a scalar component characterized by the polarizability α_S. For levels with $J > 1/2$ and $F > 1/2$ an additional tensor component with dependence on F, m has to be considered. In general, the polarizabilities depend on the oscillation frequency of the electric field. While the corrections for BBR and other AC fields near DC are small, they can become substantial when caused by lasers that off-resonantly couple the clock states to other internal states.

The root mean square (rms) electric field associated with BBR at room temperature is given by $\langle E^2(T)\rangle = (831.9\,\mathrm{V/m})^2(\mathrm{T(K)}/300)^4$. Since all strong transitions in clock ions are far detuned from the peak in the BBR spectrum at a wavelength of $\lambda = 9.7\,\mu$m, we can use the static value for the differential scalar polarizability $\Delta\alpha_S$ between the two clock states and account for dynamic effects with a correction factor η. Assuming non-polarized BBR, the tensor shift vanishes. The BBR shift is then approximated by

$$h\Delta f_{\mathrm{BBR}} = -\frac{\Delta\alpha_S\langle E^2(T)\rangle}{2}(1+\eta). \tag{7}$$

As a consequence of the strong T^4 scaling, the BBR shift can be made small by operating at cryogenic temperatures. This approach has been implemented for the Hg^+ ion optical clock and comes with the technical complications of a cryogenic set-up. All other ion clocks are operated at room temperature. Uncertainties in the systematic frequency shift can arise from uncertainties in the knowledge of $\Delta\alpha_S$ or of the temperature. The temperature seen by the clock ion consists of radiation components emitted by different parts of the ion trap (see Chapter 2) and the vacuum system (see Chapter 5). The ion trap represents a challenge in this regard, since it contains different materials with different RF properties, electrical and heat conductivities, and emissivities. Typically the trap is modeled using finite element simulations, supported by direct temperature measurements using temperature sensors or thermal imaging cameras. The differential polarizability can either be calculated or measured by applying a far-detuned laser beam with well-calibrated intensity to the ion and measuring the resulting shift [70].

The same strategy is applied for determining the dynamic differential polarizability $\Delta\alpha_S(f)$ relevant for describing the differential level shift resulting from interaction with off-resonant laser light. In this case the rms electric field is given by $\langle E^2\rangle = I_L/c\epsilon_0$, where I_L is the laser intensity. The frequency shift induced by an off-resonant laser with detuning δ from a two-level resonance with line-width Γ is given by $\Delta f_L = (2\delta\Omega_R^2)/(4\delta^2+\Gamma^2)$, where Ω_R is the on-resonance Rabi frequency. While on resonance the shift vanishes for the clock transition itself, the clock laser can induce a significant shift by coupling one or both clock states to other levels via strong transitions. This is particularly problematic for transitions with a natural line-width much smaller than the realized excitation line-width, as is the case for the Yb^+ E3 transition with a line-width of 10^{-9} Hz. The shift can be extrapolated to zero by measuring the transition frequency for two different clock laser intensities. Further cancelation of this shift can be achieved by using the so-called hyper-Ramsey interrogation scheme [8] which is an extension of well-known spin echo schemes that have been developed in the context of nuclear magnetic resonance.

3.3.3. *Electric quadrupole shift*

Atomic states with total angular momentum $J > 1/2$ (or $F > 1/2$) deviate from spherical symmetry in their electronic charge distribution and thus support multipole moments that couple to external electric field gradients. The largest energy level shift is from the electric quadrupole interacting with a field gradient. Such gradients are intrinsic to the axial confinement in linear ion traps and become larger due to the presence of neighboring ions in multi-ion traps. Spherical ion traps are ideally free of electric field gradients, but typically exhibit spurious field gradients from patch charges on electrodes and other inhomogeneous fields, resulting in field gradients as strong as 1 V/mm^2, that will lead to a level shift on the order of 1 Hz for a quadrupole moment of ea_0^2. Most ion clock candidates suffer from this shift, except the group 13 (formerly group IIIA) clock ions, since they are based on the ${}^1S_0 \leftrightarrow {}^3P_0$ transition, which is free of this shift.

The Hamiltonian describing the interaction of an external field gradient with the atomic quadrupole moment is [9]

$$H_Q = \nabla E^{(2)}.\mathbf{\Theta}^{(2)}, \tag{8}$$

where $\nabla E^{(2)}$ is a symmetric traceless tensor of second rank describing the electric field gradient at the position of the ion and $\mathbf{\Theta}^{(2)}$ is the electric-quadrupole operator for the atom.

The quadrupole shift can be treated as a small perturbation of the Zeeman shifts in the basis of states $|\,\gamma J F m_F\,\rangle$. The resulting energy shift depends on the magnitude of the elctric field gradient, the magnitude and orientation of the quadrupole with respect to this gradient and an externally applied magnetic field, and the F, m_F quantum numbers. Quadrupole moments can either be calculated or measured. In linear ion traps, it is possible to relate the trap frequency to an electric field gradient that can then be used for a precision measurement of the quadrupole moment [10]. Alternatively, one can deliberately add a well-calibrated DC electric field gradient to a spherical trapping potential and measure the resulting shift [11]. However, unavoidable drifts in the electric field gradients require cancelation schemes for this shift, taking advantage of two symmetries of the quadrupole shift. One can show that the average of the transition frequency taken for three mutually perpendicular orientations of a magnetic field of the same magnitude is free of the quadrupole shift. This method has been used in frequency standards with $^{87}Sr^+$, $^{171}Yb^+$, and $^{199}Hg^+$ [12]. The level of suppression of the quadrupole shift using this technique can reach a factor of 100 if the uncertainties of the magnetic field directions are on the order of $\pm 1°$. The second symmetry in the quadrupole shift is in its m_F dependence. The quadrupole shift vanishes when averaged overall m_F sublevels. Since the same is true for the linear Zeeman effect, both shifts may be canceled simultaneously [13]. For large F values, averaging over a subset of m_F levels will be more efficient.

3.4. *Relativistic shifts*

Clocks are subject to special and general relativistic effects that need to be evaluated. Fundamentally, they arise from different frames of reference for the clock ion compared to the probe laser or other atomic clocks. The eigentime and thus the transition frequency depend on the velocity of the atom and the gravitational potential it is located in. While motion-induced shifts are typically an integral part of the estimated systematic uncertainty of a clock, the uncertainty in the gravitational potential the clock is operated in is usually only applied when comparing to other, distant clocks.

3.4.1. *Motion-induced shifts*

According to special relativity, an atom moving with velocity v relative to the lab frame observes a frequency f' that is related to the frequency f of the laser in lab frame by the following equation:

$$f' = f\gamma\left(1 - \frac{v_\parallel}{c}\right). \tag{9}$$

Here, $\gamma = 1/\sqrt{1-(v/c)^2}$ is the Lorentz contraction factor and $v_\parallel$ is the velocity of the atom along the direction of the probe laser beam. The probe laser frequency as observed by the atom is averaged over the timescale the servo needs to stabilize it to the resonance frequency f_0 of the atom $\langle f' \rangle = f_0$. The fractional frequency shift of the stabilized laser in the laboratory frame is then given by

$$\frac{\delta f}{f_0} = \frac{f - f_0}{f_0} = \frac{1}{\langle \gamma(1 - v_{\parallel}/c) \rangle} - 1. \tag{10}$$

This expression can be expanded in powers of $v/c \ll 1$ to give

$$\frac{f - f_0}{f_0} = \frac{\langle v_{\parallel} \rangle}{c} - \frac{\langle v^2 \rangle}{2c^2} + \frac{\langle v_{\parallel} \rangle^2}{c^2} + O(v/c)^3. \tag{11}$$

The first term in Equation (11) is the first-order Doppler shift. For trapped atoms performing a periodic oscillation, this term averages to zero. However, small drifts in the mean position of the ion with respect to the laser phase, e.g. induced by charge buildup, thermal expansion, directed collisions with electrons or background gas atoms, or length changes in the optical fiber delivering the laser light, can lead to residual shifts. For example, to reach $\delta f / f_0 < 10^{-17}$, we must ensure $\langle v_{\parallel} \rangle < 3$ nm/s. These effects can be measured and compensated using the Doppler cancelation schemes discussed in Section 5.

The next two terms in Equation (11) are so-called second-order Doppler or time dilation shifts. They arise since time for a moving observer advances slower compared to a non-moving reference frame. The term containing $\langle v_{\parallel} \rangle^2$ is usually neglected, since it is orders of magnitude smaller than the first term in Equation (11). For laser cooled atoms at the Doppler limit, the remaining term containing $\langle v^2 \rangle$ is usually much smaller than 10^{-17}. It is related to the total kinetic energy E_{kin} of the ion in the trap according to $\langle v^2 \rangle / 2c^2 = E_{\text{kin}} / mc^2$. However, it can be very difficult to quantify this energy, since one usually has to make assumptions about the velocity distribution of the ion. Heating of the ion during interrogation can increase the shift and lead to additional uncertainty, making this shift one of the largest contributions to the uncertainty budget, e.g. of the Al^+ and Yb^+ clocks. There are several ways of measuring the kinetic energy of the ion in the trap. The most commonly used technique to measure the energy in one specific motional mode is based on the energy dependence of sideband transitions Rabi frequencies (see also Chapter 6 in this book). It can be shown that for a thermal energy distribution

$$Q \equiv \frac{\rho^r_{\text{rsb}}}{\rho^r_{\text{bsb}}} = \left(\frac{\bar{n}}{1 + \bar{n}} \right), \tag{12}$$

where $\rho^r_{\text{rsb,bsb}}$ are excitation probabilities of the rth-order blue and red sidebands, respectively. Remarkably, this ratio is independent of excitation time. Rearranging Equation (12) provides the mean occupation of motional excitation for a single mode. Summing overall modes with frequencies ω_j, we get the total kinetic energy

$$E_{\text{kin}} \approx \left(\frac{1}{2} + \frac{1}{2}\right) \sum_j \hbar\omega_j \left(\bar{n}_j + \frac{1}{2}\right), \tag{13}$$

where the first 1/2 in the sum is from the fact that kinetic energy makes up only half the total energy in a harmonic oscillator, and the second $\approx$1/2 is from intrinsic micromotion of the ion in the trap. It will be discussed in more detail in Section 3.5. We note in passing that the zero point energy contributes to the second-order Doppler effect and can be on the order of 10^{-19} for typical trap frequencies of a few MHz and light ion species, such as Al^+.

3.4.2. *Gravitational red shift*

According to general relativity and the equivalence principle, a clock ticks slower in a gravitational potential compared to an identical clock outside of it. The corresponding fractional frequency difference between the clocks is given by $\frac{\Delta f}{f} = -\frac{\Delta U}{c^2}$, where $\Delta U = U_1 - U_2$ is the gravitational potential difference between the positions of the clocks and $\Delta f = f_1 - f_2$ their frequency difference. On earth, the gradient of the gravitational potential results in a fractional frequency change $\Delta f/f_0 = g\Delta h/c^2$ where g is the local acceleration of gravity amounting to approximately 10^{-16} per meter height difference for clocks at rest. While heights within the same laboratory or between buildings within sight of each other may be determined to sub-mm precision, geodetic height models are required to compare distant clocks. This correction is regularly applied when comparing microwave standards via satellites or the time service provided by global navigation satellite systems (GNSS). Eventually, the insufficient knowledge about height differences between laboratories will limit the comparison of optical clocks, for some locations, such as Boulder, Colorado (USA) possibly already at a level of 3×10^{-17} [14]. However, the sensitivity of clocks to height differences may be turned into a feature in relativistic geodesy as discussed in Section 7.1.

3.5. *Shifts from micromotion*

Micromotion is a fundamental property of RF ion traps (see Chapter 2). It is a driven motion at the trap RF drive frequency Ω_{RF} on top of the slower harmonic motion (so-called secular motion) with frequency ω_j of the ion around its equilibrium position. We distinguish between excess micromotion which in principle can be nulled, and intrinsic micromotion for which this is not the case, since it is a property of the trapping concept. Both forms of micromotion contribute to the kinetic energy of the second-order Doppler effect and the ac-Stark shift arising from the differential polarizability of the clock states [15]. The classical trajectory of an ion for small micromotion amplitudes ($q_j < 1$) is given by [15]

$$u_j(t) = \left[u_{j0} + u_{j1}\cos(\omega_j t + \phi_j)\right]\left(1 + \frac{q_j}{2}\cos(\Omega_{\mathrm{RF}}t)\right), \tag{14}$$

where u_{j0} and u_{j1} are the offset from the equilibrium position and the secular motional amplitude of the considered mode j, respectively. For a trap with no DC fields along the direction of mode j (such as the radial modes in linear Paul traps), the q-parameter is given by $q_j = 2\sqrt{2}\omega_j/\Omega_{\mathrm{RF}}$. Stable trapping usually requires $q < 1$, therefore the micromotion amplitude is a small fraction of the slower secular motion. The displacement u_{j0} causes excess micromotion and can arise e.g. from stray electric fields E_{dc} and may change with time. Another source of micromotion neglected here is from a phase difference between RF electrodes that should nominally be at the same phase [15]. Usually this effect can be minimized by a careful design of the trap, its wiring, and RF drive. In the absence of excess micromotion, the intrinsic micromotion contribution doubles the second-order Doppler contribution from thermal motion. Excess micromotion adds an additional kinetic energy of

$$E_{\mathrm{kin}} = \frac{1}{m}\left(\frac{Q}{2\Omega_{\mathrm{RF}}}\right)^2 \langle E_{\mathrm{RF}}^2\rangle, \tag{15}$$

where Q is the charge of the ion and $\langle E_{\mathrm{RF}}^2\rangle$ is the average square of the RF electric field at the mean position of the ion.

According to Equation (6) the scalar differential ac-Stark shift of the clock transition experienced by the ion in a non-zero electric field is given by [16]:

$$\frac{\Delta f_S}{f_0} = -\frac{1}{2}\frac{\Delta\alpha_S\langle E^2\rangle}{hf_0} \approx -\frac{1}{2}\frac{\Delta\alpha_S}{hf_0}\left(\langle E_{\mathrm{RF}}^2\rangle + \frac{m\Omega_{\mathrm{RF}}{}^2}{Q^2}k_B T\right). \tag{16}$$

The first term is from the RF electric field induced by excess micromotion and the second term from intrinsic micromotion, since the ion's wavepacket in the trap extends into the region of micromotion. The term from intrinsic micromotion can also be expressed in terms of the mean square velocity according to $k_B T = m\langle v^2 \rangle$, where we have accounted for the fact that the kinetic energy in the micromotion doubles the contribution from secular motion (see Equation (13)). For most ion species considered for optical clocks, the second-order Doppler shift from excess micromotion dominates over the ac-Stark contribution.

AC-Stark and second-order Doppler shifts arise from harmonic motion (either secular or micromotion) extending into the region of the RF field. To relate the two quantities, we need to obtain the average square electric field expressed as a function of the average velocity square. Assuming harmonic motion $u_j = u_{1j} \cos \omega_j t$, Newton's law relates an electric field E exerting a force in the direction of motion on the ion to an acceleration $\ddot{u}_j$ by $QE = m\ddot{u}_j$. The corresponding mean square electric field is then given by

$$\langle E^2 \rangle = (m\omega_j/Q)^2 \langle v^2 \rangle. \tag{17}$$

This allows us to express ac-Stark shifts as a fraction of the second-order Doppler shift:

$$\frac{\Delta f_S}{f_0} = -\frac{1}{2} \frac{\langle v_j^2 \rangle}{2c^2} \frac{\Delta\alpha_S m^2 c^2 \omega_j^2}{h f_0 Q^2}. \tag{18}$$

Defining a "Stark shift frequency"

$$\omega_S = \sqrt{\frac{h f_0}{\Delta\alpha_S}} \frac{Q}{mc}, \tag{19}$$

we can express the combined Stark and second-order Doppler (Δf_{2D}) shifts summed overall relevant harmonic motions j of the ion (secular and micromotion) as follows:

$$\frac{\Delta f_S}{f_0} + \frac{\Delta f_{2D}}{f_0} = -\sum_j \frac{\langle v^2 \rangle}{2c^2} \left[1 + \frac{\omega_j^2}{\omega_S^2} \right]. \tag{20}$$

As an example, we calculate the Stark shift frequency for Al^+ using the calculated differential polarizability $\Delta\alpha_S = 4\pi\epsilon_0 \times 7.3(8) \times 10^{-32}$ m^3 [17], resulting in $\omega_S = 2\pi \times 574(21)$ MHz.

We note that the second-order Doppler shift and ac-Stark shift can be canceled in a spherical Paul trap if the differential polarizability is smaller than zero and a trap drive frequency $\Omega_{RF} = |\omega_S|$ is chosen. This is possible for Ca^+ and Sr^+ [13]. In linear traps with vanishing micromotion, the second-order Doppler shift from axial motion remains uncompensated.

Excess micromotion can be detected using several techniques [15,16]. Two of the four most commonly used techniques directly measure the micromotion-induced velocity $\vec{v} = \vec{v}_0 \cos(\Omega_{RF} t + \phi)$. The first-order Doppler shift from this motion along a laser probe direction $\vec{k}$ is given by $\omega_D = \vec{k}\vec{v}$. The time dependence of this shift leads to a phase modulation with modulation index $\beta = \omega_D/\Omega_{RF}$. The resulting spectrum of the laser light field observed by the ion can be approximated for small modulation indices by the first terms of a series of Bessel functions. Once the modulation index has been determined experimentally, we can use Equation (17) to obtain the mean square RF field seen by the ion:

$$\langle E_{RF}^2 \rangle = \left(\frac{m\omega^2}{2Qk} \beta^2 \right). \tag{21}$$

The simplest technique for compensating micromotion is based on observing the position of the ion as the RF potential is lowered. Any uncompensated stray electric field will push the ions away from the RF field node. By applying compensation voltages to minimize the change in position, these fields are nulled. Note that micromotion must be compensated in all three directions and that this technique is not sensitive to possible phase shifts between electrodes. However, it provides a good starting point for more quantitative techniques.

The modulation index can be obtained from probing the Rabi frequencies Ω_0 of a carrier transition and $\Omega_{+1,-1}$ of a micromotion sideband transition detuned by $\pm\Omega_{RF}$ from the carrier on a sufficiently narrow ($\Gamma < \Omega_{RF}$) optical line:

$$\frac{\Omega_{+1/-1}}{\Omega_0} = \frac{J_1(\beta)}{J_0(\beta)} \approx \frac{\beta}{2}. \tag{22}$$

This so-called *sideband technique* is only sensitive to excess micromotion, since (according to Equation (14)) all other components average to zero for small modulation index and well within the Lamb–Dicke regime [16]. Three non-coplanar directions need to be probed and minimized for full compensation of excess micromotion.

The *photon correlation technique* explores the opposite limit, in which the transition line-width is larger than the RF drive frequency ($\Gamma > \Omega_{RF}$). A probe laser excites the ion and the arrival times of fluorescence photons with respect to the RF phase are detected. The signal arises from a modulation of the ion's resonance line through the Doppler shift from micromotion. The largest signal slope is achieved for a probe laser detuning of $\Gamma/2$. The signal is then given by

$$\frac{R_d}{R_{\max}} \approx \frac{1}{2} + \frac{\beta\Omega_{\mathrm{RF}} \sin(\Omega_{\mathrm{RF}}t + \phi)}{\Gamma}, \tag{23}$$

where R_d is the detected fluorescence rate normalized to the maximum fluorescence rate $R_{\max}$. By recording the number of photons as a function of the RF phase ϕ, the modulation index can be extracted to minimize micromotion along the probe laser direction. In the more common case that $\Gamma \approx \Omega_{\mathrm{RF}}$, the correlation between laser and RF phase has to be taken into account, resulting in signals and theoretical treatments reminiscent of frequency modulation spectroscopy. In particular, the optimum detuning for maximum signal amplitude becomes larger [16].

The last technique is based on *parametric excitation* of the ion's motion in a selected mode. If the ion is displaced from its equilibrium position u_{1j} of a mode with frequency ω_j, a modulation of the RF amplitude at frequencies $2 \times \omega_j/n$, where n is an integer, will parametrically excite this motion with a rate proportional to the displacement u_{0j}. Since ion heating can be very strong and nonlinear, even resulting in ion loss, the experimental parameters for this technique need to be chosen very carefully. For the same reasons, a direct extraction of electric field amplitude or modulation index from the measurements is difficult. Therefore, this technique needs to be calibrated against one of the other micromotion measurement techniques for quantitative evaluation. While this method cannot detect possible phase shifts between electrodes, it can probe micromotion along all relevant directions by addressing the secular frequencies of the relevant (non-degenerate) modes.

4. The Clock Laser

While the atomic reference determines the inaccuracy of a trapped-ion frequency standard, its stability is mainly determined by the performance of the clock laser. As a single interrogation of a single ion only yields a single bit of information about the laser frequency, it takes tens of interrogations to obtain enough information from the ion for a reliable correction of the laser frequency error. At shorter timescales, and in particular during any single interrogation, the best available estimate of the ion's transition frequency is the clock laser frequency, as adjusted according to previous interrogations of the ion. The uncertainty of this estimate, set by the laser instability, in turn determines the resolution with which the ion's transition can be probed: the less stable the laser, the broader the range of frequencies it might have during the interrogation, and the shorter the interrogation must be to Fourier-broaden the atomic resonance to cover this range. The clock laser noise also affects the stability of the frequency standard through the Dick effect [18]: Any phase drifts during the gaps between interrogations are not seen by the ion and cannot be corrected, so they directly add to the instability of the standard. Since the instability of the frequency standard is so sensitive to the performance of the LO, clock lasers have been developed to be, at timescales of 1–10 s, the most stable classical oscillators ever constructed, with typical fractional instabilities in the range 10^{-15}–10^{-16} at one second.

To achieve this level of instability, the laser frequency is locked to a macroscopic, continuously observable reference which is very stable at the short timescales of interest. While several different types of references have been investigated, including spectral hole burning in doped crystals [19] and optical-fiber delay lines [20], the standard choice in current clocks is a Fabry–Pérot resonator. The stability of the laser then derives from the dimensional stability of the resonator cavity.

The lock of the laser to the cavity resonance generally uses the Pound–Drever Hall technique [21], in which light from the laser is phase-modulated with an electro-optic modulator before impinging on the resonator. The light undergoes a frequency-dependent phase shift as it reflects from the resonator, converting the phase modulation to amplitude modulation whose magnitude and phase depends on the laser's detuning from cavity resonance. This amplitude signal can be detected with a photodiode, demodulated with a phase detector and used to generate the error signal for a high-bandwidth laser frequency servo. As the laser must be locked to within less than a thousandth of a cavity line-width, electronic and optical imperfections that shift the servo's lock point must be relentlessly eliminated. Particular care must be taken to avoid so-called residual amplitude modulation (RAM), fluctuations in the intensity of the *incident* light at the same frequency as the phase modulation, as such fluctuations mimic a detuning of the laser from resonance and disturb the lock. Common sources of RAM include parasitic cavities formed between weakly reflecting surfaces on the beam path from EOM to resonator, polarization modulation caused by the voltage-dependent birefringence of the EOM, and pointing noise caused by voltage-dependent refraction in the EOM.

As well as careful alignment of the optical set-up to minimize these effects passively, active cancelation of RAM by feedback to the EOM can be used to help improve the stability of the lock [22].

Given a good lock of the laser to the cavity resonance, the problem of laser stabilization reduces to keeping constant the optical path length between the cavity mirrors. First, one must eliminate length changes due to mechanical forces on the resonator spacer, which fluctuate as low-frequency acoustic or seismic noise accelerates the set-up. Where possible, the resonator should be passively isolated from such environmental accelerations by a compliant, vibration-damping mounting system, such as suspending the optical set-up with surgical tubing [23] or mounting it on a vibration-isolation platform. The geometry of the spacer that holds the mirrors is even more important: by choosing the mounting points with careful attention to symmetries and by avoiding over-determined mounting geometries that impose unnecessary additional forces on the spacer, one can ensure that the deformations induced by accelerations of the set-up do not change the distance between the mirrors [24–26]. State-of-the-art designs can yield acceleration sensitivities on the order of $10^{-11}/g$. When this acceleration sensitivity has been accurately characterized, one can further suppress the effect of seismic noise by measuring it with nearby accelerometers and applying a feed-forward correction to compensate for the known residual response of the cavity [27].

To avoid optical path-length changes caused by the pressure-dependent refractive index of air, the reference cavity is kept in a high-vacuum enclosure. This vacuum environment is also essential to suppress convective heat exchange between the cavity and the fluctuating laboratory environment, which would produce unacceptable length changes by simple thermal expansion and contraction. Indeed, avoidance of thermal expansion is one of the chief design considerations of the whole reference cavity system. Thus, the spacer is generally made from a glass or ceramic whose coefficient of thermal expansion (CTE) has a zero-crossing, i.e. a temperature at which the material's dimensions are first-order insensitive to temperature changes [28, 29]. Even so, suppressing the second-order dependence of cavity length on temperature generally requires millikelvin-level temperature stabilization. Besides the vacuum environment already described, this is usually achieved using several concentric layers of metal shielding, polished or electroplated to reduce its emissivity and thus to reduce the radiative coupling between layers. The whole system acts as a low-pass filter for laboratory temperature fluctuations, often with a time constant of several days. In addition to suppressing temperature fluctuations from the laboratory environment, one must also control local temperature fluctuations in the mirror coating due to the power they absorb from the clock laser itself. This can lead to shifts of the cavity resonance of order 100 Hz/μW, so that one must ensure that the clock laser power transmitted through the cavity is stabilized at the nanowatt level [23,25].

Even with a perfectly isolated clock laser system, however, certain fundamental noise processes would remain. The most important of these, for cavity-stabilized lasers, is the intrinsic Brownian motion of the atoms in the cavity spacer, mirror substrates, and mirror coatings at any fixed non-zero temperature. It follows from the fluctuation-dissipation theorem that this thermal noise grows together with the damping, or internal friction, in the materials comprising the cavity [30, 31]. On the other hand, the effect of thermal fluctuations decreases as one increases the number of atoms in the relevant mechanical modes, as the Brownian motion then gets averaged over a greater number of particles. Improvements to clock laser performance thus come, broadly speaking, from two approaches: the use of crystalline materials supporting higher-Q mechanical resonances than glasses or amorphous mirror coatings, and increasing size.

Increasing the mechanical quality is the principal motivation for machining cavities and mirror substrates from a single crystal of pure silicon [32]. Being much stiffer than glass, and with an ordered structure that reduces dissipation, crystalline silicon exhibits much less Brownian motion. However, unlike glasses, whose thermal expansion behavior can be adjusted by doping, the temperature for which the monocrystalline material's thermal expansion coefficient vanishes is fixed and the cavity must therefore be operated at 124 K. Operating the cavity at this temperature while maintaining control of vibrations and other technical perturbations requires a substantial engineering effort, but the reward is a clock laser whose stability, at 1×10^{-16}, is entirely dominated by the thermal fluctuations in the mirror coatings. This thermal noise could, in turn, be suppressed by another order of magnitude using newly developed monocrystalline mirror coatings [33] instead of traditional ion-beam-sputtered amorphous coatings. While the optical qualities of the monocrystalline coatings do not yet match those of amorphous coatings, they have improved dramatically in recent years and should soon be sufficient to allow the reliable production of reference cavities with substantially improved thermal noise. This would bring the stability of the clock laser into the low 10^{-17} range.

The other approach to suppressing thermal noise in reference cavities has been simply to make the cavities longer. This has two principal benefits. First, for a longer cavity the same thermal fluctuations of the mirror surface represent a smaller fraction of the cavity length, and thus a smaller fractional fluctuation of the cavity resonance frequency. Second, for a given cavity geometry and laser wavelength, the modes of a longer cavity will have a larger area at the mirrors, so that the effective length fluctuations of the cavity mode will be an average over a greater number of atoms in the mirror coatings [34]. Historically, the length of cavities was limited by practical concerns: difficulties in obtaining and machining large blocks of ULE glass with the necessary accuracy, and the problem of controlling the effect of vibrations and temperature gradients on long and comparatively floppy spacers. As better machining and more symmetric mounting designs have evolved, so reference cavities have gotten longer, reaching 40–50 cm in recent designs whose stability rivals that of the cryogenic silicon cavity [35]. Such long cavities are, however, bulky and generally too fragile to transport. Clocks intended to be portable must use more compact, rigidly mounted spacers for their clock laser reference cavities [26,27]. As they are shorter (typically ~5 cm), these cavities suffer much more from thermal fluctuations in the mirror coatings, with a typical thermal noise floor in the 10^{-15} range. The development of monocrystalline coatings will therefore also play a crucial role in improving the stability of portable clocks.

5. Counting and Distributing the Clock Frequency

A laser-beam that is known to oscillate within a few millihertz of an ion's unperturbed resonance frequency is an impressive achievement but does not, on its own, constitute a useful measurement. Optical frequency standards become practically useful when it is possible to *compare* their frequencies to that of other signals, and thus to measure frequency ratios and differences, or when it is possible to count the cycles of the laser oscillation and thus use them to establish a timescale. This generally requires the ability to transfer the accuracy and stability of the standard to an electromagnetic signal of a different frequency, whether to compare different types of standards or to bring the signal into the RF frequency range where digital electronics can count oscillations. It also requires the ability to transmit the signal from one laboratory to another without increasing its instability or inaccuracy. The first problem is solved by optical frequency combs, the second by noise-canceled optical frequency transfer links, and we will discuss each of these in turn in this section.

The heart of an optical frequency comb is a mode-locked femtosecond pulsed laser, in which a short pulse of light, typically no more than a few tens of wavelengths long, circulates around the laser cavity. Nonlinearities in the cavity keep the pulse short, counteracting the dispersion which would tend to lengthen it. Such a laser produces a burst of light every time the circulating pulse hits the output mirror, thus producing a pulse train with a delay between pulses equal to the round-trip time in the oscillator cavity. The corresponding frequency is known as the *repetition rate* f_{rep}. Importantly, there is always light in the cavity, even between pulses, and this persistent intracavity field acts as a phase memory, ensuring that the phase of the light field does not change randomly from pulse to pulse but rather drifts at a predictable rate. This rate is characterized by the *carrier-envelope offset frequency* f_{CEO}, which describes the rate of change of the optical phase relative to the peak of the pulse envelope.

This steady train of phase-coherent pulses can be viewed, in the frequency domain, as a comb of frequency components. The same nonlinearities which, in the time domain, kept the pulses short, in the frequency domain enforce a constant spacing of f_{rep} between the frequency components. Thus, even though the longitudinal modes of the laser cavity, in the absence of gain, would be unevenly spaced due to dispersion (wavelength-dependent phase shifts), once mode-locked they lase simultaneously with a rigidly regular spectrum

$$f_n = nf_{\text{rep}} + f_{\text{CEO}}, \quad n \in \mathbb{N}. \tag{24}$$

Here, f_{CEO} corresponds to an overall frequency offset, the only remaining degree of freedom (DoF) for a comb of evenly spaced lasing modes. The range of comb teeth $\{n\}$ that are actually observable depends on the shape, and in particular on the duration, of individual comb pulses, which sets the overall envelope of the comb spectrum. This spectrum typically contains hundreds of thousands of usable comb teeth. Thus, given control of the two frequencies f_{rep} and f_{CEO}, a comb is effectively a battery of hundreds of thousands of reference lasers with known frequency relationships, which can be compared with other optical signals by a simple heterodyne beat measurement [36].

The repetition rate of the pulses, which typically lies in the range of tens to hundreds of megahertz, can be measured directly with a photodetector. The carrier-envelope offset frequency is more challenging to observe, but provided the comb spectrum contains teeth at wavelengths separated by a factor of two, $f_{\rm CEO}$ can be obtained from a heterodyne beat measurement between the short-wavelength comb teeth and frequency-doubled light from the long-wavelength teeth:

$$2 \times f_n - f_{2n} = 2 \times (nf_{\rm rep} + f_{\rm CEO}) - (2nf_{\rm rep} + f_{\rm CEO}) = f_{\rm CEO}. \tag{25}$$

With tools to monitor the two parameters that determine the frequencies of all the comb teeth, the comb can be used in any of three ways. First, one can lock $f_{\rm rep}$ and $f_{\rm CEO}$ to specified RF references derived, directly or indirectly, from the ^{133}Cs standards that define the SI second. One then obtains comb teeth whose frequencies are known in SI units, enabling absolute optical frequency spectroscopy. The stability and accuracy of the comb is then typically limited by the available RF references, which can be as good as $\sim 10^{-15}$ when locking the comb to a hydrogen maser. Second, one can instead lock a particular comb tooth to an optical reference, thus taking advantage of the superior stability and accuracy of optical frequency standards. The beat of a second laser with the comb can then be used to compare it to the frequency standard [37]. By avoiding an intermediate comparison with a microwave-frequency standard, such optical-to-optical frequency ratio measurements can have lower inaccuracy than current realizations of the SI second [38]. Indeed, the repetition rate of such an optically-stabilized comb is a superb low-noise microwave source, competitive with the best sapphire oscillators [39]. The third option is to lock the comb loosely or not at all, and to feed correction signals derived from the measured comb parameters forward. Typically, the beat between one comb tooth (n) and an optical frequency reference is measured and used, together with $f_{\rm CEO}$, to produce a signal with the same frequency fluctuations as another comb tooth (m). This signal can then be mixed with the measured beat between another laser and the comb tooth m to produce a virtual transfer beat that, ideally, depends only on the relative frequency of the two lasers without being sensitive to comb noise at all [40]. This technique is now widely used for optical frequency comparisons.

So much for transferring optical signals from one frequency to another. What about transmitting them from one location to another? Whether sharing signals between set-ups in a single lab or between standards laboratories in different countries, one must overcome a host of environmental effects that perturb the optical frequency even if its source has been carefully stabilized to an atomic transition. Acoustic and seismic vibrations, temperature drifts and atmospheric pressure fluctuations are just some of the effects that can modify either the length or the index of refraction of the optical path between two experiments, and thus introduce a time-dependent phase shift, i.e. a frequency error. To suppress these errors, optical frequency transfer links use noise-cancelation strategies in which the phase-drifts in the link are measured and corrected. Although noise-canceled free-space links are possible [41], here we focus on the much more common case of noise-canceled fiber links [42].

The essential ingredient in a noise-canceled link is a reciprocal optical path, one in which light travels back to the source after reaching the destination. It is important that the returning light see exactly the same phase perturbations that affected the outbound light. One must, for instance, ensure that it uses the same polarization mode when polarization maintaining fiber is used, and in long-haul links one cannot use separate amplifiers (with possibly different phase shifts) for the two propagation directions, but must rather resort to symmetric bidirectional amplifiers. Given such a reciprocal optical path, the source of the link can detect phase drifts in the link by comparing the returning light with the original, unperturbed signal in a heterodyne beat. Since the returning light has traveled the link twice, the fluctuations in the beat frequency are twice as large as the fluctuations seen at the destination end, and so they can be corrected by applying *half* of the observed frequency fluctuation to the outbound light with an AOM. In long-distance links, the bandwidth of this corrective feedback is severely limited by the round-trip delay due to the finite speed of light, sometimes to as little as 20 Hz, but for accurate frequency comparisons lasting minutes or hours this is not a major limitation as the relevant noise frequencies are then within a few millihertz of the optical carrier signal. By such methods it is possible to transmit light over several thousand kilometers of telecom fiber with an added inaccuracy that is consistent with zero at the 10^{-19} level, which is entirely negligible for current frequency standards [43]. For such long links the Allan deviation at 1 s may be around 10^{-13}, due to the difficulty of suppressing seismic noise with a limited feedback bandwidth. However, as the link keeps continuous track of the phase its Allan deviation typically improves as $1/\tau$ at long times, so the link stability catches up with the stability of the optical frequency standard by the time the latter has averaged down to its systematic uncertainty. For shorter noise-canceled links (up to a few tens of kilometers), the instability can be below 10^{-17}, better than the stability of the clock laser [44], so that the link adds negligible instability to remote comparisons of optical frequency standards.

6. Examples of Ion-Based Optical Clocks

6.1. *Aluminium quantum logic clock*

Already in the 70's and 80's Dehmelt has realized that the group 13 (formerly group IIIA) singly-charged ions are excellent candidates for optical clocks, since their $^1S_0 \leftrightarrow {}^3P_0$ transition is free of the electric quadrupole shift and features small magnetic field shifts. The two main representatives of that group are In^+ and Al^+. The major challenges for building a clock based on these two species is their lack of an accessible laser cooling transition (see Figure 3). Much later it was realized that for the same reason black-body radiation shifts are very small for these species, since all strong transitions are deep in the UV and therefore far detuned from the peak of the black-body spectrum at room temperature. Dave Wineland proposed to use quantum logic techniques in which a co-trapped cooling or logic ion provides sympathetic cooling and state readout usually performed on a Doppler cooling transitions. This way the best features of two ion species could be combined to implement clocks based on Al^+ with excellent accuracy. This "quantum logic spectroscopy technique" is a powerful concept and applicable to many other spectroscopy ion species.

6.2. *Quantum logic spectroscopy of* Al^+

6.2.1. *Clock operation*

Quantum logic spectroscopy technique using Be^+ as the cooling or logic ion was first implemented for the Al^+ $^1S_0 \leftrightarrow {}^3P_1$ transition [45] and is

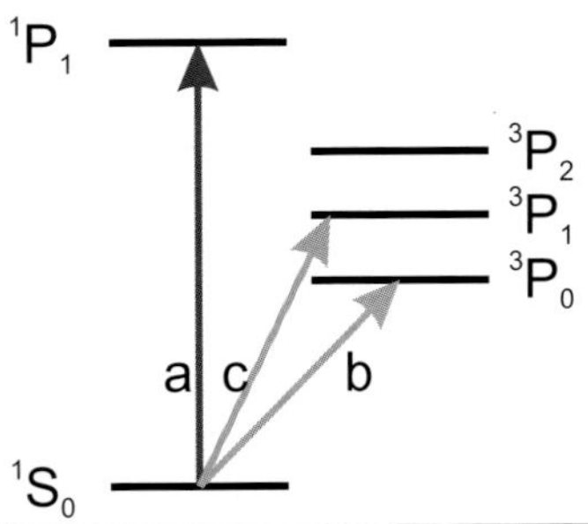

	Al^+	In^+
a: VUV cooling	167.1 nm, 233 MHz	159 nm, 1.5 GHz
b: clock	267.4 nm, 7.7 mHz	236.5 nm, 0.8 Hz
c: narrow cooling/quantum logic	266.9 nm, 520 Hz	230.6 nm, 360 kHz

Fig. 3. Schematic level structure of Al^+ and In^+ ion, together with a table of the most relevant transition wavelengths and line-widths. Energy levels are not to scale.

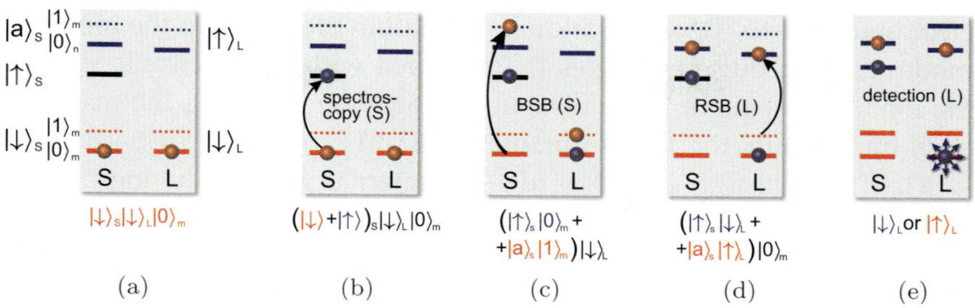

Fig. 4. Quantum logic spectroscopy sequence. Shown are two long-lived electronic states of the clock ion (clock states $|\downarrow\rangle_S, |\uparrow\rangle_S$) and an auxiliary metastable state $|a\rangle_S$ together with the logic ion (qubit states $|\downarrow\rangle_L, |\uparrow\rangle_L$). In addition, two vibrational levels ($|0\rangle_m, |1\rangle_m$) of a common motional mode of the ions in the trap are shown. (a) Initially, both ions are prepared in the electronic and motional ground state. (b) After clock interrogation, the spectroscopy ion is in a superposition of the two clock states. (c) Resolved-sideband pulse on the blue sideband [BSB] of the clock ion to the auxiliary state, mapping the ground state amplitude onto the first excited motional state. (d) Resolved-sideband pulse on the red sideband (RSB) of the logic ion, mapping the first excited motional state amplitude to the electronically excited state of the logic ion. (e) Detection of the logic ion's internal state via the electron shelving technique. Energy levels are not to scale. Adapted from Ref. [4].

the read-out scheme for the aluminum clock [46]. A simplified quantum logic spectroscopy scheme for interrogating the Al^+/Be^+ clock is shown in Figure 4. The clock ion is represented by a three-level system with the two clock states ${}^1S_0 \equiv |\downarrow\rangle_S$, ${}^3P_0 \equiv |\uparrow\rangle_S$ and an auxiliary state ${}^3P_1 \equiv |a\rangle_S$, whereas the logic ion is represented as a two-level system with generic qubit states $|\downarrow\rangle_L, |\uparrow\rangle_L$. Both ions share an axial normal mode m denoted by the state vector $|n\rangle_m$ with excitation n. The system is initialized in the electronic and motional ground state $|\downarrow\rangle_C\,|\downarrow\rangle_S\,|0\rangle_m$ (we neglect motional heating for the moment) (a). After interrogation of the clock transition (b), the internal state of the clock ion is in a superposition $\alpha|\downarrow\rangle_C + \beta|\uparrow\rangle_C$ with $|\alpha|^2 + |\beta|^2 = 1$. In a "normal" ion clock, state-dependent fluorescence projects the clock ion in either of the two states providing information about the excitation probability. In a quantum logic clock, the state detection is performed on the co-trapped logic ion. The internal state amplitudes are mapped from the spectroscopy onto the logic ion through a series of resolved sideband pulses. These are implemented using the auxiliary state in the clock ion, since it allows faster pulses. A BSB transition on the ${}^1S_0 \leftrightarrow {}^3P_1$ transition implements the mapping $(\alpha|\downarrow\rangle_C + \beta|\uparrow\rangle_C)|\downarrow\rangle_L|0\rangle_m \rightarrow (\alpha|a\rangle_S|1\rangle_m + \beta|\uparrow\rangle_C|0\rangle_m)|\downarrow\rangle_S$, changing the electronic state to $^3\text{P}_1$, while adding a quantum of motion to the motional mode (c). This pulse entangles the motional with the electronic state of the ion. A subsequent RSB pulse on the logic ion reversing the mapping step, implements the transformation $(\alpha|a\rangle_\text{S}|1\rangle_\text{m} + \beta|\uparrow\rangle_\text{C}|0\rangle_\text{m})|\downarrow\rangle_\text{S} \rightarrow (\alpha|a\rangle_\text{S}|\uparrow\rangle_\text{L} + \beta|\uparrow\rangle_\text{C}|\downarrow\rangle_\text{L})|0\rangle_\text{m}$ (d). The internal state of the logic ion is then detected using the usual electron shelving technique on the logic ion, projecting the system in either $|\downarrow\rangle_\text{C}|\uparrow\rangle_\text{L}$ or $|\uparrow\rangle_\text{C}|\downarrow\rangle_\text{L}$ (e). The lifetime of the $^3\text{P}_1$ state is on the order of 300 μs, whereas the excited clock state lifetime is on the order of 21 s. After a few ms, spontaneous emission has brought all population from the $|a\rangle_\text{S}$ in the clock ion back to $|\downarrow\rangle_\text{C}$, whereas the excited clock state population suffers only negligible loss of population: $(\alpha|a\rangle_\text{S}|\uparrow\rangle_\text{L} + \beta|\uparrow\rangle_\text{C}|\downarrow\rangle_\text{L})|0\rangle_\text{m} \rightsquigarrow (\alpha|\downarrow\rangle_\text{C}|\uparrow\rangle_\text{L} + \beta|\uparrow\rangle_\text{C}|\downarrow\rangle_\text{L})|0\rangle_\text{m}$. Imperfections limit the fidelity of single-cycle state readout. Since we have now recovered the situation just before the state mapping started (beginning of Figure 4(c)), except that the ions have been projected onto one of the two possible outcomes of the state detection, we can repeat the readout cycle several times. This way, state discrimination with up to 99.94% fidelity using Bayesian inference has been demonstrated for 10 detection repetitions [47].

Several additional steps are required to operate a clock using this scheme, which we will discuss in the following. A typical probe sequence containing approximate durations for the different steps is outlined in Figure 5. Every few seconds, the initial Zeeman state of the clock is changed via optical pumping using polarized light on the $(^1\text{S}_0, m_F = \pm 5/2 \rightarrow {}^3\text{P}_1, F = 7/2, m_F = \pm 7/2)$ transition. Recording the center frequencies $f_{+5/2}, f_{-5/2}$ of both streched states $(^1\text{S}_0, m_F = \pm 5/2 \leftrightarrow {}^3\text{P}_0, m_F' = \pm 5/2)$ allows the calculation of a linear-Zeeman-shift-free transition frequency from the average $(f_{+5/2} + f_{-5/2})/2$ of both frequencies as discussed in Section 3.3.1. The difference frequency $f_1 = f_{+5/2} - f_{-5/2}$ provides a direct measure of the magnetic field, which is then used to compute the dc component of the quadratic Zeeman shift [46]. The total duration of a single interrogation cycle is approximately 120 ms of which 100 ms are used for probing [48]. Not shown in Figure 5 are "service cycles" to evaluate slowly-varying parameters, such as micromotion compensation, and the calibration of motional and Rabi frequencies. The additional overhead from calibration effectively reduces the fraction of time spent on probing the transition (duty cycle) to between 45% and 65%, depending on the details of the implementation. This parameter is relevant for the Dick effect as discussed in Section 4.

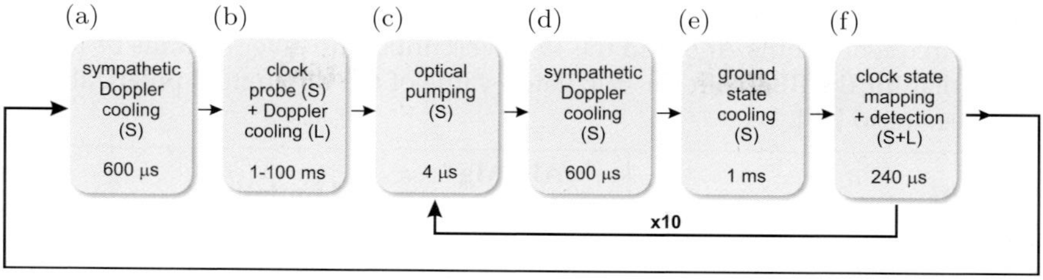

Fig. 5. Quantum logic clock interrogation cycle [46]. The following sequence describes interrogation of the $^1S_0$, $m_F = 5/2 \longrightarrow {}^3P_0$, $m_F = 5/2$ state. A similar protocol is used for the other ($m_F = -5/2$) stretched state interrogation. (a) Sympathetic Doppler cooling, reaching $\bar{n} \approx 3$ in all modes with tilted ion crystal. (b) Probing of the Al^+ clock transition $^1S_0 \leftrightarrow {}^3P_0$ with simultaneous application of cooling light to maintain steady-state motional occupation. (c) Optical pumping on the $^1S_0 \leftrightarrow {}^3P_1$ transition to $^1S_0$, $m_F = 5/2$ state. (d) Sympathetic Doppler cooling followed by ground state cooling of a selected axial mode to a mean motional excitation of $\bar{n} \approx 0.05$ (e). (f) Quantum logic state detection (see Figure 4 for details). Steps (c) through (f) are repeated 10 times for improved readout fidelity. Adapted from Ref. [4].

6.2.2. *Systematic shifts of the* Al^+ *clocks*

In Section 3, we have given an overview of physics behind different systematic frequency shifts. In the following, we will summarize the evaluation techniques and mitigation strategies of some of the important systematic shifts for the Al^+/Mg^+ clock using Mg^+ as the logic ion species that has been operated at NIST [49]. This clock can be viewed as a prototypical system for a high-accuracy frequency standard. However, each clock ion species has its unique features and dominating shifts that need to be carefully addressed and may require more advanced mitigation strategies and evaluation techniques than presented here. Table 1 provides a summary of the shifts and their uncertainty for the Al^+/Mg^+ clock. The largest shift is caused by the quadratic Zeeman effect. Since this shift can be evaluated with very low uncertainty, it does not limit the accuracy of the clock at the current level. The dominant uncertainty is from micromotion and secular motion induced time dilation shifts. Micromotion was measured using the sideband technique (see Section 3.5) and compensated by applying static compensation fields. The magnitude of this shift is typically bounded by the error in nulling it. However, the trap used for this Al^+/Mg^+ clock showed strong axial micromotion that could be compensated only for a singular point where the Al^+ ion should be located to minimize the effect. Background gas collisions can change the order of the ion crystal. As a

Table 1. Systematic shifts and uncertainties for the Al^+/Mg^+ [49] clock. The fractional frequency shifts $\Delta f/f$ and the 1σ uncertainties are given in units of 10^{-18}. Note that for the BBR shift the calculated value of the differential polarizability has been used [17].

Shift	**Al^+/Mg^+**		**Limitation**
	$\Delta f/f$	σ	
Micromotion	−9	6	Static electric fields
Secular motion	−16.3	5	Doppler cooling
Black-body radiation	−3.8	0.4	dc polarizability
Cooling laser Stark	−3.6	1.5	Polarizability, intensity
Clock laser Stark	0	0.2	Polarizability, intensity
quadratic Zeeman	−1079.9	0.7	*B*-field calibration
First-order Doppler	0	0.3	Statistical imbalance
Background gas collisions	0	0.5	Collision model
AOM phase chirp	0	0.2	RF power
Total	−1112.6	8.0	

consequence, the Al^+ ion may experience a larger micromotion field for a fraction of the interrogation time, resulting in an increased uncertainty. Charging of material near the ion from the 267 nm UV radiation for clock and logic operations can cause temporal changes in micromotion, further increasing the uncertainty of the shift. As discussed in Section 3.5, the associated ac-Stark shift from penetration of the ion's wavepacket into the RF field is on the few percent level of the time dilation shift for typical RF drive frequencies of 20–100 MHz.

The non-zero kinetic energy in the secular motional modes during interrogation causes second-order Doppler shifts. Motional heating from electric field noise at the position of the ions during the clock interrogation times of typically 150 ms can lead to a dynamic change in kinetic energy. This effect can be counteracted in quantum logic clocks by simultaneous sympathetic cooling via the logic ion, which is not possible with single-ion clocks. The steady-state temperature of each mode depends on the heating and cooling rates during Doppler cooling. In the absence of external heating mechanisms, the Doppler temperature is reached in all modes. However, for some of the modes the Doppler cooling rate is smaller than for others as a consequence of the small amplitude of motion for the cooling ion in these modes. A constant external heating rate will therefore result in an increased steady-state kinetic energy of these modes. Since we can assume the electric field of the noise process to be constant across the ion crystal, the heating rate will also depend on the relative mode amplitudes and phases of the two ions. For example, for two ions of the same mass and charge, the in-phase modes should experience a heating rate, whereas the out-of-phase modes should not. For ions of different mass, it turns out that the effect of steady-state temperature increase is largest for radial modes and that it is advantageous to have a cooling ion with lower mass than Al^+. In this situation, the least efficiently cooled modes are the ones experiencing the smallest external heating rate [50]. This is one of the few systematic effects where the choice of logic ion plays a role. In the presence of large heating rates, Mg^+ is the ideal partner for Al^+ due to its near-perfect mass match, significantly reducing their effect on the kinetic energy. However, Mg^+ also has a large natural line-widths of around 40 MHz, resulting in twice the Doppler cooling temperature compared to most other ion species. The magnitude of the shift was measured using the ratio between blue- and red-sideband excitation as described in Section 3.4. The uncertainty of this shift is given by the experimental error of 30% in determining it.

Several sources of linear Doppler shifts can potentially play a role and need to be investigated. Ejection of photo-electrons by the clock laser that collide with the ion correlated to the direction of the clock laser may lead to such linear Doppler shifts. This has been checked in the Al^+/Mg^+ clock by probing the ion from two opposing directions with separate frequency locks. Another shift that can be interpreted as a linear Doppler shift arises from phase chirps of the interrogation laser during the probe time. They can arise from instabilities in the optical set-up that do not average to zero for long times [51]. The major contribution typically originates from ringing and thermal expansion of the acousto-optical modulators (AOMs) used for switching the probe beam [52]. It can be significantly reduced by applying only a very small RF power (e.g. 1 mW for Al^+/Mg^+).

Several shifts arise from interaction of the clock states with external electric fields. The most recent value for the differential polarizability between the two clock states has been derived from *ab initio* calculations to be $\Delta\alpha_S = \alpha(P) - \alpha(S) = 0.82(8) \times 10^{-41} \mathrm{Jm^2/V^2}$ [17], resulting in a relative frequency shift of only $3.8(4) \times 10^{-18}$ at 300 K. This value was experimentally confirmed by the NIST group through a measurement of the dynamic polarizability at a wavelength of 976 nm. This is the smallest BBR shift of an electronic transition in neutral or singly-charged atoms considered for optical clocks. As a consequence, a temperature calibration corresponding to an uncertainty of 15 K is sufficient to reach 10^{-18} relative frequency uncertainty.

The simultaneous Doppler cooling on the logic ion during clock interrogation imposes an additional Stark shift on the clock transition that depends on the cooling laser wavelength and intensity. The intensity of the cooling laser beam was calibrated through off-resonant excitation of the Mg^+ dark state $|F = 2, m_F = -2\rangle$ and applying the model for the BBR shift extrapolated to the cooling laser wavelength of 280 nm. This shift can be further reduced by focusing the laser beam onto the cooling ion, or by using a logic ion species with smaller saturation intensity and further wavelength detuning, such as Ca^+.

The linear Zeeman shift of $\Delta f_{M1} = -82884(5)B$ Hz/mT [46] in the Al^+/Mg^+ clock is canceled by averaging the stretch state transition frequencies as described above. The remaining quadratic Zeeman effect is proportional to the average of the square of the magnetic field $\langle B^2 \rangle = \langle B_{dc} \rangle^2 + B_{ac}^2$, consisting of a static and dynamic contribution, B_{dc} and B_{ac}, respectively. The clock is operated at a small static field of $B_{dc} \approx 0.1$ mT to provide a quantization axis for cooling. Slow drifts of this field can directly be deduced from the difference of the Al^+ stretched state frequencies f_1 as described above. The quadratic shift of $\Delta f_{M2} = -7.1988(48) \times 10^7$ Hz/T^2 has been calibrated by deliberately varying the static field and measuring the transition frequency against another frequency standard [38]. It arises mostly from charge/discharge currents of the RF trap electrodes at the RF drive frequency. They can be calibrated from hyperfine spectroscopy on the logic ion using states with a large and well-known linear Zeeman shift.

Although collision shifts between cold and localized trapped ions are absent, collisions with background gas can result in a differential shift between the ground and excited clock state. Estimating the shift for a worst case scenario of an undetected $\pi/2$-phase shift during clock interrogation, the resulting fractional shift is 0.5×10^{-18} [38]. A recent study of background gas atoms with cold ions indicates that the shift is much smaller than this conservative estimate [53].

7. Clock Applications

7.1. *Relativistic geodesy*

As discussed in Section 3.4, two relativistic effects influence the frequency comparison of two or more clocks: the second-order Doppler effect and the gravitational red shift. Both effects are absent in the frame of the atomic reference. Therefore, they only arise when comparing clocks, possibly in different reference frames. The usual relativistic transformation prescriptions work only for inertial frames. The earth-centered earth-fixed (ECEF) frame is rotating with the earth and therefore no inertial frame. The safest approach to compare the frequency between two optical clocks (fixed to the rotating surface of the earth), is therefore to transform their reading into a non-rotating earth-centered inertial (ECI) reference frame. Following [54,55], we can write the scalar interval in a non-rotating, freely-falling coordinate system with origin at the center of mass of the earth, assuming a static Newtonian potential U as

$$ds^2 \approx \left(1 - \frac{2U}{c^2}\right) c^2 dt^2 - (dx^2 + dy^2 + dz^2). \tag{26}$$

Here, we have neglected terms of order $(1/c)$ and higher, where (x, y, z) are the coordinates, c is the speed of light, and t is coordinate time in this frame in the absence of gravitational sources (at infinity). Proper time of a clock in this frame is given by $d\tau = ds/c$. The ratio between proper time and coordinate time is then given by

$$\frac{d\tau}{dt} = \frac{\Delta f}{f_0} = \sqrt{1 - \frac{2U}{c^2} - \frac{v^2}{c^2}} \approx 1 - \frac{U}{c^2} - \frac{v^2}{2c^2}, \tag{27}$$

where $v^2 = (dx^2 + dy^2 + dz^2)/dt^2$ is the square of the velocity of the clock within the inertial frame. The first term in Equation (27) is the gravitational redshift of a clock in the Newtonian gravitational potential of the earth, $U \approx GM_E/r$, where $G \approx 6.67384 \times 10^{-11}$ m^3 kg^{-1} s^{-2} is the gravitational constant and $M_E \approx 5.97219 \times 10^{24}$ kg is the mass of the earth. The second term is the second-order Doppler or time dilation shift from the clock's finite velocity. These expressions are valid for a clock fixed (non-moving) on the surface of the earth as observed from the non-rotating reference frame. We can explicitly account for the rotation of the earth by going to spherical coordinates (r, θ, ϕ) and performing the transformation $t = t'$, $r = r'$, $\theta = \theta'$, and $\phi = \phi' + \omega_E t'$ into the rotating frame with primed variables:

$$\frac{d\tau}{dt} = \frac{\Delta f}{f_0} \approx 1 - \frac{U}{c^2} - \frac{(\omega_e r' \sin\theta')^2}{2c^2} = 1 - \frac{\Phi}{c^2}, \tag{28}$$

where we have defined the effective gravitational potential Φ in the rotating frame. From the term containing the rotation of the earth we see that the clock experiences a second-order Doppler shift that is different for a clock on the equator compared to a clock near the poles. In reality, the earth is deformed and inhomogeneous, resulting in a potential $U(r,\theta,\phi)$ that depends on the position of the clock on the surface of the earth. In a clock comparison on earth we have to account for both effects. We will observe a frequency difference $\Delta f = f_1 - f_2$ between two clocks at fixed positions $\vec{r}_1$ and $\vec{r}_2$ on earth of $\Delta f/f = (\Phi(\vec{r}_2) - \Phi(\vec{r}_1))/c^2$. Another consequence of these effects is that a timescale within the ECEF, such as atomic time international (TAI) or Universal coordinated time (UTC) needs to be defined with reference to an equipotential surface. Consequently, an effective gravitational potential $\Phi_0 = 6.969290134 \times 10^{-10}c^2$ [56] has been defined as the reference for these timescales. It corresponds to the equipotential surface in the rotating frame of the earth in which all clocks tick with the same rate. This notion is closely related to the definition of the geoid in geodesy, which is defined as a specific reference surface on which no tangential forces exist (a plumb line is always perpendicular to the geoid). It is defined as the sum of the Newtonian gravitational potential U and the centrifugal potential $U_c = v^2/2$: $\Phi_g = U + U_c$ roughly corresponding to the distance of mean sea level from the earth's center of mass. Comparison with Equation (28) reveals that the geoid and the effective gravitational potential scale exactly the same way. While Φ_0 is well-defined, the same is not true for Φ_g [57], however, we have $\Phi_0 \approx \Phi_g$.

The geoid plays an important role in geodesy and geophysics, since it provides a vertical reference frame. The height above the geoid is called orthometric height H_p and tells us in which direction water flows. It has applications in engineering, coastal protection, and water resource management. It is to be distinguished from the ellipsometric height, e.g. provided by GNSS, such as GPS, which is defined as the height above a perfect ellipse approximating the oblate shape of the earth. Differences between the two height systems can amount to hundreds of meters and can only be determined through involved measurement campaigns. Within a country a height system is typically established through geometric leveling with theodolites supported by local gravimetry along leveling lines (see Figure 6). This is performed in loops with a total length of more than 30,000 km for a country such as Germany with an area of 360,000 km^2. Establishing such a height network with typical single-set-up distances of around 50 m is a time-consuming and costly task. Most importantly, errors in single measurements accumulate, compromising the overall height system to an accuracy of a few centimeters within a country. This is where optical clocks with accuracies on the order of 10^{-17} or better, corresponding to a height resolution of $\Delta r \approx r_E^2 c^2/(GM_E)\Delta f/f \approx 10$ cm, can play a decisive role.

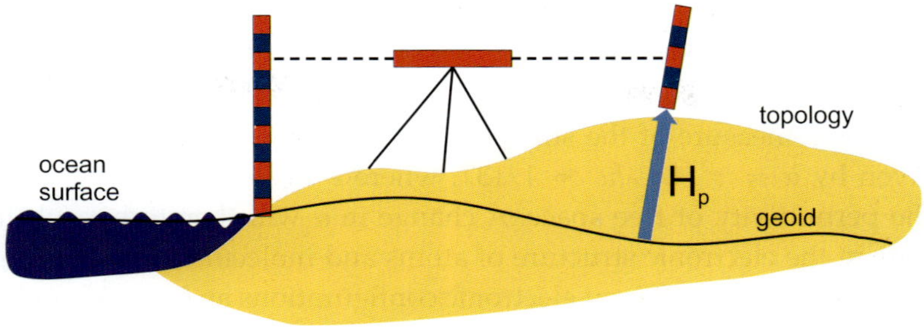

Fig. 6. Establishing a height system. Leveling along loops provides orthometric heights H_p above the geoid to establish a height system.

Clock comparisons e.g. via long-haul optical fibers as described in Section 5 provide directly a differential height measurement between remote locations [58].

Geodesy and timescales are inextricably linked through the reference potential Φ_0 of the timescale. The height above this reference potential needs to be known to better precision than the optical clock uncertainty. This can already be a limitation when comparing clocks at a level of 10^{-17} [14]. A world-encompassing network of optical clocks operating at a level of 10^{-18} with a suitable infrastructure for high-level frequency comparison would not only provide a more accurate time standard, but also form the basis for a unified, long-term stable geodetic height reference frame [56,59].

7.2. *Variation of fundamental constants*

The high accuracy of optical clocks makes them prime candidates to investigate the foundations of physics by probing subtle deviations from theoretical expectations. Comparing clocks over the course of several years allows us to put bounds on possible tiny variations in their level structure. One such deviation could be a change in fundamental constants, which is forbidden by the Standard Model of Particle Physics (SM), but in principle allowed by several models beyond the SM. The basic idea originating from String theory is, that fundamental constants are given by vacuum expectation values of scalar fields [60]. These fields can exhibit temporal and spatial variations, resulting in temporal and/or spatial variations of fundamental constants. One can also assume that the values of fundamental constants are coupled to other fields, e.g. the gravitational field [61] or dark matter [62]. Unfortunately, there is no prediction at which level one should be able to observe such changes, since all models are also compatible with space–time fixed constants.

An example for such a fundamental constant is the fine-structure constant. It is a measure of the strength of electromagnetic interactions and is given by $\alpha = e^2/4\pi\epsilon_0\hbar c \approx 1/137$, where e is the electric charge and ϵ_0 the permittivity of free space. A change in α will therefore result in a change in the electronic structure of atoms and molecules. These changes will be different for different electronic configurations and species and can be estimated from atomic structure calculations with high accuracy. They are usually characterized by sensitivity factors q_j relating a relative change in α to a change in the frequency of a transition j with nominal frequency ω_j according to

$$\omega_j(\alpha) \approx \omega_j + 2q_j \frac{\Delta\alpha}{\alpha}. \tag{29}$$

Sometimes the sensitivity is given as a relative change in transition frequency according to $\frac{\Delta\omega_j}{\omega_j} \approx K_j \frac{\Delta\alpha}{\alpha}$, with $K_j = 2q_j/\omega_j$.

Two complementary approaches using this relation are being pursued. The first is based on quasar absorption spectroscopy, in which the spectral fingerprint of atoms and molecules in interstellar clouds on light emitted by bright quasars is recorded by spectrometers connected to large telescopes. By comparing the (red-shifted) absorption spectra with current laboratory data for many species and transitions using Equation (29) in a multi-dimensional fit analysis, velocity components, redshift, and the value of the fine-structure constant some 10^{10} years ago can be extracted. Such an analysis has provided a non-zero result of $\Delta\alpha/\alpha = -5.4(1.2) \times 10^{-6}$ [63], resulting in $\dot{\alpha}/\alpha = -6.4(1.4) \times 10^{-16}$ yr^{-1} when linearly extrapolated, whereas others have found a null result [64]. An analysis combining data from two telescope observing different areas of the universe is best compatible with a spatial variation of α along a certain direction [65]. This highly disputed result has become known as the "Australian dipole", which may be compromised by undiscovered systematic effects. Since the earth is moving through this gradient, it would appear as a temporal change of $\dot{\alpha}/\alpha \sim 10^{-19}$/year.

While the quasar absorption spectroscopy technique takes advantage of the long distances and cosmological timescales, comparisons between high-accuracy optical clocks with different sensitivity coefficients probe a possible variation of fundamental constants in the current epoch. Table 2 shows the sensitivity factors for some of the important species.

Table 2. Table with sensitivity coefficients q for different atomic systems. The entries with a grey background have been proposed, but as of the writing of this manuscript not yet contributed to a measurement.

system	q (cm^{-1})
Sr	443
Dy	−24000, 6000
Yb^+ E2	10397
Yb^+ E3	−63752
Hg^+	−52200
Al^+	146
Ho^{14+}	−186000
Ir^{17+}	−385367, 367161
Cf^{*16+}	−370928, 465293
Th* nuclear	$\sim 10^8$

A recent compilation of all results from optical spectroscopy gives an upper bound of $\dot{\alpha}/\alpha = -0.7(2.1) \times 10^{-17}$ $yr^{-}1$ [66] (see also Ref. [67]), compatible with no variation. Improvements in optical clock stability and accuracy will push these limits further down, verifying/falsifying the astronomical observations and possibly revealing deviations from SM predictions.

8. Future Trends: Multi-Ion Clocks

While the inaccuracy (systematic uncertainty) of ion-based optical frequency standards continues to improve, their stability has progressed much more slowly. This means that longer and longer averaging times are required to realize a frequency whose total uncertainty reflects the systematic uncertainty. For a clock with an instability of 2×10^{-15} at 1 s, it takes more than 11 days of averaging to reach a statistical uncertainty of 2×10^{-18}, testing the reliability of the experiments and the patience of the experimentalists. Considerable effort is therefore being invested in finding ways to improve the stability of ion-based optical clocks.

All ion-based optical standards to date have used only a single trapped ion as their atomic reference, and their instability has thus been strictly limited by the poor signal-to-noise ratio of a measurement that yields only one bit of information per interrogation cycle. The stability of such single-ion standards can only be improved by extending interrogation times, which requires hard-won improvements in clock laser stability. However, the technical obstacles to operating multi-ion clocks are gradually being overcome. New methods of trap fabrication based on stacks of laser-machined wafers, combined with careful engineering of the electrode geometry to minimize boundary effects, have allowed the construction of traps with micromotion-induced Doppler shifts below 1×10^{-18} for strings of tens of ions [68], while efficient schemes for the simultaneous readout of the internal state of multiple clock ions have been devised [69]. Thus, although a multi-ion optical clock has yet to run in the lab, it is already interesting to consider how best to use multiple ions once they become available.

The simplest way to operate a multi-ion clock is to probe the N available ions in parallel with the clock laser, read out their final state independently, and average the resulting estimates of the laser frequency error. Such parallel, independent operation improves the stability at a given averaging time by the usual statistical factor of $\sqrt{N}$, corresponding to a reduction by a factor of N in the time required to average down to a target statistical uncertainty. Even this simple strategy, implemented in a modest 10-ion string, would suffice to turn a week-long measurement campaign into a one-day task.

One can do better, however, by taking advantage of the fact that all the ions see the same laser phase noise, so that measurements done on a subset of the available ions can be used to correct for the laser phase noise seen by the others. This leads to the idea of separating the ions in the clock into a hierarchy of subensembles. The first such subensemble is interrogated as usual, with a probe time shorter than the coherence time of the laser. The measurements on this first subensemble are used to stabilize the laser coarsely, extending its coherence time and thus allowing the second ensemble to be probed with a longer probe time. The measurements from the second subensemble can, in turn, be used to correct for laser phase noise during the even longer interrogation of a third subensemble, and so forth. The interrogation time used by the last subensemble, and hence the stability of the clock, improves exponentially with the number of available ions [71, 72]. Of course, at some point the interrogation time reaches the excited-state lifetime of the clock ions, laser phase noise ceases to limit the clock stability and the exponential improvement stops. The value of this strategy thus depends on a separation of timescales, between the phase-coherence time due to *correlated* noise which acts similarly on each ion (such as laser phase noise) and the coherence time due to *independent* noise which disrupts each ion individually (such as spontaneous decay). As long as the former is shorter than the latter, correlated interrogation strategies can be useful. As there are clock transitions, such as the octupole transition in Yb^+, whose excited-state lifetime exceeds the duration of any reasonable experiment, there is scope for several orders of magnitude of stability improvement by this approach.

Multi-ion clocks also offer the opportunity of exploiting quantum entanglement between ions to improve stability, an approach studied under the banner of quantum metrology. It is known that quantum entanglement can be used to improve the phase resolution of the comparison between local oscillator and ions, either by preparing squeezed spin states with reduced phase fluctuations [73] or maximally entangled GHZ states with increased phase sensitivity [74]. In the absence of decoherence and in the limit of small phase fluctuations, either approach can reduce the phase uncertainty of a single Ramsey measurement from $1/\sqrt{N}$ to $1/N$. However, the ions in a real experiment do suffer from decoherence, and the interrogation time in an optical frequency standard is generally extended until the assumption of small phase fluctuations breaks down, in order to improve the frequency resolution associated with a given phase uncertainty. Thus, while some microwave frequency standards have demonstrated improved frequency stability for fixed interrogation time by using entangled states [75,76], it is not yet clear whether entangled states can provide a useful stability enhancement in an optical frequency standard under realistic operating conditions. It is likely that the aforementioned separation of timescales between correlated noise and uncorrelated decoherence plays a critical role here as well. Entanglement-based strategies are known to provide only a small constant-factor improvement in stability in the presence of uncorrelated noise or decoherence [77]. Thus, for a technically perfect system in which the dominant decoherence was spontaneous decay of the excited state, the fundamental stability limit would be essentially the same with entanglement as it would be for the simplest classical strategy of interrogating each ion independently with an interrogation time equal to the excited-state lifetime. However, when correlated laser noise limits the interrogation time, then quantum correlations between ions may be helpful. Numerical simulations using a realistic noise model for a clock laser limited by thermal noise [78] suggest that the use of highly symmetric partially-entangled states [79] can provide a useful stability improvement over conventional Ramsey spectroscopy with independent atoms for a plausible clock ensemble of tens of ions. Thus, the exceptional level of quantum control developed in the trapped-ion community may yet help improve the stability of trapped-ion optical frequency standards, allowing the full use of their exceptional frequency accuracy in practical applications.

9. Practice Problems

9.1. *Problems*

(1) Show that the stability limit set by QPN for a clock using independent, parallel interrogation of N atoms is

$$\sigma_y(\tau) = \frac{1}{\omega T}\sqrt{\frac{T_c}{N\tau}},$$

where ω is the transition frequency, T the interrogation time, T_c the experiment cycle time, and τ the total averaging time. Assume a perfect system with no technical noise and ideal Ramsey interrogation with quasi-instantaneous $\pi/2$ pulses. Note that projection noise is white frequency noise, uncorrelated from cycle to cycle of the clock's operation, and thus the Allan deviation $\sigma_y(\tau)$ resulting from projection noise is equal to the conventional standard deviation. (*Hints*: How does the excitation probability for each atom after the Ramsey sequence depend on the phase $\phi = \delta T$ accumulated between the two $\pi/2$ pulses, where δ is the detuning of the LO? How well can this excitation probability be determined from a single read-out of the N atoms, and thus what fraction of a cycle can be resolved by the measurement?)

(2) To better understand the motivation for moving from microwave to optical frequency standards, compare the (projection-noise-limited) stability of a microwave atomic fountain to that of a single-ion optical frequency standard. In your estimate, take into account the far greater number of atoms in the fountain and the longer interrogation times allowed for microwave standards by the long coherence time of microwave oscillators as well as the difference in operating frequencies.

9.2. *Solutions*

(1) For an ideal Ramsey interrogation whose duration T is much longer than that of the individual $\pi/2$ pulses that start and end it, the probability P that an atom is excited at the end of the interrogation depends on the phase accumulated between the pulses $\phi = \delta T$ as

$$P = \frac{1}{2}(1 + \cos\phi) = \frac{1}{2}(1 + \cos\delta T). \qquad (30)$$

At read out, each atom yields a binary measurement result: either the atom was excited or it was not. This leads to a binomial distribution of measurement results, so that the standard deviation of the number of excited atoms is $\sqrt{NP(1-P)}$. If P is estimated from the fraction of excited atoms, the statistical error on the estimate is then

$$\Delta P = \sqrt{\frac{P(1-P)}{N}} = \frac{1}{2}\sqrt{\frac{1-\cos^2 \delta T}{N}}. \tag{31}$$

Converting this to a frequency uncertainty using standard error propagation techniques yields

$$\Delta\delta = \frac{\Delta P}{|\partial P/\partial \delta|} = \frac{\frac{1}{2}\sqrt{\frac{1-\cos^2 \delta T}{N}}}{\frac{1}{2}T\,|\sin \delta T|} = \frac{1}{T\sqrt{N}}. \tag{32}$$

Thus, the fractional frequency uncertainty after a single interrogation is

$$\Delta y = \frac{\Delta\delta}{\omega} = \frac{1}{\omega T\sqrt{N}}. \tag{33}$$

If the standard has a cycle time $T_c \geq T$ and is allowed to operate for a time τ, so that τ/T_c measurements of the ion can be averaged, then the statistical uncertainty on the frequency of the standard averages down to

$$\sigma_y(\tau) = \frac{1}{\omega T}\sqrt{\frac{T_c}{N\tau}}.$$

(2) A typical atomic fountain might operate with an effective (detected) atom number of $N \approx 10^5$ and an interrogation time $T \approx 0.7$ s (limited by the flight time in the fountain) in a total cycle time of around one second. With a microwave oscillation frequency of 9.2 GHz (for the transition that defines the SI second), this yields an instability $\sigma_y(\tau) \approx 5 \times 10^{-13}\,\text{s}^{1/2}/\sqrt{\tau}$. An optical standard based on a single ion has a phase resolution more than two orders of magnitude worse ($1/\sqrt{N} = 1$ instead of 0.003) and a shorter (laser-limited) interrogation time (typically around 0.1 s), but the five-order-of-magnitude increase in the transition frequency (to 1 PHZ for Al^+), and thus in the rate at which frequency errors become detectable, more than compensates for these drawbacks, allowing an instability $\sigma_y(\tau) \approx 3 \times 10^{-15}\,\text{s}^{1/2}/\sqrt{\tau}$.

References

1. P. Gill, When should we change the definition of the second?, *Philos. T. R. Soc. A.* **369**(1953), 4109–4130 (2011).
2. F. Riehle, Towards a Re-definition of the second based on optical atomic clocks, *Comptes Rendus Physique* **16**, 506–515 (2015).
3. N. Poli *et al.*, Optical atomic clocks, *Riv. Nuovo Cimento.* **36**(12), 555–624 (2013).
4. A. D. Ludlow *et al.*, Optical atomic clocks, *Rev. Mod. Phys.* **87**, 637 (2015).
5. C. Audoin and B. Guinot, *The Measurement of Time: Time, Frequency and the Atomic Clock*, Cambridge, Cambridge University Press, (2001).
6. F. Riehle, *Frequency standards: Basics and Applications*, Wiley-VCH, Weinheim (2004).
7. A. Jones, *Splitting The Second: The Story of Atomic Time*, Boca Raton, Florida, CRC Press (2000).
8. N. Huntemann *et al.*, Generalized Ramsey excitation scheme with suppressed light shift, *Phys. Rev. Lett.* **109**(21), 213002 (2012).
9. W. M. Itano, External-field shifts of the $^{199}Hg^{+}$ optical frequency standard, *J. Res. Nat. Inst. Stand. Tech.* **105**(6), 829–837 (2000).
10. C. F. Roos *et al.*, 'Designer atoms' for quantum metrology, *Nature.* **443**(7109), 316–319 (2006).
11. N. Huntemann *et al.*, High-accuracy optical clock based on the octupole transition in $^{171}Yb^{+}$, *Phys. Rev. Lett.* **108**(9), 090801 (2012).
12. W. Oskay *et al.*, Single-atom optical clock with high accuracy, *Phys. Rev. Lett.* **97**(2), 020801 (2006).
13. P. Dubé *et al.*, Evaluation of systematic shifts of the $^{88}Sr^{+}$ single-ion optical frequency standard at the 10^{-17} level, *Phys. Rev. A.* **87**(2), 023806 (2013).
14. N. K. Pavlis and M. A. Weiss, The relativistic redshift with 3×10^{-17} uncertainty at NIST, *Metrologia.* **40**(2), 66–73 (2003).
15. D. J. Berkeland *et al.*, Minimization of ion micromotion in a Paul trap, *J. Appl. Phys.* **83**(10), 5025–5033 (1998).
16. J. Keller *et al.*, Precise determination of micromotion for trapped-ion optical clocks, *J. Appl. Phys.* **118**, 104501 (2015).
17. M. S. Safronova *et al.*, Precision calculation of blackbody radiation shifts for optical frequency metrology, *Phys. Rev. Lett.* **107**(14), 143006 (2011).
18. G. J. Dick. Local oscillator induced instabilities in trapped ion frequency standards. In *Proceedings Precise Time and Time Interval Meeting*, pp. 133–147 (1987).
19. S. Cook *et al.*, Laser-frequency stabilization based on steady-state spectral-hole burning in $Eu^{3+}:Y_2SiO_5$, *Phys. Rev. Lett.* **114**, 253902 (2015).
20. F. Kefelian *et al.*, Ultralow-frequency-noise stabilization of a laser by locking to an optical fiber-delay line, *Opt. Lett.* **34**(7), 914–916 (2009).
21. E. D. Black, An introduction to Pound–Drever–Hall laser frequency stabilization, *Am. J. Phys.* **69**(1), 79–87 (2001).
22. W. Zhang *et al.*, Reduction of residual amplitude modulation to 1×10^{-6} for frequency-modulation and laser stabilization, *Opt. Lett.* **39**, 1980–1983 (2014).
23. B. C. Young *et al.*, Visible lasers with subhertz linewidths, *Phys. Rev. Lett.* **82**(19), 3799–3802 (1999).

24. T. Nazarova *et al.*, Vibration-insensitive reference cavity for an ultra-narrow-linewidth laser, *Appl. Phys. B.* **83**(4), 531–536 (2006).
25. A. D. Ludlow *et al.*, Compact, thermal-noise-limited optical cavity for diode laser stabilization at 1×10^{-15}, *Opt. Lett.* **32**, 641 (2007).
26. S. Webster and P. Gill, Force-insensitive optical cavity, *Opt. Lett.* **36**(18), 3572–3574 (2011).
27. D. R. Leibrandt *et al.*, Field-test of a robust, portable, frequency-stable laser, *Opt. Express.* **19**(11), 10278–10286 (2011).
28. P. Dubé *et al.*, A narrow linewidth and frequency-stable probe laser source for the Sr-88(+) single ion optical frequency standard, *Appl. Phys. B.* **95**(1), 43–54 (2009).
29. T. Legero *et al.*, Tuning the thermal expansion properties of optical reference cavities with fused silica mirrors, *J. Opt. Soc. Am. B: Opt. Phys.* **27**(5), 914–919 (2010).
30. K. Numata *et al.*, Thermal-noise limit in the frequency stabilization of lasers with rigid cavities, *Phys. Rev. Lett.* **93**(25), 250602 (2004).
31. T. Kessler *et al.*, Thermal noise in optical cavities revisited, *J. Opt. Soc. Am. B: Opt. Phys.* **29**(1), 178–184 (2012).
32. T. Kessler *et al.*, A sub-40-mHz-linewidth laser based on a silicon single-crystal optical cavity, *Nat Photon.* **6**, 687–692 (2012).
33. G. D. Cole *et al.*, Tenfold reduction of Brownian noise in high-reflectivity optical coatings, *Nat Photon.* **7**(8), 644–650 (2013).
34. S. Amairi *et al.*, Reducing the effect of thermal noise in optical cavities, *Appl. Phys. B.* **113**(2), 233–242 (2013).
35. S. Häfner *et al.*, 8×10^{-17} fractional laser frequency instability with a long room-temperature cavity, *Opt. Lett.* **40**(9), 2112–2115 (2015).
36. S. T. Cundiff and J. Ye, Colloquium: Femtosecond optical frequency combs, *Rev. Mod. Phys.* **75**(1), 325–342 (2003).
37. L.-S. Ma *et al.*, Optical frequency synthesis and comparison with uncertainty at the 10^{-19} level, *Science* **303**(5665), 1843–1845 (2004).
38. T. Rosenband *et al.*, Frequency comparison of Al^+ and Hg^+ optical standards. In *Proceedings of the XVIII International Conference: ICOLS 2007: Telluride, Colorado, USA, 24–29 June 2007*, p. 297 (2008). ISBN 9812813195.
39. T. M. Fortier *et al.*, Generation of ultrastable microwaves via optical frequency division, *Nat Photon.* **5**(7), 425–429 (2011).
40. J. Stenger *et al.*, Ultraprecise measurement of optical frequency ratios, *Phys. Rev. Lett.* **88**(7), 073601 (2002).
41. F. R. Giorgetta *et al.*, Optical two-way time and frequency transfer over free space, *Nat Photon.* **7**(6), 434–438 (2013).
42. L.-S. Ma *et al.*, Delivering the same optical frequency at two places: accurate cancellation of phase noise introduced by optical fiber or other time-varying path, *Opt. Lett.* **19**(21), 1777 (1994).
43. S. Droste *et al.*, Optical-frequency transfer over a single-span 1840 km fiber link, *Phys. Rev. Lett.* **111**(11), 110801 (2013).
44. S. M. Foreman *et al.*, Coherent optical phase transfer over a 32-km fiber with 1s instability at 10^{-17}, *Phys. Rev. Lett.* **99**, 153601 (2007).

45. P. O. Schmidt *et al.*, Spectroscopy using quantum logic, *Science* **309**(5735), 749–752 (2005).
46. T. Rosenband *et al.*, Observation of the $^1S_0$ –> $^3P_0$ clock transition in $^{27}Al^+$, *Phys. Rev. Lett.* **98**(22), 220801 (2007).
47. D. Hume *et al.*, High-fidelity adaptive qubit detection through repetitive quantum nondemolition measurements, *Phys. Rev. Lett.* **99**(12), 120502 (2007).
48. T. Rosenband *et al.*, Frequency ratio of Al^+ and Hg^+ single-ion optical clocks; metrology at the 17th decimal place, *Science* **319**(5871), 1808–1812 (2008).
49. C. W. Chou *et al.*, Frequency comparison of two high-accuracy Al^+ optical clocks, *Phys. Rev. Lett.* **104**(7), 070802 (2010).
50. J. B. Wübbena *et al.*, Sympathetic cooling of mixed-species two-ion crystals for precision spectroscopy, *Phys. Rev. A.* **85**(4), 043412 (2012).
51. S. Falke *et al.*, Delivering pulsed and phase stable light to atoms of an optical clock, *Appl. Phys. B.* **107**(2), 301–311 (2012).
52. C. Degenhardt *et al.*, Influence of chirped excitation pulses in an optical clock with ultracold calcium atoms, *IEEE Trans. Instrum. Meas.* **54**(2), 771–775 (2005).
53. K. Gibble, Scattering of cold-atom coherences by hot atoms: Frequency shifts from background-gas collisions, *Phys. Rev. Lett.* **110**(18), 180802 (2013).
54. T. D. Moyer, Transformation from proper time on Earth to coordinate time in solar system barycentric space-time frame of reference, *Celestial Mechanics.* **23** (1), 33–56 (1981).
55. N. Ashby, Relativity in the global positioning system, *Living Reviews in Relativity.* **6**, 1 (2003).
56. M. Soffel *et al.*, The IAU 2000 Resolutions for Astrometry, Celestial Mechanics, and Metrology in the Relativistic Framework: Explanatory Supplement, *Astron. J.* **126**(6), 2687 (2003).
57. J. Müller *et al.*, Geodesy and relativity, *J. Geodesy.* **82**(3), 133–145 (2008).
58. P. Delva and J. Lodewyck, Atomic clocks: New prospects in metrology and geodesy, arXiv: e-print 1308.6766 (2013).
59. R. Lehmann, Altimetry–gravimetry problems with free vertical datum, *J. Geodesy.* **74**(3–4), 327–334 (2000).
60. J.-P. Uzan, Varying constants, gravitation and cosmology, *Living Reviews in Relativity.* **14**(2), 1–155 (2011).
61. S. Blatt *et al.*, New limits on coupling of fundamental constants to gravity using Sr87 optical lattice clocks, *Phys. Rev. Lett.* **100**, 140801 (2008).
62. A. Derevianko and M. Pospelov, Hunting for topological dark matter with atomic clocks, *Nat Phys.* **10**(12), 933–936 (2014).
63. M. T. Murphy *et al.*, Further evidence for a variable fine-structure constant from Keck/HIRES QSO absorption spectra, *Monthly Notices RAS.* **345**(2), 609–638 (2003).
64. R. Srianand *et al.*, Limits on the time variation of the electromagnetic fine-structure constant in the low energy limit from absorption lines in the spectra of distant quasars, *Phys. Rev. Lett.* **92**, 121302 (2004).
65. J. K. Webb *et al.*, Indications of a spatial variation of the fine structure constant, *Phys. Rev. Lett.* **107**(19), 191101 (2011).

66. N. Huntemann *et al.*, Improved limit on a temporal variation of mp/me from comparisons of Yb+ and Cs atomic clocks, *Phys. Rev. Lett.* **113**(21), 210802 (2014).
67. R. M. Godun *et al.*, Frequency ratio of two optical clock transitions in Yb+171 and constraints on the time variation of fundamental constants, *Phys. Rev. Lett.* **113**(21), 210801 (2014).
68. K. Pyka *et al.*, A high-precision segmented Paul trap with minimized micromotion for an optical multiple-ion clock, *Appl. Phys. B.* **114**(1–2), 231–241 (2014).
69. M. Schulte *et al.*, Quantum algorithmic readout in multi-ion clocks, arXiv:1501.06543v2 (2015).
70. T. Rosenband *et al.*, Blackbody radiation shift of the 27Al$^+$ 1S0 − 3P0 transition, In *Proceedings of the 20th European Frequency and Time Forum*, pp. 289—291 (2006).
71. T. Rosenband and D. R. Leibrandt. Exponential scaling of clock stability with atom number, arXiv:1303.6357 (2013).
72. J. Borregaard and A. S. Sørensen, Efficient atomic clocks operated with several atomic ensembles, *Phys. Rev. Lett.* **111**(9), 090802 (2013).
73. V. Meyer *et al.*, Experimental demonstration of entanglement-enhanced rotation angle estimation using trapped ions, *Phys. Rev. Lett.* **86**(26), 5870–5873 (2001).
74. T. Monz *et al.*, 14-Qubit entanglement: Creation and coherence, *Phys. Rev. Lett.* **106**(13), 130506 (2011).
75. A. Louchet-Chauvet *et al.*, Entanglement-assisted atomic clock beyond the projection noise limit, *New J. Phys.* **12**(6), 065032 (2010).
76. I. Leroux *et al.*, Orientation-dependent entanglement lifetime in a squeezed atomic clock, *Phys. Rev. Lett.* **104**, 250801 (2010).
77. S. F. Huelga *et al.*, Improvement of frequency standards with quantum entanglement, *Phys. Rev. Lett.* **79**(20), 3865–3868 (1997).
78. T. Rosenband. Numerical test of few-qubit clock protocols, arXiv:1203.0288 (2012).
79. V. Bužek *et al.*, Optimal quantum clocks, *Phys. Rev. Lett.* **82**(10), 2207–2210 (1999).

INDEX

G

H

I

J

K

L

M

N

O

P

Q

R